TOP TRAILS™

Sequoia and Kings Canyon National Parks

64 MUST-DO HIKES FOR EVERYONE

Written by

Mike White

WILDERNESS PRESS ... *on the trail since 1967*

Top Trails Sequoia and Kings Canyon National Parks: 64 Must-Do Hikes for Everyone
1st EDITION 2009
2nd EDITION 2016

Copyright © 2009, 2016 by Mike White

All photos, except where noted, © by Mike White
Maps: Mike White
Cover design: Frances Baca Design and Scott McGrew
Text design: Frances Baca Design

Library of Congress Cataloging-in-Publication Data

Names: White, Michael C., 1952-
Title: Sequoia and Kings Canyon National Parks : must-do hikes for everyone /
   written by Mike White.
Description: Second Edition. | Birmingham, AL : Wilderness Press, [2016] |
   Series: Top Trails | "Distributed by Publishers Group West"—T.p. verso. |
   Includes index.
Identifiers: LCCN 2016000573| ISBN 9780899978055 | ISBN 9780899978062 (eISBN)
Subjects: LCSH: Hiking—California—Sequoia National Park—Guidebooks. |
   Hiking—California—Kings Canyon National Park—Guidebooks. | Trails—California—
   Sequoia National Park—Guidebooks. | Trails—California—Kings Canyon National Park—
   Guidebooks. | Sequoia National Park (Calif.)—Guidebooks. | Kings Canyon National Park
   (Calif.)—Guidebooks.
Classification: LCC GV199.42.C22 S4698 2016 | DDC 796.510979486—dc23
LC record available at http://lccn.loc.gov/2016000573

ISBN 978-0-89997-805-5; eISBN 978-0-89997-806-2

Manufactured in the United States of America

Published by: 🦌 **WILDERNESS PRESS**
   An imprint of AdventureKEEN
   2204 First Avenue South, Suite 102
   Birmingham, AL 35233
   800-443-7227
   info@wildernesspress.com
   wildernesspress.com

Visit our website for a complete listing of our books and for ordering information.

Distributed by Publishers Group West

Cover photo: Kearsarge Lakes (see Trail 54) © Mike White

SAFETY NOTICE: Although Wilderness Press and the author have made every attempt to ensure that the information in this book is accurate at press time, they are not responsible for any loss, damage, injury, or inconvenience that may occur to anyone while using this book. You are responsible for your own safety and health while in the wilderness. The fact that a trail is described in this book does not mean that it will be safe for you. Be aware that trail conditions can change from day to day. Always check local conditions, know your own limitations, and consult a map.

The Top Trails™ Series

Wilderness Press

When Wilderness Press published *Sierra North* in 1967, no other trail guide like it existed for the Sierra backcountry. The first print run sold out in less than two months, and its success heralded the beginning of Wilderness Press. Since we were founded almost 50 years ago, we have expanded our territories to cover California, Alaska, Hawaii, the US Southwest, the Pacific Northwest, the Midwest, the Southeast, New England, Canada, and Baja California.

Wilderness Press continues to publish comprehensive, accurate, and readable outdoor books. Hikers, backpackers, kayakers, skiers, snowshoers, climbers, cyclists, and trail runners rely on Wilderness Press for accurate outdoor adventure information.

Top Trails

In its Top Trails guides, Wilderness Press has paid special attention to organization so that you can find the perfect hike each and every time. Whether you're looking for a steep trail to test yourself on or a walk in the park, a romantic waterfall or a city view, Top Trails will lead you there.

Each Top Trails guide contains trails for everyone. The trails selected provide a sampling of the best that the region has to offer. These are the must-do hikes, walks, runs, and bike rides, with every feature of the area represented.

Every book in the Top Trails series offers:

- The Wilderness Press commitment to accuracy and reliability
- Ratings and rankings for each trail
- Distances and approximate times
- Easy-to-follow trail notes
- Map and permit information

TRAIL FEATURES TABLE

Sequoia and Kings Canyon National Parks

TRAIL NUMBER AND NAME	Page	Difficulty -12345+	Length in Miles	Type	Day Hiking	Backpacking	Running	Horses	Dogs Allowed	Wheelchair	Children
1. The Foothills											
1 Putnam and Snowslide Canyons	35	3	6.8	Out-and-back	Day Hiking		Running	Horses			
2 Ladybug Trail	39	3	3.5	Out-and-back	Day Hiking	Backpacking	Running	Horses			
3 Potwisha Pictographs Loop	43	1	0.5	Loop	Day Hiking						Children
4 Marble Falls	49	3	6.8	Out-and-back	Day Hiking						
5 Paradise Creek Trail	53	3	4.4	Out-and-back	Day Hiking		Running				
6 Middle Fork Trail to Panther Creek	57	3	5.6, 8.2	Out-and-back	Day Hiking	Backpacking	Running				
2. Mineral King											
7 Paradise Peak	71	4	9.6	Out-and-back	Day Hiking		Running	Horses			
8 East Fork Grove	77	3	5.0	Out-and-back	Day Hiking		Running	Horses			
9 Cold Springs Trail	81	1	1.2	Point-to-point	Day Hiking						Children
10 Mosquito Lakes	85	4	7.6	Out-and-back	Day Hiking	Backpacking	Running	Horses			
11 Eagle Lake	89	4	6.5	Out-and-back	Day Hiking	Backpacking	Running	Horses			
12 White Chief Bowl	95	5	7.5	Out-and-back	Day Hiking	Backpacking					
13 Crystal Lake	101	4	7.6	Out-and-back	Day Hiking	Backpacking	Running	Horses			
14 Monarch Lakes	105	4	6.5	Out-and-back	Day Hiking	Backpacking	Running	Horses			
3. Giant Forest and Lodgepole											
15 Moro Rock	121	2	0.6	Out-and-back	Day Hiking						
16 Huckleberry Meadow Loop	125	2	3.8	Loop	Day Hiking		Running				
17 Bobcat Point Loop	131	1	1.25	Loop	Day Hiking		Running				
18 High Sierra Trail to Eagle View and Panther Creek	137	2	5.4	Out-and-back	Day Hiking	Backpacking	Running				
19 Crescent and Log Meadows Loop	141	2	2.4	Loop	Day Hiking						Children
20 Trail of the Sequoias Loop	147	3	5.8	Loop	Day Hiking		Running				
21 Hazelwood Nature Trail	153	1	1.3	Loop	Day Hiking						Children

---

USES & ACCESS	TYPE	TERRAIN	FLORA & FAUNA	OTHER
Day Hiking	Loop	Canyon	Fall Colors	Great Views
Backpacking	Out-and-back	Mountain	Wildflowers	Camping
Running	Point-to-point	Summit	Giant Sequoias	Swimming
Horses	DIFFICULTY -12345+ less more	Lake		Secluded
Dogs Allowed		Stream		Steep
Child Friendly		Waterfall		Fishing
Wheelchair-Access				Historical Interest

TRAIL FEATURES TABLE

Canyon	Mountain	Summit	Lake	Stream	Waterfall	Fall Colors	Wildflowers	Giant Sequoias	Great Views	Camping	Swimming	Secluded	Steep	Fishing	Historical Interest
									TERRAIN		FLORA & FAUNA			OTHER	
✓				✓			✓	✓	✓	✓		✓			
✓				✓			✓	✓		✓		✓			
				✓						✓	✓				✓
✓				✓	✓		✓		✓			✓			
✓				✓	✓		✓				✓	✓			
✓				✓	✓		✓		✓	✓		✓			
	✓	✓					✓	✓	✓			✓	✓		
✓				✓			✓	✓				✓			✓
				✓			✓				✓			✓	✓
	✓		✓							✓	✓			✓	
	✓		✓	✓			✓		✓	✓	✓			✓	
✓	✓		✓	✓			✓		✓	✓					
	✓		✓	✓			✓		✓	✓	✓				
			✓	✓			✓		✓	✓	✓	✓			
		✓							✓						✓
							✓	✓							✓
									✓						✓
				✓				✓	✓	✓					
					✓	✓	✓	✓							✓
							✓	✓							✓
							✓	✓							

Sequoia and Kings Canyon National Parks

TRAIL NUMBER AND NAME	Page	Difficulty -12345+	Length in Miles	Type	Day Hiking	Backpacking	Running	Horses	Dogs Allowed	Wheelchair	Children
3. Giant Forest and Lodgepole (continued)											
22 Big Trees Trail	157	1	1.2	Loop	Day Hiking					Wheelchair	Children
23 General Sherman Tree	161	1	0.9	Out-and-back	Day Hiking					Wheelchair	
24 Congress Trail	165	2	3.1	Loop	Day Hiking						Children
25 Alta Peak	171	5	13.4	Out-and-back	Day Hiking	Backpacking		Horses			
26 Heather, Aster, Emerald, and Pear Lakes	179	4	11.5	Out-and-back	Day Hiking	Backpacking		Horses			
27 Tokopah Falls	187	2	4.1	Out-and-back	Day Hiking			Horses			
28 Twin Lakes	191	4	13.0	Out-and-back	Day Hiking	Backpacking		Horses			
29 Little Baldy	197	3	3.5	Out-and-back	Day Hiking						
30 Muir Grove	201	3	4.2	Out-and-back	Day Hiking						
4. Grant Grove and Redwood Mountain											
31 Big Stump Grove	215	1	2.0	Loop	Day Hiking						Children
32 Sunset Loop Trail	221	3	6.4	Loop	Day Hiking		Running				
33 General Grant Tree Trail	229	1	0.5	Loop	Day Hiking					Wheelchair	Children
34 North Grove Loop	233	2	1.5	Loop	Day Hiking		Running				
35 Panoramic Point and Park Ridge Lookout	237	3	5.6	Loop	Day Hiking		Running				
36 Big Baldy	243	3	4.4	Out-and-back	Day Hiking		Running				
37 Buena Vista Peak	247	2	2.0	Out-and-back	Day Hiking		Running				
38 Hart Tree Loop	251	3	7.25	Loop	Day Hiking	Backpacking	Running				
39 Sugar Bowl Loop	257	3	6.6	Loop	Day Hiking	Backpacking	Running				
40 Mitchell Peak	263	4	6.6	Out-and-back	Day Hiking		Running				
5. Kings Canyon											
41 Sheep Creek and Lookout Peak	275	3 and 4	1.8, 10.0	Out-and-back	Day Hiking		Running				
42 Roaring River Falls	281	1	0.5	Out-and-back	Day Hiking						Children

USES & ACCESS	TYPE	TERRAIN	FLORA & FAUNA	OTHER
Day Hiking	Loop	Canyon	Fall Colors	Great Views
Backpacking	Out-and-back	Mountain	Wildflowers	Camping
Running	Point-to-point	Summit	Giant Sequoias	Swimming
Horses	DIFFICULTY - 1 2 3 4 5 + less more	Lake		Secluded
Dogs Allowed		Stream		Steep
Child Friendly		Waterfall		Fishing
Wheelchair-Access				Historical Interest

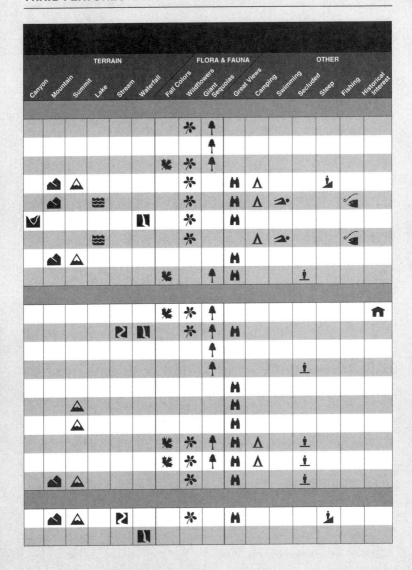

TRAIL FEATURES TABLE

Sequoia and Kings Canyon National Parks

Trail Number and Name	Page	Difficulty -12345+	Length in Miles	Type	Day Hiking	Backpacking	Running	Horses	Dogs Allowed	Wheelchair	Children
5. Kings Canyon (continued)											
43 Zumwalt Meadow Nature Trail	285	1	1.5	Loop	Day Hiking						Child Friendly
44 Kanawyer Loop Trail	289	2	4.7	Loop	Day Hiking		Running	Horses			Child Friendly
45 Mist Falls	293	3	7.8	Out-and-back	Day Hiking		Running	Horses			
46 Rae Lakes Loop	296	4 and 5	41.6	Loop		Backpacking	Running				
47 Hotel and Lewis Creeks Loop and Cedar Grove Overlook	309	4	4.8, 6.4	Loop, Out-and-back	Day Hiking		Running	Horses			
6. Eastern Sierra: Mount Whitney Ranger District											
48 Chicken Spring Lake	325	3	8.2	Out-and-back	Day Hiking	Backpacking	Running	Horses			
49 Long and High Lakes	329	3	13.0	Out-and-back	Day Hiking	Backpacking	Running	Horses	Dogs Allowed		
50 Cottonwood Lakes	335	3	11.8	Out-and-back	Day Hiking	Backpacking	Running	Horses	Dogs Allowed		
51 Meysan Trail	341	4	9.0	Out-and-back	Day Hiking	Backpacking	Running				
52 Mount Whitney	345	5	22.0	Out-and-back	Day Hiking	Backpacking	Running				
53 Robinson Lake	355	3	3.0	Out-and-back	Day Hiking	Backpacking	Running		Dogs Allowed		
54 Flower Lake and Kearsarge Lakes	359	3 and 4	5.0, 12.2	Out-and-back	Day Hiking	Backpacking	Running	Horses	Dogs Allowed		
55 Golden Trout Lakes	367	3	4.4	Out-and-back	Day Hiking	Backpacking	Running	Horses	Dogs Allowed		
7. Eastern Sierra: White Mountain Ranger District											
56 Brainerd Lake	383	4	10.0	Out-and-back	Day Hiking	Backpacking	Running	Horses	Dogs Allowed		
57 Big Pine Lakes	389	4	11.4	Loop	Day Hiking	Backpacking	Running	Horses	Dogs Allowed		
58 Long, Saddlerock, and Bishop Lakes	401	3	8.6	Out-and-back	Day Hiking	Backpacking	Running	Horses	Dogs Allowed		
59 Chocolate Lakes Loop	407	3	7.2	Loop	Day Hiking	Backpacking	Running	Horses	Dogs Allowed		
60 Treasure Lakes	413	3	7.6	Out-and-back	Day Hiking	Backpacking	Running	Horses	Dogs Allowed		
61 Tyee Lakes	419	3	6.5	Out-and-back	Day Hiking	Backpacking	Running	Horses	Dogs Allowed		
62 Sabrina Basin Lakes	425	3	13.6	Out-and-back	Day Hiking	Backpacking	Running	Horses	Dogs Allowed		
63 Lamarck Lakes	433	4	5.4	Out-and-back	Day Hiking	Backpacking	Running	Horses	Dogs Allowed		
64 Piute Lake and Humphreys Basin	439	3 and 4	6.6, 14.4	Loop	Day Hiking	Backpacking	Running	Horses	Dogs Allowed		

USES & ACCESS	TYPE	TERRAIN	FLORA & FAUNA	OTHER
Day Hiking	Loop	Canyon	Fall Colors	Great Views
Backpacking	Out-and-back	Mountain	Wildflowers	Camping
Running	Point-to-point	Summit	Giant Sequoias	Swimming
Horses	DIFFICULTY -12345+ less more	Lake		Secluded
Dogs Allowed		Stream		Steep
Child Friendly		Waterfall		Fishing
Wheelchair-Access				Historical Interest

TRAIL FEATURES TABLE

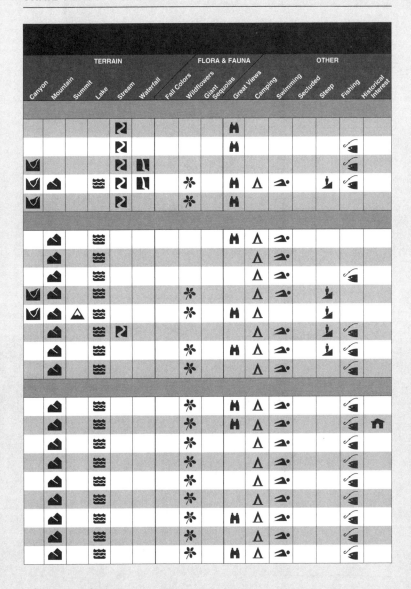

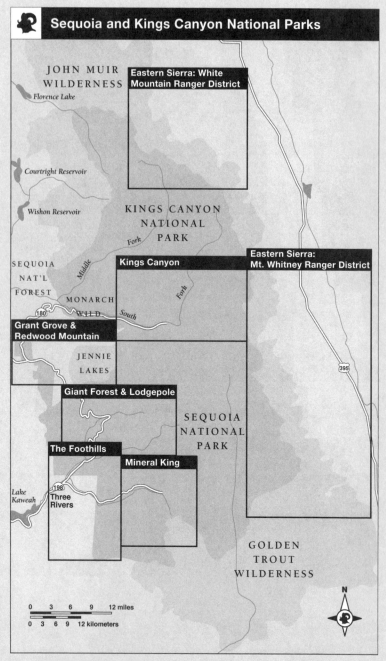

Sequoia and Kings Canyon National Parks

JOHN MUIR
WILDERNESS

Florence Lake

Eastern Sierra: White
Mountain Ranger District

Courtright Reservoir

Wishon Reservoir

KINGS CANYON
NATIONAL
PARK

Fork

SEQUOIA
NAT'L
FOREST

Middle

Kings Canyon

Eastern Sierra:
Mt. Whitney Ranger District

Fork

MONARCH
WILD.

180

South

Grant Grove &
Redwood Mountain

JENNIE
LAKES

395

Giant Forest & Lodgepole

SEQUOIA
NATIONAL
PARK

The Foothills

Mineral King

*Lake
Kaweah*

198

Three
Rivers

GOLDEN
TROUT
WILDERNESS

0   3   6   9   12 miles

0 3 6 9   12 kilometers

N

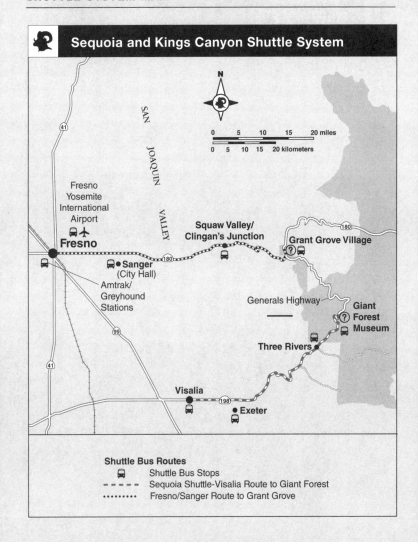

Sequoia and Kings Canyon Shuttle System

Shuttle Bus Routes

🚌 Shuttle Bus Stops

– – – – Sequoia Shuttle-Visalia Route to Giant Forest

· · · · · · · · · Fresno/Sanger Route to Grant Grove

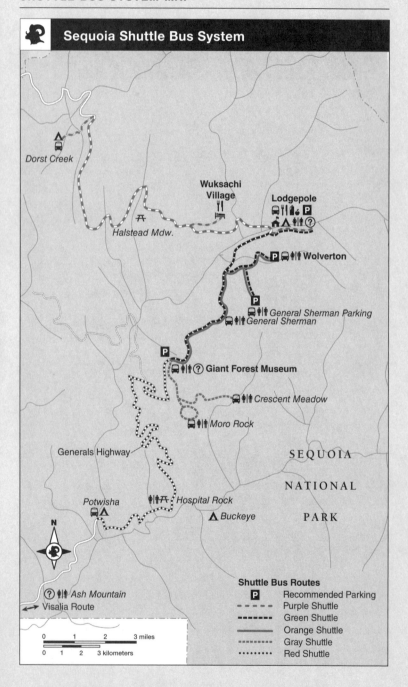

Sequoia Shuttle Bus System

Dorst Creek

Wuksachi
Village

Lodgepole

Halstead Mdw.

Wolverton

General Sherman Parking
General Sherman

Giant Forest Museum

Crescent Meadow

Moro Rock

Generals Highway

SEQUOIA

NATIONAL

PARK

Potwisha

Hospital Rock

Buckeye

N

Ash Mountain
Visalia Route

0   1   2   3 miles
0   1   2   3 kilometers

Shuttle Bus Routes

🅿 Recommended Parking
- - - - Purple Shuttle
------- Green Shuttle
——— Orange Shuttle
········ Gray Shuttle
•••••••• Red Shuttle

Contents

CHAPTER 1
The Foothills

CHAPTER 2
Mineral King

CHAPTER 3
Giant Forest and Lodgepole

Map Legend

Trail	———	River/Stream	～～～
Other Trail	··········	Seasonal Stream	- - - -
Road	———	Park Headquarters	⌂
Railroad	+—+—+	Water Feature and Dam	
Information	⑦	Marsh/Swamp	⸜⸜⸜
Tunnel	⌒	Restaurant	ⵘ
Cabin	⌂	Peak	▲
Fire Tower	⛴	Park/Forest	
Gate	•–•	Store	
Trailhead	🚶	Overlook	
Shuttle Bus Stop	🚌	Pack Station	
Pass	‿		

Using Top Trails™

Organization of Top Trails

Top Trails is designed to make identifying the perfect trail easy and enjoyable, and to make every outing a success and a pleasure. With this book you'll find it's a snap to find the right trail, whether you're planning a major hike or just a sociable stroll with friends.

The Region

At the very front of this guide, the Sequoia and Kings Canyon National Parks Trail Features Table (pages iv–ix) lists every trail covered in this guide, along with attributes for each trail.

The Sequoia and Kings Canyon National Parks Overview Map (page x) provides a geographic overview of the entire region and shows the areas covered by each chapter. A quick reading of the regional map and the trail features table gives you a quick overview of the entire region covered by the guide.

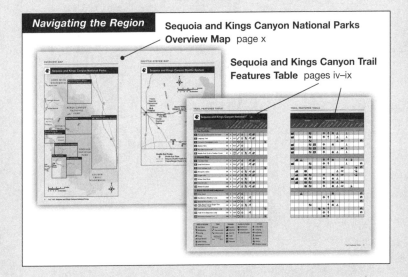

Navigating the Region

Sequoia and Kings Canyon National Parks Overview Map page x

Sequoia and Kings Canyon Trail Features Table pages iv–ix

The Areas

The region covered in each book is divided into areas, with each chapter corresponding to one area in the region.

Each area chapter starts with information to help you choose and enjoy a trail every time out. Use the table of contents or the regional map to identify an area of interest, and then turn to the area chapter to find the following:

- An overview of the area, including park and permit information
- An area map with all trails clearly marked
- A trail features table providing trail-by-trail details
- Trail summaries written in a lively, accessible style

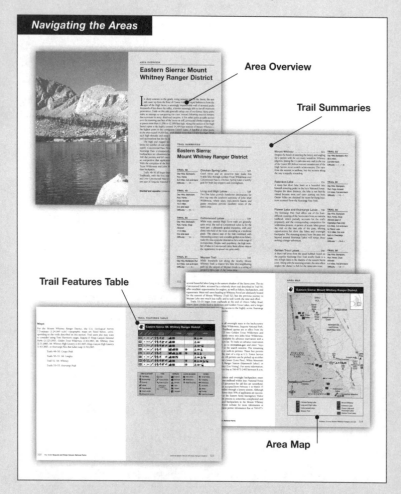

Navigating the Areas

Area Overview

Trail Summaries

Trail Features Table

Area Map

The Trails

The basic building block of each Top Trails guide is the trail entry. Each one is arranged to make finding and following the trail as simple as possible, with all pertinent information presented in this easy-to-follow format:

- A trail map
- Trail descriptors covering difficulty, length, and other essential data
- A written trail description
- Trail milestones providing easy-to-follow, turn-by-turn trail directions

Some trail descriptions offer additional information:

- An elevation profile
- Trail options
- Trail highlights

In the margins of the trail entries, keep your eyes open for graphic icons that signal passages in the text.

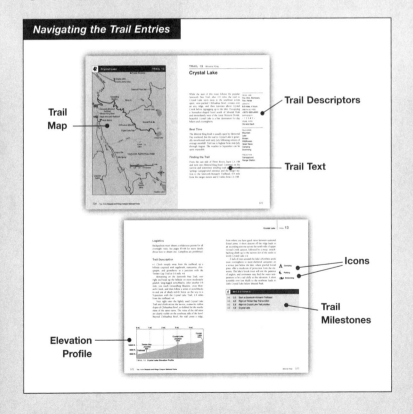

Choosing a Trail

Top Trails provides several different ways of choosing a trail, all presented in easy-to-read tables, charts, and maps.

Location

If you know in general where you want to go, Top Trails makes it easy to find the right trail in the right place. Each chapter begins with a large-scale map showing the starting point of every trail in that area.

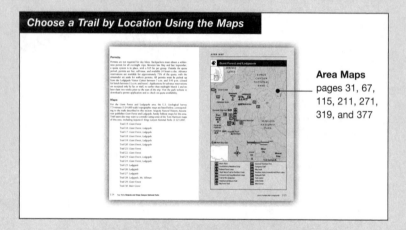

Choose a Trail by Location Using the Maps

Area Maps
pages 31, 67, 115, 211, 271, 319, and 377

Features

This guide describes the top trails of the Sequoia and Kings Canyon National Park region. Each trail has been chosen because it offers one or more features that make it interesting. Using the trail descriptors, summaries, and tables, you can quickly examine all the trails for the features they offer, or seek a particular feature among the list of trails.

Season and Condition

Time of year and current conditions can be important factors in selecting the best trail. For example, an exposed grassland trail may be a riot of color in early spring, but an oven-baked taste of hell in midsummer. Wherever relevant, Top Trails identifies the best and worst conditions for the trails you plan to hike.

Difficulty

Each trail has an overall difficulty rating on a scale of 1 to 5, which takes into consideration length, elevation change, exposure, trail quality, and more, to create one (admittedly subjective) rating.

The ratings assume you are an able-bodied adult in reasonably good shape using the trail for hiking. The ratings also assume normal weather conditions—clear and dry.

Readers should make an honest assessment of their own abilities and adjust time estimates accordingly. Also, rain, snow, heat, and poor visibility can all affect the pace on even the easiest of trails.

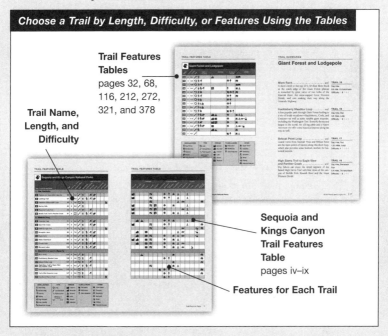

Choose a Trail by Length, Difficulty, or Features Using the Tables

Trail Features Tables
pages 32, 68, 116, 212, 272, 321, and 378

Trail Name, Length, and Difficulty

Sequoia and Kings Canyon Trail Features Table
pages iv–ix

Features for Each Trail

Vertical Feet

This important measurement is often underestimated by hikers and bikers when gauging the difficulty of a trail. The Top Trails measurement accounts for all elevation change, not simply the difference between the highest and lowest points, so that rolling terrain with lots of ups and downs will be identifiable.

The calculation of vertical feet in the Top Trails series is accomplished by a combination of trail measurement and computer-aided estimation. For routes that begin and end at the same spot—that is, loop or out and back—the vertical gain exactly matches the vertical descent. With a point-to-point route, the vertical gain and loss will most likely differ, and both figures will be provided in the text.

For one-way trips, the elevation gain is listed first, and the loss figure follows. For loops or out-and-back trips, the elevation figures are the total gain and loss for the entire trip. The last number is the total gain plus loss for the entire trip.

Finally, some trail entries in the Top Trails series have an elevation profile, an easy means for visualizing the topography of the route. These profiles graphically depict the elevation throughout the length of the trail.

Top Trails Difficulty Ratings

1. A short trail, generally level, which can be completed in one hour or less.

2. A route of 1 to 3 miles, with some up and down, which can be completed in one to two hours.

3. A longer route, up to 5 miles, with uphill and/or downhill sections.

4. A long or steep route, perhaps more than 5 miles, or with climbs of more than 1,000 vertical feet.

5. The most severe route, both long and steep, more than 5 miles long, with climbs of more than 1,000 vertical feet.

Introduction to Sequoia and Kings Canyon National Parks

Somewhat less well known by tourists than neighboring Yosemite, Sequoia and Kings Canyon are nonetheless revered by outdoor enthusiasts from around the globe as containing some of the most coveted backcountry in the world. A large portion of the distinguished John Muir Trail and all of the High Sierra Trail lies within the parks, as does the Lower 48's highest mountain, Mount Whitney, and the world's largest tree, General Sherman. As one of North America's deepest gorges, Kings Canyon is another important feature of the region that draws a host of sightseers, campers, hikers, backpackers, equestrians, and anglers. Protecting a large area of prime Sierra Nevada topography, Sequoia and Kings Canyon leave a lasting impression on all who are fortunate enough to experience these marvelous national treasures.

The spectacular terrain within the current configuration of Sequoia and Kings Canyon was not fully set aside as national parkland until fairly recently. Although the first legislation to protect any of these lands was approved as far back as 1880, when Theodore Wagner, then U.S. Surveyor General for California, suspended 4 square miles of Grant Grove from application for land claims. The next 85 years saw various threats to the preservation of the Sequoia and Kings Canyon area from water, timber, mining, and development interests. After decades of advocacy from private citizens and government servants alike, including such notables as John Muir himself, the stunning landscape we know today was mostly set aside as Sequoia and Kings Canyon National Parks in 1965. However, national-park status failed to confer complete protection to all these lands until 1978 when, after the Sierra Club successfully defeated the Walt Disney Company's bid to develop a destination ski resort, the Mineral King area was added to the parklands.

Geography and Topography

The Sequoia–Kings Canyon region is blessed with some of the most magnificent scenery in North America, including one of the deepest canyons,

1

Whirlwind Tour

Although this book is primarily a hiking guide, if you plan to visit the parks for just one day, you'll hardly have time to get out of your vehicle. Higher gas prices have greatly limited the appetite of the masses for the old-fashioned Sunday drive, but, if you don't mind the expense, you can sample some of the wonders of Sequoia and Kings Canyon on a one-day auto tour.

From the town of Three Rivers on CA 198, with a full tank of gas, drive into Sequoia National Park via the Ash Mountain Entrance and the Generals Highway to the **Foothills Visitor Center,** where you can get acclimatized to the park and obtain information about roads and facilities.

Continue on the Generals Highway along Middle Fork Kaweah River until the road eventually makes a stiff, winding climb out of the canyon and up to the Giant Forest. Park your vehicle in the large lot across from the **Giant Forest Museum** and take a tour of the museum before boarding the free shuttle bus to Moro Rock. Hike the short, steep, quarter-mile-long path to the top of **Moro Rock** for the incredible view. Afterward, ride the shuttle back to Giant Forest, transfer to the free shuttle to the Sherman Tree bus stop, and walk the very short loop around the **General Sherman Tree.** From there, ride the shuttle bus back to the Giant Forest and pick up your vehicle.

Continue on Generals Highway away from the Giant Forest. By now you should be ready for lunch, which you can procure either at the Watchtower Deli or Harrison BBQ & Grill in **Lodgepole,** or the dining room at **Wuksachi Village.** If you prefer to picnic, pack a basket beforehand and enjoy lunch at **Halstead picnic area.**

After lunch, follow Generals Highway past Lost Grove and proceed through Giant Sequoia National Monument to Kings Canyon National Park. At the intersection of Highway 180, veer right and drive a short distance to **Grant Grove Village.** Just past the visitor center, turn right and follow Panoramic Point Road 2.3 miles to the parking area at the end of the road. Take the quarter-mile path to the viewpoint for a superb vista of the Great Western Divide and Sierra Crest from **Panorama Point.** Afterward, return to Highway 180.

Bound ultimately for the deep cleft of Kings Canyon, proceed out of the park on Highway 180, cresting the road's high point at Cherry Gap, before starting the long descent into the canyon. Stop at **Boyden Cavern** for the 45-minute guided tour for which you must pay a fee.

From the cavern, drive Highway 180 along the South Fork Kings River back into Kings Canyon National Park and up Kings Canyon past Cedar Grove to the turnout for **Roaring River Falls**. Walk the very short paved path to the falls viewpoint and return to the parking area. From there, continue up the highway to the **Zumwalt Meadow Nature Trail** and take the 1.5-mile, nearly level path around the meadow, which offers good views of the river from a bridge and the vertical, Yosemite-like canyon walls. Back at the car, drive up the canyon to Roads End and then loop back to **Cedar Grove Village.** At Cedar Grove, you can grab a burger at the restaurant or pick up deli items from the market and enjoy a picnic on the grounds nearby.

Conclude your long day by driving Highway 180 back to Grant Grove and then out of the park toward Fresno.

8,000-foot-deep Kings Canyon, and the tallest mountain in the Lower 48, Mount Whitney at 14,494 feet. The Kern, San Joaquin, Kaweah, and Kings rivers all begin here, flowing westward through dramatic canyons on their way to the plain of the agriculturally verdant San Joaquin Valley below. Along with Mount Whitney, the High Sierra offers up numerous peaks topping out at 12,000 to 14,000 feet. The range rises gradually out of the San Joaquin Valley, first through the characteristic oak woodland of the foothills and then a grand belt of forest on the way to the towering, glacial-sculpted alpine crest of granite peaks along the spine of the High Sierra. From there, the landscape tumbles steeply in dramatic fashion toward the basin of the Owens Valley. The vertical relief of this eastern escarpment as measured from the top of Mount Whitney to the town of Lone Pine at the mountain's base is a staggering 10,760 feet (all in a mere 13 air miles) and is the greatest relief in the continental United States.

The two parks, managed by the National Park Service as one unit, have a combined area of 862,103 acres, more than 90 percent of which is managed as wilderness. With more than 800 miles of trail, the parks are a virtual nirvana for hikers, backpackers, and equestrians. Adding in the acreage and trail mileage of the neighboring John Muir, Golden Trout, Jennie Lakes, Monarch, and Dinkey Lakes wilderness areas, the region is one of the largest roadless areas in the West. Fortunate visitors will find towering granite peaks, picturesque mountain lakes, dramatic glacier-carved canyons with clear running streams and cascading waterfalls, lush meadows filled with colorful wildflowers, and

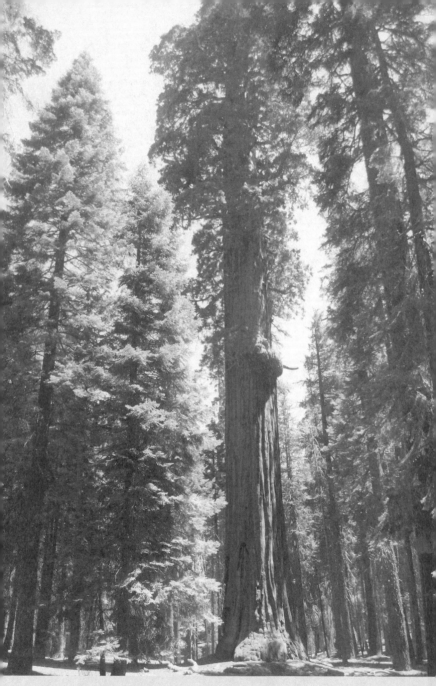

McKinley Tree (*Trail 24*)

dense forests of magnificent trees. Pockets of those forests include the most magnificent tree of all, the giant sequoia, touted as the largest living species of tree in the world. While having some areas of focused visitation, namely Giant Forest, Lodgepole, Grant Grove, and Cedar Grove, the two parks escape the concentration of tourists so common to Yosemite National Park to the north.

Geology

Most of the land within the greater Sequoia–Kings Canyon region is granitic. These light-colored, salt-and-pepper speckled, coarse-grained rocks include granite, granodiorite, and tonalite (formerly referred to as quartz diorite). A large mass of granitic rock, 300 miles long and at points more than 50 miles wide, which geologists call the Sierra Nevada Batholith, was uplifted and exposed over a long period of geologic time to transform into the characteristic granite landscape known today as the Sierra Nevada. In addition to the overwhelming amount of granite, a small percentage of the rock in the Sierra is metamorphic. Darker in color and variegated in appearance, these metamorphic rocks are older than the granitic rocks. Remnants of these older rocks are scattered across the Sequoia–Kings Canyon region. An even smaller amount of the area's composition includes volcanic rock, although within the park's boundaries volcanic rock is almost nonexistent. The most extensive area of volcanic rock in the region is located just east of Kings Canyon National Park in the Big Pine Volcanic Field, visible by motorists from US 395.

The Sequoia–Kings Canyon region is home to some of the most impressive canyons in North America. Both stream erosion and glaciation have greatly influenced these canyons. At lower elevations, the power of water is clearly evident in the carving of V-shaped canyons. In the higher elevations, classic U-shaped canyons bear the evidence of glacial formation.

Speculation about the role of glaciers in the sculpting of the Sierra Nevada dates back to John Muir's day. Whatever their importance in the past, glaciers in today's Sierra Nevada are nearly insignificant in size and depth and will certainly be even more so in the future thanks to climate change. Despite their lack of volume, the small number of remaining glaciers found at high elevations on shady north- and east-facing slopes add touches of alpine beauty to the rocky summits and dramatic faces of the High Sierra.

Flora and Fauna

Since the greater Sequoia–Kings Canyon region encompasses elevations from 2,000 to more than 14,000 feet, you can expect to see a diverse cross section of plant and animal life. Heading from west to east, the first zone encountered is the Sierra **foothills,** a low-elevation area that begins just east of the San

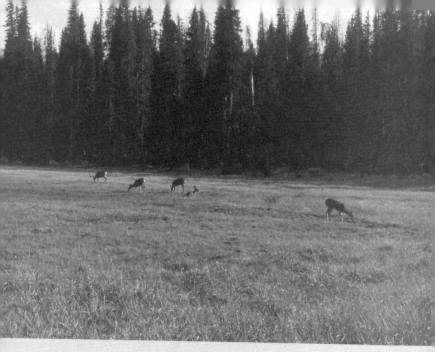

Deer grazing *in Hockett Meadow*

Joaquin Valley and extends upward to around 4,500 to 5,000 feet. Characterized by a Mediterranean climate, the foothills include areas of grasslands, oak woodland, and chaparral. Poison oak is common here and you should be equipped to identify and avoid this three-leaved plant. A wide range of critters call the foothills home, including a variety of amphibians and reptiles. Although the western rattlesnake lives in the foothills, you're not likely to see one on the trail. Common small to medium mammals include rabbits, squirrels, rats, mice, raccoons, skunks, and coyotes. Mule deer and the seldom-seen bobcat and mountain lion make up the larger mammals in this zone. Numerous birds reside in the foothills—far too many to list even the most common species. Raptors include the red-tailed hawk, golden eagle, American kestrel, and great horned owl.

The next zone on your eastward journey through the Sierra Nevada is the **montane forest**. Ranging in elevation from 4,500 to 7,000 feet, the area is composed of both conifers, such as ponderosa pine, Jeffrey pine, white fir, sugar pine, and incense cedar, and deciduous trees, such as black oak and dogwood. Along streams, the montane forest supports a diverse array of riparian foliage. Amphibians and reptiles are common here, as they are in the foothills. In addition to many of the mammals of the foothill zone, the montane forest is home to black bears, porcupines, and weasels. A wide assortment of birds includes songbirds, woodpeckers, and raptors.

In areas of moist soil between 4,500 and 8,400 feet, 75 groves of **giant sequoias** are found sprinkled along the west side of the Sierra Nevada, the only place in the world to witness these monarchs of the forest. The highest concentration of giant sequoias is found within Sequoia and Kings Canyon National Parks. The groves are not pure stands, but include white fir, incense cedar, sugar pine, and dogwood. Mature giant sequoias can reach heights of 150 to 300 feet and widths of 5 to 30 feet. Although quite massive in height and width, giant sequoias have very shallow root systems. The most common cause of death is not disease, infestation, or fire (thanks to their thick bark) but simply toppling over. Animal life in the giant sequoia groves is similar to that in the montane forest.

Moving up in elevation, between 7,000 and 9,000 feet is the **red fir forest**, where the namesake tree is frequently the sole species of this climax forest. Pure stands of red fir can be so dense that competitors and understory plants cannot survive if they aren't shade-tolerant. Where red firs are less dense, lodgepole pines, western white pines, Jeffrey pines, western junipers, and quaking aspens may join the forest. In addition, white fir may intermingle with red fir along the lower edge of this zone. The red-fir zone receives the highest amounts of precipitation in the Sierra, which falls mainly as snow during the winter. Animals must adapt to the harsher conditions in this zone, which consequently limits the number of amphibians and reptiles. However, a wide variety of mammals seems to flourish here, including mice, gophers, voles, shrews, pikas, chipmunks, squirrels, rabbits, marmots, foxes, porcupines, coyotes, weasels, wolverines, badgers, pine martens, mule deer, and black bears. A diverse number of birds live in the red-fir forest; some of the more interesting birds include blue grouse, dipper, and mountain bluebird.

Between 8,000 and 11,000 feet is the **lodgepole-pine forest**. This two-needled pine is one of the most common trees of the American West. Commonly found in pure stands, lodgepoles do intermix in areas with western white pines and, in the higher elevations, whitebark pines. Where abundant groundwater is present, quaking aspens also may be found with lodgepoles. Animal life is similar to that in the red-fir forest.

Occurring between 9,500 and 12,000 feet, the **subalpine zone** straddles the Sierra Crest and bridges the gap between the mighty forests of the lower altitudes and the much more austere realm above timberline. The most dominant conifer is the foxtail pine, a five-needled pine with pendulous branches, similar in appearance to the bristlecone pine. The most common associate is the whitebark pine, a multitrunked tree that grows in the harsh conditions just below timberline, oftentimes in the form of a windblown shrub. Mountain lakes, craggy peaks, and granite slabs and boulders fill breaks in the forest, as well as numerous meadows carpeted with lush grasses, sedges, and wildflowers. Animal life is similar to that in the red-fir forest.

The **alpine zone** carpets the uppermost elevations of the High Sierra, where the growing season is measured in weeks rather than months. Lower temperatures and cloudier skies allow snow patches to linger here throughout the summer, despite the fact that the alpine zone actually receives less precipitation than zones below. With altitudes above 12,000 feet, frost can occur at any point in the summer, and cool temperatures and nearly constant winds combine with the lack of moisture to produce desertlike conditions. The generally poor, granitic soil further limits the ability of plant species to adapt to this environment. Most plants in the alpine zone are perennial and have developed a low-growing, compact, and drought-tolerant form, which allows them to avoid the strongest winds, grow closer to the warmth of the soil, and survive on small amounts of moisture.

The alpine zone can be subdivided into two classifications: alpine meadow and alpine rock. Alpine meadows are common where a sufficient layer of soil is present. Composed principally of sedges and a limited number of grasses, colorful wildflowers put on a showy display in alpine meadows during the brief summer. Unlike the broad swaths of foliage in alpine meadows, small patches of vegetation make up the plant life in the alpine rock community, where open gravel flats produce a smattering of alpine plants, and protected areas in boulder fields host a wide array of wildflowers.

Aside from insects and invertebrates, few other animals find a suitable home in the alpine zone, where both food and shelter are severely limited. The only common residents are voles, marmots, and pikas. Sierra bighorn sheep may venture to these heights, but they generally prefer realms below timberline. Although many different species of birds fly through the alpine zone, the rosy finch is the only common member.

Continuing east over the Sierra Crest, below the alpine and subalpine zones, you will encounter forest zones similar to those on the west side with one major distinction. The great barrier of the Sierra Nevada insures that the precipitation falling on the **east side** of the range will be much less than what falls on the west side. Consequently, trees and plants found east of the crest have adapted to the drier conditions, which results in a more scattered forest and shorter individual trees. Trees common to the eastside montane forest include white fir, western white pine, Sierra juniper, lodgepole pine, Jeffrey pine, and incense cedar.

Below the montane forest belt, at elevations roughly between 6,000 and 9,000 feet, is the **pinyon-juniper woodland,** composed primarily of widely scattered, singleleaf pinyon pine, Sierra juniper, and curl-leaf mountain mahogany. These trees can withstand the dry conditions east of the crest, where only 5 to 15 inches of precipitation falls each year. Open areas are often filled with sagebrush, rabbitbrush, and bitterbrush. Many eastside trails into the High

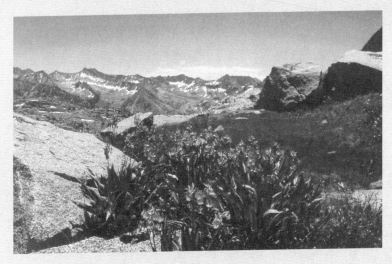

Wildflowers *near Thunderbolt Pass, Knapsack Pass cross-country*

Sierra begin in this zone. Animals common to the pinyon-juniper woodland include a wide variety of amphibians, reptiles, birds, and insects. Mammals include mice, squirrels, voles, rabbits, shrews, chipmunks, coyotes, skunks, badgers, and mule deer.

When to Go: Weather and Seasons

The low-elevation foothills region of Sequoia National Park does offer some off-season hiking opportunities. Chapter 1 includes six hikes in this zone. **Spring** is the best time of year for the foothills, when the higher elevations are still locked in the deep freeze of winter's snowpack. During this time, foothills wildflowers are ablaze with color, the grasses are lush and green, the oaks are budding out, and temperatures are mild.

Above the foothills, snow-free hiking in the montane zone on the western side of the parks generally begins sometime in May, when the road into Kings Canyon is opened and trails in Giant Forest and Grant Grove shed winter's mantle. Once the spring thaw is underway, the snow line steadily recedes up the mountainside, opening more trails along the way. By June, most west-side paths make the frontcountry accessible, but the High Sierra typically remains buried in snow until early to mid-July, depending on the depth of the previous winter's snowpack and the late spring and early summer weather.

If you're a typical hiker using this guidebook, you'll probably visit the parks and surrounding backcountry during the **summer**. Unlike most mountain ranges in the United States, the Sierra Nevada summer is dry, receiving only about 1.5 inches of precipitation, most of which falls from random thunderstorms. About 95 percent of the moisture that falls on the Sierra Nevada usually comes between November and March in the form of rain in the foothills and snow in the higher elevations. Summer temperatures are generally mild, although they vary considerably between the lowlands and alpine heights. By midsummer all trails in the greater Sequoia–Kings Canyon region should be snow-free, although the high passes may still hold patches of snow.

Hiking season begins in earnest during the month of July, but this period also brings a couple of concerns: Mosquitoes reach their zenith of irritation for about a two-week period, and thunderstorms become a distinct possibility. Effective insect repellent, long-sleeved shirts and pants, and possibly a mosquito headnet should help to keep pesky mosquitoes at bay. If you're backpacking, be sure to include a tent with adequate mosquito netting in your pack. Thunderstorms usually occur from midafternoon until sunset but are typically short-lived and localized. However, they can be quite severe, drenching an area with wind-driven rain and shooting out bolts of lightning. When

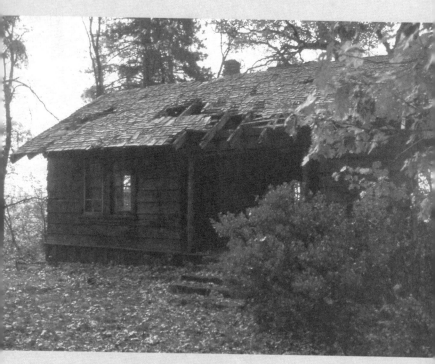

Old Colony Mill Ranger Station, *Colony Mill Road*

thunderheads start to develop, seek lower ground and find a spot within a large stand of forest. Avoid open areas and isolated or small groves of trees.

The first half of August generally provides the best conditions for hikers in the Sierra, as chances of a major frontal storm (possibly with snow at the higher elevations) or an isolated thunderstorm are minimal, and the mosquito population has dwindled to the point of being only a minor irritation. Also, lakes, which typically reach maximum temperatures by late July (low to mid-70s for lower lakes and mid- to high 60s for higher lakes), are still almost as warm, providing pleasant swimming opportunities. September can often be a great time to visit the High Sierra, when the number of visitors to the parks drops dramatically after Labor Day weekend. During this period, backpackers should always check the weather forecast for possible storms. Tents are highly recommended during this time as well.

Fall can be a pleasant time for a visit to the foothills, when the heat of summer has abated and autumn provides a touch of color. Pleasant weather can oftentimes persist in the high country well into October, with chilly nights but mild daytime temperatures. However, backpackers must be prepared for the possibility of encountering the season's first storm during this time. The hiking season finally comes to a close with significant snowfall from the first major storm, usually by the end of the month, but occasionally not until sometime in November.

December ushers in the quiet **winter** season, when access along the east side of the greater Sequoia–Kings Canyon region is severely limited by snow-covered roads. However, the National Park Service does a good job of maintaining access into the west side of the parks via Highway 180 and the Generals Highway, closing roads only during and immediately after substantial storms. Some lodging facilities remain open during the winter months, providing fine basecamps for cross-country skiers and snowshoers seeking to enjoy the solitude and serenity of the season without having to camp in the snow. Lodgepole Campground remains open all year, although winter campers must be prepared for snow camping. Giant Forest, Wolverton, and Grant Grove all offer marked trails for skiers and snowshoers.

Trail Selection

Several criteria were used to arrange this assortment of Sequoia and Kings Canyon's 64 best trails. Only the premier hikes were included, based upon beautiful scenery, access, trail quality, and diversity of experience. Because these trips occur in two of the nation's most magnificent national parks and two of the region's most desirable wilderness areas, most of the trails selected are highly popular, although a handful of routes should offer some level of solitude (hikers willing to step off maintained trails will find lots of lonely backcountry). Anyone fortunate enough to complete all the trips described in this guide would have a comprehensive appreciation for the natural beauty of one of the West's most scenic areas.

About two-thirds of the trails included in this guide are classified as out-and-back trips, requiring you to retrace your steps back to the starting trailhead. The remaining one-third are primarily loops, with some semiloops, and one point-to-point trip.

Features and Facilities

Top Trails books contain information about "features" for each trail, such as lakes, great views, summits, waterfalls, or wildflowers. These features are listed in the margin of each trail description. Beneath the list of features is a list of facilities, including such amenities as restrooms, nearby phones, running water, or campgrounds.

Trail Safety

Although most of the trails in this book are very obvious routes, getting lost is a remote possibility. In the granite-rich High Sierra, it can be easy to lose a trail across a lengthy stretch of bedrock when it's inadequately marked by a line of rocks or low piles of stones, called ducks. In early season, patches of snow may obscure a route as well. Frequently noting landmarks along the way will help you to stay on route—if you find yourself uncertain about your location, simply backtrack to your last known landmark.

Elevations in the Sequoia–Kings Canyon region vary dramatically from the lowland foothills to alpine heights above 14,000 feet. Hikers who reside at or near sea level who recreate at the higher elevations in this range may experience symptoms of altitude sickness, which include headache, fatigue, loss of appetite, shortness of breath, nausea, vomiting, dizziness, drowsiness, memory loss, and loss of mental acuity. Untreated, altitude sickness may lead to the much more severe acute mountain sickness (AMS), requiring immediate medical assistance, without which victims may die.

To avoid altitude sickness, acclimatize slowly, drink plenty of fluids, and eat a diet high in carbohydrates just prior to your trip. Spending the night before your trip at a campground near the trailhead is a good way to get a jump on the acclimatization process. A rapid descent to lower elevations is usually enough to alleviate any symptoms should they develop. A severe case of AMS is unlikely in the Sierra but not impossible—AMS-caused deaths have occurred here.

At higher altitudes, there is less atmosphere with which to filter the sun's rays, increasing the risks of exposure. Always wear an appropriate sunblock on exposed skin and reapply often, as necessary. Sunburns can occur even on cloudy days. A decent pair of sunglasses will protect the eyes, an especially important precaution when you're around reflective snow-covered slopes and granite bedrock.

Dehydration is another potential hazard while recreating in the backcountry. Carry and drink plenty of fluids while on the trail. An electrolyte replacement drink can be quite restorative during periods of intense exertion. Check your route for water sources along the way, plan accordingly, and always filter any water acquired in the field to prevent giardia.

Although the summer weather in the High Sierra is usually fair, conditions can change radically and rapidly at any time. Pack along the appropriate gear to endure any significant climate change. Even if the weather is pleasant, temperatures can be significantly different between the trailhead and your destination. Dousing rains from thunderstorms can leave the ill prepared soaked and cold, potentially leading to hypothermia. Cold fronts have produced snow during every month of the year in the High Sierra. Lightning strikes during infrequent but not uncommon afternoon thunderstorms can be quite dangerous. If thunderclouds start to develop, do not venture above the forest cover. If you find yourself near or above treeline, beat a hasty retreat to lower elevations. Thankfully, most thunderstorms pass rather quickly in the Sierra.

The animal kingdom may provide additional safety issues. Mosquitoes can be major irritants during midsummer, when long pants, long-sleeved shirts, and mosquito netting may be good choices of apparel. These pests are most prevalent around meadows and lakeshores and in moist lodgepole pine forests. Before August, backpacking with a tent is highly advisable. Application and reapplication of an effective repellent (usually with plenty of DEET or Picaridin, and avoiding direct contact with your skin) should help keep the winged pests at bay when you are on the trail or in camp. Such repellent usually is effective on ticks as well, although in the High Sierra ticks are typically much less of a nuisance than mosquitoes (watch for ticks at lower elevations, particularly in spring). However, there exists the remote possibility that a tick can infect you with a number of ailments, including Lyme disease and Rocky Mountain spotted fever. When in tick country, inspect your body regularly and check your clothes for any loose bugs. If a tick bites you, use a pair of good tweezers to firmly grasp the pest, applying firm but gentle traction in order to remove the tick from your flesh, making sure not to leave the head behind. After removal, wash the affected area thoroughly with antibacterial soap and apply an antibiotic ointment. Consult a physician if flulike symptoms such as headache, rash, joint pain, or fever develop.

Black bears are the largest animals you might possibly see in the Sierra. (Grizzly bears were exterminated from the Sierra early in the 20th century.) Thanks to recent efforts by the National Park Service and U.S. Forest Service to require bear canisters in some areas and encourage their use in others, encounters between bears and humans in the backcountry have been greatly reduced (although injuries have occurred and several human-food-conditioned bears were put to death). Backpackers can rent bear canisters at visitor centers and stores within the parks and at U.S. Forest Service ranger stations. Day hikers need not worry too much about bear encounters, as bears usually search for food at campsites at night.

Whereas omnivorous bears see humans as bearers of food, exclusively carnivorous mountain lions, also referred to as cougars, see you as food. Therefore, avoid hiking alone, and if you have children along, keep them close by. Although the likelihood of an attack is extremely remote, if attacked you should fight back. Trying to run away is merely inviting pursuit; such behavior is exactly what prey does when threatened. Make yourself appear as large as possible, hold your ground, wave your arms, and make noise.

Nearly as remote a possibility as meeting up with a mountain lion is the likelihood of encountering a rattlesnake on the trail. The chance of being bitten is even more remote, and the odds of dying from such a bite are incredibly low. Rattlers are not aggressive and will seek an escape route unless cornered. If you happen upon one (chances are highest in the western foothills and below 6,000 feet in the pinyon-juniper zone on the east side of the Sierra), quickly back away to allow the snake a safe path of escape.

The most common large animals you should expect to see are deer. While the general public seems inclined to treat these wild animals like Bambi, they are potentially dangerous (a young child was once killed in Yosemite Valley by a startled deer). All animals, big and small, within Sequoia, Kings Canyon, and the surrounding wilderness should be seen as wild. Do not attempt to touch or feed them. The survival of any animal that becomes familiar with human food is put at risk when fed by those who have learned about them from cartoons.

Marmots are generally seen as cute and furry rodents that produce a high-pitched whistle when approached. However, the marmots of Mineral King have developed a quirky and occasionally destructive tendency to munch on radiator hoses, brake lines, and fan belts. Fortunately, this odd behavior is usually confined to late spring and early summer. If you're planning an early season trip to Mineral King, check with the rangers about current conditions.

Fees, Camping, and Permits

Entrance to Sequoia and Kings Canyon National Parks is subject to a fee. The most common fee is a seven-day pass costing $20 per vehicle. An annual pass is $30 per vehicle. An America the Beautiful Pass is $80 per year and provides admission for one vehicle to all national parks, national monuments, and national recreation areas. Seniors 62 and older can purchase a lifetime pass with similar access for $10. Permanently disabled citizens or permanent residents can acquire a similar pass free with the proper documentation.

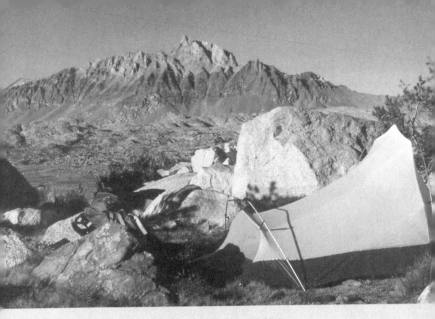

Campsite *near Mount Humphreys, Humphreys Basin (Trail 64)*

Many hikers prefer to stay in campgrounds during their visit. Information about the campgrounds nearest to a trailhead is included near the end of each trail's Finding the Trail section. During the height of the summer season, many campgrounds will be full. Only five of the National Park Service campgrounds (Potwisha, Buckeye Flat, Lodgepole, Dorst Creek, and Sunset) accept reservations. The other nine campgrounds are first come, first served. Approximately half of the U.S. Forest Service campgrounds surrounding the parks will accept reservations. Reservations can be made for both the park and national forest campgrounds at **recreation.gov.**

In addition to campgrounds, nearby resorts are also mentioned (where applicable) in each hike's Finding the Trail section. The parks offer several lodging options, from rustic cabins to finely appointed hotel rooms. Reservations and information for facilities within the parks, operated by the Delaware North Company, and privately run options outside the parks can be obtained at **visitsequoia.com.**

Permits are not required for day hikes (except for trips in the Mount Whitney Zone). Backpackers must have a valid wilderness permit for entry into the backcountry of both the parks and wilderness areas. For overnight trips beginning in the parks, trailhead quotas are in effect from about the end of May through the end of September. Approximately 75 percent of the daily quota is available by advance reservation between March 1 and September 15. A permit application can be downloaded from the park website (**nps.gov /seki**) and, when completed, submitted by mail (Sequoia and Kings Canyon

National Parks, Wilderness Permit Reservations, 47050 Generals Highway 60, Three Rivers, CA, 93271) or fax (559-565-4239). A $10 reservation fee is assessed per reservation, plus $5 per person, and can be made by credit card, check, or money order. Successful applicants will receive a reservation confirmation by mail, which must then be turned in to the nearest issue station to your departure trailhead for the actual wilderness permit. You must confirm or pick up the permit before 9 a.m. on the departure day, otherwise the permit is canceled and becomes available for walk-ins. Free walk-in permits may be obtained after 1 p.m. on the day before departure, and unclaimed reserved permits become available after 9 a.m. on the day of departure.

For all overnight trips beginning on national forest lands, except those entering the Mount Whitney Zone, trailhead quotas are in effect for John Muir Wilderness from May 1 through November 1 and the last Friday in June through September 15 in Golden Trout Wilderness. About 60 percent of the daily quota is available by advance reservation from six months to two days prior to the start of your trip. To make an advance reservation, go to **recreation.gov**, enter "inyo national forest wilderness permit" in the search window, and follow the instructions. A $6 fee is charged per reservation, along with an additional $5 per person. Successful applicants will receive a reservation confirmation by mail, which must then be turned into an Inyo National Forest contact station no more than two days before departure to receive the actual wilderness permit. Permits must be picked up before 10 a.m. on the departure day, unless other arrangements are made by calling the reservation office. Free walk-in permits can be obtained starting at 11 a.m. the day before departure, and unclaimed advance reservations are made available for walk-in permits after 10 a.m. on the day of departure.

Permits for entry into the Mount Whitney Zone are required year-round for both day hikes and overnight backpacks, and daily quotas are in effect. Due to high demand, all permits are obtainable through a lottery process. Applications are accepted by mail beginning on February 1, and the lottery is drawn on February 15. Any remaining permits can be applied for after February 15 up to two days before the day of departure. If any leftover space remains, walk-in permits will be made available. Lottery applications can be made at **recreation.gov**. Additional information on the lottery process is available on the Inyo National Forest's website (**www.fs.usda.gov/inyo**) or by calling the wilderness permit information line at 760-873-2483 between 8 a.m. and 4:30 p.m.

Topographic Maps

An assortment of topographic maps at various scales cover the greater Sequoia and Kings Canyon region, as well as some specific areas within the region, such as Mount Whitney and Mineral King. Taken along on the trail, a small-scale map covering a large area is particularly useful for identifying distant peaks, canyons, lakes, and other geographic features. The U.S. Forest Service, Tom Harrison Maps, and National Geographic Maps are good resources for maps in the Sequoia–Kings Canyon region.

I recommend that hikers and backpackers carry a more detailed map while on the trail. The 7.5-minute topographic quadrangles (1:24,000 scale) published by the U.S. Geological Survey (USGS) fill this bill well. In the introductory material for each chapter under "Maps," there is a list of the pertinent USGS 7.5-minute maps needed for each trip. These maps can be ordered online at **store.usgs.gov** ($8 per map), or purchased from U.S. Forest Service or National Park Service ranger stations. Computer software that you may purchase allows you to customize and print topographic maps from your home computer (although the map is limited to the size of paper your printer can handle).

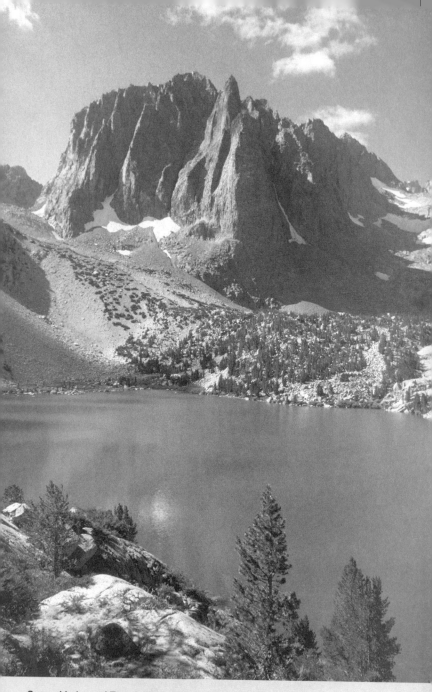

Second Lake and Temple Crag (*Trail 57*)

On the Trail

Every outing should begin with proper preparation, which usually takes just minutes. Even the easiest trail can turn up unexpected surprises. Hikers never think that they will get lost or suffer an injury, but accidents do happen. Simple precautions can make the difference between a good story and a dangerous situation.

Use the Top Trails ratings and descriptions to determine if a particular trail is a good match with your fitness and energy level, given current conditions and time of year. Pay particular attention to the **Best Time** description given for each trail.

Have a Plan

Choose Wisely The first step to enjoying any trail is to match the trail to your abilities. It's no use overestimating your experience or fitness—know your abilities and limitations, and use the Top Trails Difficulty Rating that accompanies each trail.

Leave Word The most basic of precautions is leaving word of your intentions with family or friends. Many people will hike the backcountry their entire lives without ever relying on this safety net, but establishing this simple habit is free insurance.

It's best to leave specific information—location, trail name, intended time of travel—with a responsible person. However, if this is not possible or if plans change at the last minute, you should still leave word. If there is a registration process available, make use of it. If there is a ranger station or park office, check in.

Prepare and Plan

- Know your abilities and your limitations.
- Leave word about your plans.
- Know the area and the route.

Review the Route Before embarking on any trail, be sure to read the entire description and study the map. It isn't necessary to memorize every detail, but it is worthwhile to have a clear mental picture of the trail and the general area.

If the trail and terrain are complex, augment the trail guide with a topographic map; Top Trails points out when this could be useful. Maps as well as current weather and trail condition information are often available from local ranger and park stations.

Check Before Going It's a good idea to check in with the local ranger or land management agency to determine the status of the trail and the roads to the trailhead, particularly just after a storm. Roads and trails may be washed out by floods.

Carry the Essentials

Proper preparation for any type of trail use includes gathering certain essential items to carry. Trip checklists will vary tremendously by trail and conditions.

Clothing When the weather is good, light, comfortable clothing is the obvious choice. It's easy to believe that very little spare clothing is needed, but a prepared hiker has something tucked away for any emergency from a surprise shower to an unexpected overnight stay in a remote area.

Clothing includes proper footwear, essential for hiking and running trails. As a trail becomes more demanding, you will need footwear that performs. Running shoes are fine for many trails. If you will be carrying substantial weight or encountering sustained rugged terrain, step up to hiking boots.

In hot, sunny weather, proper clothing includes a hat, sunglasses, long-sleeved shirt and sunscreen. In cooler weather, particularly when it's wet, carry waterproof outer garments and quick-drying undergarments (avoid cotton). As general rule, whatever the conditions, bring layers that can be combined or removed to provide comfort and protection from the elements in a wide variety of conditions.

Food

While not as critical as water, food is energy and its importance shouldn't be underestimated. Avoid foods that are hard to digest, such as candy bars and potato chips. Carry high-energy, fast-digesting foods: nutrition bars, dehydrated fruit, gorp, jerky. Bring a little extra food—it's good protection against an outing that turns unexpectedly long, perhaps due to weather or losing your way.

Trail Essentials

- Spare cold-weather clothing
- Plenty of water
- Adequate food (plus a little more)

Also, long pants and long-sleeved shirts are a useful first line of defense against poison oak, ticks, and mosquitoes.

Water Never embark on a trail without carrying water. At all times, particularly in warm weather, adequate water is of key importance. Experts recommend at least 2 quarts of water per day, and when hiking in heat, a gallon or more may be more appropriate. At the extreme, dehydration can be life threatening. More commonly, inadequate water brings fatigue and muscle aches.

For most outings, unless the day is very hot or the trail very long, you should plan to carry sufficient water for the entire trail. Unfortunately, natural water sources are usually questionable, and may be contaminated with bacteria, viruses, and other pollutants.

Water Treatment If it's necessary to make use of trailside water, you should filter or treat it. There are three methods for treating water: boiling, chemical treatment, and filtering. Boiling is best, but often impractical—it requires a heat source, a pot, and time. Chemical treatments, available in sporting goods stores, handle some problems, including the troublesome giardia parasite, but will not combat many chemical pollutants. The preferred method is filtration, which removes giardia and other contaminants and doesn't leave any unpleasant aftertaste.

If this hasn't convinced you to carry all the water you need, one final admonishment: Be prepared for surprises. Water sources described in the text or on maps can change course or dry up completely. Never run your water bottle dry in expectation of the next source; fill up when water is available and always keep a little in reserve.

Pests and Hazards

As much as we like to think of the outdoors as our home, it can surprise us with some annoyances and pests like poison oak, ticks, mosquitoes, and rattlesnakes.

A number of the trails may support thickets of trailside poison oak. People susceptible to poison oak should wear long pants and long-sleeved shirts to avoid poison oak rash. If you suspect that poison oak has touched your skin, rinse off in a nearby stream or lake and be sure to shower as soon as you get home. Consult your doctor about treatments to help you avoid and heal from poison oak rash.

Trails may also harbor ticks lurking in the trailside vegetation. As a precaution against Lyme disease, which is spread by ticks, it is a good idea to avoid getting a tick bite by wearing a long-sleeved shirt. Tuck your pant legs into your boots. Check your appendages frequently for ticks. Wear light-colored clothing to spot ticks more easily. If you are bitten by a tick, clutch it firmly between two fingers and pull it out. Even though most ticks are not disease carriers, it is best to save the tick in a baggie or film canister. If your tick bite becomes inflamed, acquires a suspicious bull's-eye-like ring around it, or if you come down soon after the bite with flulike symptoms, consult your doctor immediately, and be sure to bring the tick for identification. The long-term affects of Lyme disease can be both permanent and debilitating.

Depending on the time of the year, you may encounter mosquitoes, which can, in rare instances, carry encephalitis or the West Nile virus. But typically, you simply have to be concerned about the obnoxious itching bite of these pests. Again, a long-sleeved shirt is a good first line of defense, along with mosquito repellent.

Rattlesnakes are common on many of the Sierra foothills trails. Despite these snakes' bad rap, rattlesnake bites are rare in California, and rattlers and other snakes perform an important ecosystem function by eating rats, mice, and other small mammals that would soon strip most of the vegetation from our outdoor areas if they were not kept in check. Snakes are cold-blooded and may be found in the middle of a trail or in other open spaces sunning themselves. Just be sure to look ahead of you as you walk along a trail and be alert for the telltale rattling. Be sure to look on the other side before stepping over or sitting on logs and rocks. Rattlesnakes want nothing more than to be left alone, so avoid harassing, following, or poking at a rattler.

Attacks by mountain lions and bears on humans are very rare in California. The smaller and usually nonaggressive California black bear is more of a threat to your camping food than to anything else.

Thunderstorm-derived lightning is a concern at higher elevations. Peaks, ridgetops, and tall trees may attract lightning strikes. It's best to get to lower elevations and avoid being the highest object in your area during thunderstorms.

Less Than Essential, But Useful, Items

Map and Compass (And the Know-How to Use Them) Many trails don't require much navigation, meaning a map and compass aren't always as essential as water or food—but it can be a close call. If the trail is remote or infrequently visited, a map and compass should be considered necessities. As

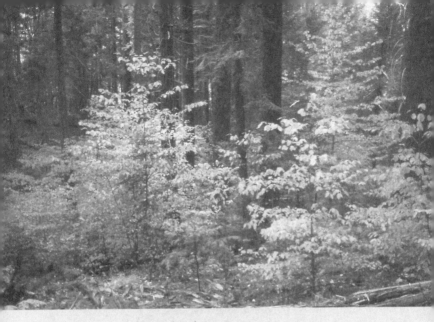

Dogwoods *in autumn, Sunset Rock Trail, Giant Forest*

the budgets of federal and state land management agencies have declined, so have the frequency and reliability of trail signs, as well as maintenance of the trails themselves.

A hand-held GPS receiver is also a useful trail companion, but is really no substitute for a map and compass; knowing your longitude and latitude is not much help without a map.

Cell Phone Most parts of the country, even remote destinations, have some level of cellular coverage, particularly on peaks and ridgetops. In extreme circumstances, a cell phone can be a lifesaver. But don't depend on it; coverage is unpredictable, and batteries fail.

Gear Depending on the remoteness and rigor of the trail, there are many additional useful items to consider: pocketknife, flashlight, fire source (waterproof matches, lighter, or flint), and a first-aid kit. Always carry some toilet paper and a light plastic trowel in case there is a need to go in the woods. Bury your waste at least 6 inches deep and more than 300 feet away from all water sources. Also, bring extra plastic bags to carry your used toilet paper out for proper disposal. A hiking staff or walking poles may enhance your experience by reducing the load on your feet and legs. Small binoculars are useful for viewing and identifying wildlife.

Every member of your party should carry the appropriate essential items described above; groups often split up or get separated along the trail. Solo

Trail Etiquette

- Leave no trace—never litter.
- Stay on the trail—never cut switchbacks.
- Share the trail—use courtesy and common sense.
- Leave it there—don't disturb wildlife.

hikers should be even more disciplined about preparation, and carry more gear. Traveling solo is inherently more risky. This isn't meant to discourage solo travel, simply to emphasize the need for extra preparation. Solo hikers should make a habit of carrying a little more gear than absolutely necessary.

Trail Etiquette

The overriding rule on the trail is "leave no trace." Interest in visiting natural areas continues to increase in North America, even as the quantity of unspoiled natural areas continues to shrink. These pressures make it ever more critical that we leave no trace.

Never Litter If you carried it in, it's easy enough to carry it out. Leave the trail in the same (if not better) condition that you find it. Try picking up any litter you encounter and packing it out if possible.

Stay on the Trail Paths have been created, sometimes over many years, for many purposes: to protect the surrounding natural areas, to avoid dangers, and to provide the best route. Leaving the trail can cause damage that takes years to undo. Never cut switchbacks. Shortcutting rarely saves energy or time, and it takes a terrible toll on the land, trampling plant life and hastening erosion. Moreover, safety and consideration intersect on the trail. It's hard to get truly lost if you stay on the trail.

Share the Trail The best trails attract many visitors, and you should be prepared to share the trail with others. Do your part to minimize impact.

Many of the trails in this book are used by hikers, mountain bikers, and equestrians. Some of the non-wilderness trails are even open to motorized use. Commonly accepted trail etiquette dictates that motor vehicles and bike riders yield to both hikers and equestrians, hikers yield to horseback riders, downhill hikers yield to uphill hikers, and everyone stays to the right. Not everyone knows these rules of the trail, so let common sense and good humor be the final guide.

Leave It There Destruction or removal of plants and animals, or historical, prehistoric, or geological items, is certainly unethical and almost always illegal.

Follow Campfire Rules Many of the higher-elevation areas are off-limits to campfires due to high use and impacts on local vegetation from wood gathering. Lower-elevation areas may have seasonal campfire prohibitions during dry periods to reduce the chance of starting a wildfire. Check with the management agency before your outing for permanent and seasonal rules.

Getting Lost If you become lost on the trail, stay on the trail. Stop and take stock of the situation. In many cases, a few minutes of calm reflection will yield a solution. Consider all the clues available; use the sun to identify directions if you don't have a compass. If you determine that you are indeed lost, remain on the main trail and stay put. You are more likely to encounter other people if you stay in one place.

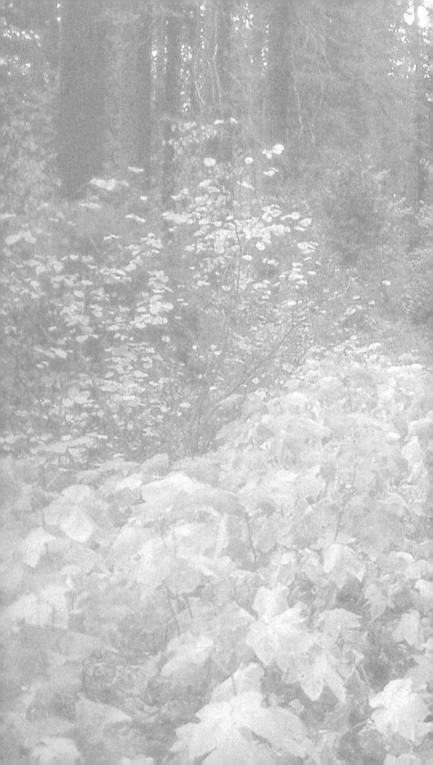

CHAPTER 1

The Foothills

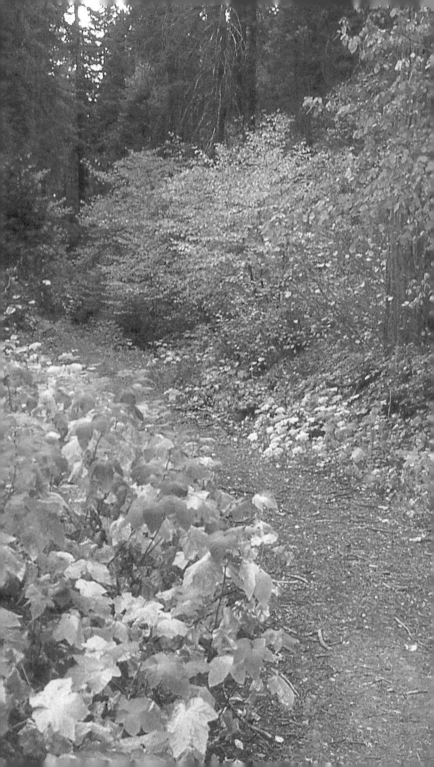

The Foothills

The west side of the Sierra Nevada rises slowly but steadily from the broad plain of the San Joaquin Valley toward the federally protected lands of Sequoia National Park. Traveling east, the usually verdant and productive agricultural lands of the valley gradually transition into the oak-dotted grasslands and chaparral of the foothills zone, where visitors have a unique opportunity to experience a slice of California's lower-elevation terrain in an undeveloped setting—a definite rarity throughout most of the rest of the state. Due to the low elevation and correspondingly mild Mediterranean climate, year-round hiking is possible within the drainages of the South Fork and Middle Fork Kaweah Rivers.

All six of the trips described in this chapter follow low-elevation trails into Sequoia National Park's frontcountry, providing off-season hiking opportunities when the higher elevations are customarily buried in snow. The first two entries begin from the end of the South Fork Road, following stream canyons into the beginnings of the montane forest zone. Native American history is the primary focus of the Potwisha Pictographs Loop along the banks of Middle Fork Kaweah River. Trails 4 and 5 follow tributaries up steep canyons to waterfalls, while Trail 6 is along a section of the Middle Fork Trail with fine views of the surrounding terrain.

Permits

Permits are not required for day hikes. Backpackers must obtain a wilderness permit for all overnight trips. Between late May and late September, a quota system is in place, with a $15 fee per group. Outside the quota period, permits are free, self-issue, and available 24 hours a day. Advance reservations are available for approximately 75% of the quota, with the remainder set aside for walk-in permits. Monday through Friday, all permits must be picked up from the Wilderness Office below the Foothills Visitor Center between 8 a.m. and 4 p.m. (credit cards or checks only). On Saturday and

---

Overleaf and opposite: *Autumn foliage along the old Colony Mill Road in the Foothills zone of Sequoia National Park*

Sunday, permits can be picked up at the Foothills Visitor Center between 8 a.m. and 4:30 p.m. Applications for advance reservations are accepted only by fax or mail, no earlier than midnight March 1 and no later than two weeks prior to the start of the trip. Visit the park website to download a permit application and to check on quota availability.

Maps

For The Foothills, the U.S. Geological Survey 7.5-minute (1:24,000 scale) topographic maps are listed below, corresponding to the trails described in this section. Trail users also may want to consider using some of the Tom Harrison maps of this area, including *Sequoia & Kings Canyon National Parks* (1:125,000).

Trail 1: *Dennison Peak and Moses Mountain*

Trail 2: *Dennison Peak and Moses Mountain*

Trail 3: *Giant Forest*

Trail 4: *Giant Forest*

Trail 5: *Giant Forest*

Trail 6: *Giant Forest*

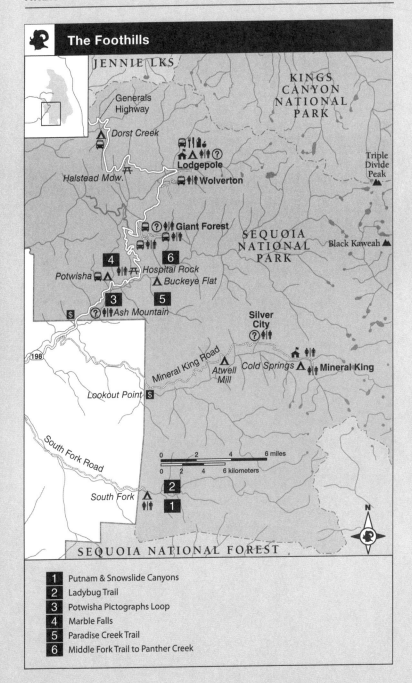

The Foothills

JENNIE LKS

KINGS CANYON NATIONAL PARK

Generals Highway

Dorst Creek

Halstead Mdw.

Lodgepole

Wolverton

Triple Divide Peak

Giant Forest

SEQUOIA NATIONAL PARK

Black Kaweah

4

Potwisha

6

Hospital Rock

Buckeye Flat

3

5

Ash Mountain

Silver City

198

Mineral King Road

Atwell Mill

Cold Springs

Mineral King

Lookout Point

South Fork Road

0   2   4   6 miles
0   2   4   6 kilometers

South Fork

2

1

N

SEQUOIA NATIONAL FOREST

1	Putnam & Snowslide Canyons
2	Ladybug Trail
3	Potwisha Pictographs Loop
4	Marble Falls
5	Paradise Creek Trail
6	Middle Fork Trail to Panther Creek

The Foothills

TRAIL	DIFFICULTY	LENGTH	TYPE	USES & ACCESS	TERRAIN	FLORA & FAUNA	OTHER
1	3	6.8	⟋	🥾 🏃 🐎	Canyon, Stream	Wildflowers, Giant Sequoias	Great Views, Camping, Secluded
2	3	3.5	⟋	🥾 🎒 🏃 🐎	Canyon, Stream	Wildflowers, Giant Sequoias	Camping, Secluded
3	1	0.5	↻	🥾 👪	Stream		Camping, Swimming, Historical Interest
4	3	6.8	⟋	🥾	Canyon, Stream, Waterfall	Wildflowers	Great Views, Secluded
5	3	4.4	⟋	🥾 🏃	Canyon, Stream, Waterfall	Wildflowers	Swimming, Steep
6	3	5.6, 8.2	⟋	🥾 🎒 🏃 🐎	Canyon, Stream, Waterfall	Wildflowers	Great Views, Camping, Secluded

USES & ACCESS	TYPE	TERRAIN	FLORA & FAUNA	OTHER
🥾 Day Hiking	↻ Loop	Canyon	Fall Colors	Great Views
🎒 Backpacking	⟋ Out-and-back	Mountain	Wildflowers	Camping
🏃 Running	⟍ Point-to-point	Summit	Giant Sequoias	Swimming
🐎 Horses	DIFFICULTY	Lake		Secluded
🐕 Dogs Allowed	- 1 2 3 4 5 +	Stream		Steep
👪 Child Friendly	less more	Waterfall		Fishing
♿ Wheelchair-Access				Historical Interest

The Foothills

Putnam and Snowslide Canyons 35

A fine early-season hike to a pair of canyons above South Fork Kaweah River. Colorful wildflowers spice up early spring, but the views of Homers Nose and Dennsion Mountain are excellent year-round. As with all hikes in the foothills, be on the alert for poison oak, ticks, and rattlesnakes.

TRAIL 1

Day Hike, Run, Horse
6.8 miles, Out-and-back
Difficulty: 1 2 **3** 4 5

Ladybug Trail. 39

Vibrant wildflowers and the rushing waters of South Fork Kaweah River will delight in spring, while autumn colors reward fall visitors. As with all hikes in the foothills, be on the alert for poison oak, ticks, and rattlesnakes.

TRAIL 2

Day Hike, Backpack,
Run, Horse
3.5 miles, Out-and-back
Difficulty: 1 2 **3** 4 5

Potwisha Pictographs Loop 43

This short and easy hike, suitable for just about anyone, leads to the banks of Middle Fork Kaweah River, passing Native American bedrock mortars and pictographs along the way. Within the foothills zone, the trail offers the possibility of an early-season hike. Later in the summer, the diminished flow in the river makes swimming an attractive proposition.

TRAIL 3

Day Hike, Child Friendly
0.5 mile, Loop
Difficulty: **1** 2 3 4 5

Marble Falls. 49

A 3-plus-mile climb through a foothills canyon provides a year-round opportunity to stretch your legs on the way to a series of cascades known collectively as Marble Falls.

TRAIL 4

Day Hike
6.8 miles, Out-and-back
Difficulty: 1 2 **3** 4 5

TRAIL 5

Day Hike, Run
4.4 miles, Out-and-back
Difficulty: 1 2 **3** 4 5

Paradise Creek Trail 53

A mostly shaded route, suitable for just about any time of the year, follows Paradise Creek to a 15-foot-high waterfall. Wildflowers provide an added bonus in spring. As with all hikes in the foothills, be on the alert for poison oak, ticks, and rattlesnakes.

TRAIL 6

Day Hike, Backpack,
Run, Horse
5.6 miles (9.2 miles
when road is closed),
Out-and-back
Difficulty: 1 2 **3** 4 5

Middle Fork Trail to Panther Creek . . 57

Mild temperatures, colorful wildflowers, and the swollen Middle Fork Kaweah River make spring the best time to journey along the initial stretch of the Middle Fork Trail. Additionally, along the way are good views of Moro Rock, Castle Rocks, Alta Peak, and the Great Western Divide, followed by a dramatic waterfall at Panther Creek.

Putnam and Snowslide Canyons

The short journey to Putnam and Snowslide Canyons offers hikers early- and late-season opportunities to enjoy the foothills zone on the western fringe of Sequoia while the higher elevations are buried in snow. Wildflowers offer splashes of color in early spring, and views of Homers Nose and Dennison Mountain are excellent throughout the hiking season. The journey to Putnam Canyon passes through oak woodland, while continuing on to Snowslide Canyon exposes hikers to a mixed coniferous forest, including a small grove of giant sequoias.

TRAIL USE
Day Hike, Run, Horse
LENGTH
6.8 miles, 3–4 hours
VERTICAL FEET
+2690/-460/±6300
DIFFICULTY
– 1 2 **3** 4 5 +
TRAIL TYPE
Out-and-back

FEATURES
Canyon
Stream
Wildflowers
Giant Sequoias
Camping
Great Views
Secluded

FACILITIES
Campground

Best Time

With a location in the foothills, the first 2-plus miles of trail to Putnam Canyon can be hiked year-round. Snow may blanket the trail between Putnam Canyon and Snowslide Canyon during the winter months, but the trail should be snow-free from March to December.

Finding the Trail

Drive CA 198 eastbound from Visalia to the town of Three Rivers and turn right onto South Fork Road, approximately 7 miles west of the Ash Mountain Entrance. Follow South Fork Road for about 9 miles to the end of the pavement, and continue another 3 miles on narrow, dirt road to the South Fork Campground (pit toilets, no water, and no fee). Pass through the campground and leave your vehicle in the small, shady parking area.

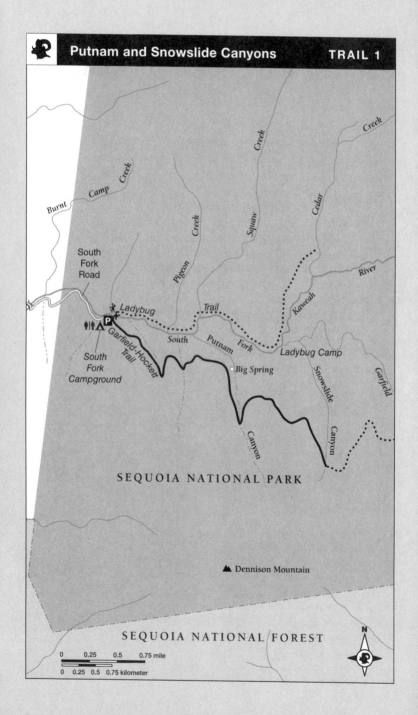

SEQUOIA NATIONAL PARK

SEQUOIA NATIONAL FOREST

Logistics

In the foothills zone, hikers should be on the look-out for poison oak, ticks, and rattlesnakes.

Trail Description

▶1 The signed Garfield-Hockett Trail begins at the campground access road, a short distance before the parking area. Climb moderately across an oak-dotted hillside amid lush trailside vegetation, including colorful wildflowers and a rather healthy population of poison oak. Enter a side canyon about 1 mile from the trailhead and hop across the first of many small rivulets slicing down the lower slopes of Dennison Mountain. The extra moisture in these diminutive nooks creates a dramatic change in vegetation, as ferns, thimbleberry, maples, nutmegs, alders, dogwoods, and cedars line the shady streambanks.

Continue a steady climb through oak woodland to Putnam Canyon. ▶2 The sound of rushing water out of sight below the trail, coursing down the canyon from Big Spring, will be quite noticeable, but chances are the creek at trail level will be dry following the conclusion of snowmelt. The steep and narrow canyon is filled with boulders and low

> Wildflowers offer splashes of color in early spring, and views of Homers Nose and Dennison Mountain are excellent throughout the hiking season.

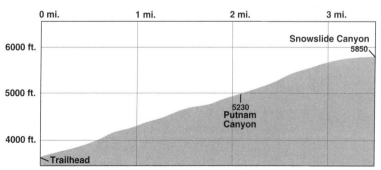

TRAIL 1   Putnam and Snowslide Canyons Elevation Profile

shrubs, allowing a cross-canyon view of the bulbous granite dome dubbed Homers Nose.

Beyond Putnam Canyon, the steady climb continues as a smattering of ponderosa pines, white firs, and incense cedars begin to intermix with the deciduous trees. Fortunately the arrival of the conifers coincides with the departure of the poison oak, although the innocuous flowers and plants from the lush understory below start to disappear as well. A mile from Putnam Canyon, the oak woodland is left behind for good, as the trail bends southeast into a canyon near the western fringe of Garfield Grove. A bit farther up the trail, a dozen or so giant sequoias dwarf smaller conifers on the way to a crossing of the vigorous creek that flows down Snowslide Canyon. ▶3 Hikers will find the canyon to be a worthy early-season goal, as the winter snowpack generally covers the trail beyond here until summer.

 Wildflowers

Giant Sequoias

Canyon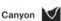

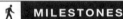 MILESTONES

▶1	0.0	Start at Garfield-Hockett Trailhead
▶2	2.1	Putnam Canyon
▶3	3.4	Snowslide Canyon

Ladybug Trail

While the High Sierra is still cloaked in winter's mantle, those seeking an off-season alternative will find satisfaction on this short foothills hike to Ladybug Camp. Spring visitors will enjoy both a fine display of colorful wildflowers and the full force of the tumbling South Fork Kaweah River filled with melting snows. After the heat of summer and before winter returns, dashes of color will delight autumn travelers.

Best Time

Early spring is when the oak trees start to leaf out, wildflowers begin to blossom, and the grassy hillsides turn green along the Ladybug Trail, providing a fine complement to the snowmelt-swollen South Fork Kaweah River.

Finding the Trail

Drive CA 198 eastbound from Visalia to the town of Three Rivers and turn right onto South Fork Road, approximately 7 miles west of the Ash Mountain Entrance. Follow South Fork Road about 9 miles to the end of the pavement, and continue another 3 miles on narrow, dirt road to the South Fork Campground (pit toilets, no water, and no fee). Pass through the campground and leave your vehicle in the small, shady parking area.

TRAIL USE
Day Hike, Backpack, Run, Horse

LENGTH
3.5 miles, 2 hours

VERTICAL FEET
+960/-180/±2280

DIFFICULTY
– 1 2 **3** 4 5 +

TRAIL TYPE
Out-and-back

FEATURES
Canyon
Stream
Wildflowers
Giant Sequoias
Camping
Secluded

FACILITIES
Campground

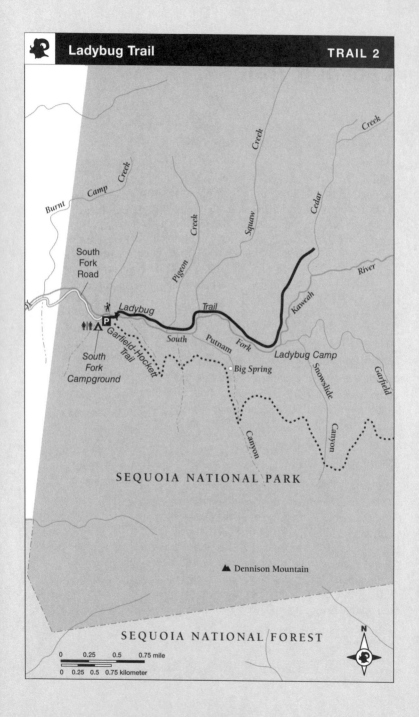

South Fork Road

Burnt

Camp Creek

Creek

Creek

Pigeon Creek

Squaw Creek

Cedar Creek

River

Ladybug Trail

Kaweah

South Fork

Putnam Fork

Ladybug Camp

South Fork Campground

Garfield-Hockett Trail

Big Spring

Canyon

Snowslide Canyon

Garfield

SEQUOIA NATIONAL PARK

▲ Dennison Mountain

SEQUOIA NATIONAL FOREST

N

0   0.25   0.5   0.75 mile

0   0.25   0.5   0.75 kilometer

Logistics

In the foothills zone, hikers should be on the lookout for poison oak, ticks, and rattlesnakes.

Trail Description

▶1 Head east away from the parking area and proceed upstream on a broad path, soon reaching a wood bridge ▶2 spanning the river. On the far side of the bridge, begin a moderate ascent through oak woodland and scattered boulders, climbing high above the South Fork. Springtime visitors will experience a fine display of wildflowers in sunny areas. Immediately before you cross the normally dry channel of Pigeon Creek, you may observe the faint track of an abandoned trail that once climbed steeply to Homers Nose. Past the creek, the trail eventually breaks out of the trees, offering a fine view of the river below and the cascading stream coursing down Putnam Canyon upstream. From there, gently ascending tread leads back into the forest and continues to a log-and-boulder crossing of Squaw Creek at 0.9 mile.

A moderate, 0.75-mile climb away from the creek swings back into the main canyon and continues upstream through alternating stretches of

 Wildflowers

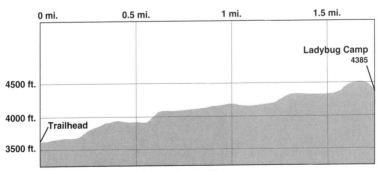

TRAIL 2 Ladybug Trail Elevation Profile

shady oak woodland and sun-drenched slopes of chaparral. More gently graded tread precedes your arrival at the level spot known as Ladybug Camp, ▶3 so dubbed for a wintering population of the namesake beetles. Positioned picturesquely next to the swirling waters of the river, backpackers may find a couple of campsites beneath the shade of oaks, incense cedars, and a few ponderosa pines.

Camping ▲

Those with extra time and energy may continue beyond Ladybug Camp, following the somewhat obscure main trail another mile or so to Cedar Creek, where a handful of giant sequoias are scattered about the drainage. On the way is a fine view of Homers Nose.

Giant Sequoias 🌲

🚶 MILESTONES

▶1	0.0	Start at South Fork Trailhead
▶2	0.1	Bridge
▶3	1.75	Ladybug Camp

Potwisha Pictographs Loop

Although the Potwisha Pictographs Loop is not much of a hike by most standards, visitors of all ages will enjoy this very short trip to the banks of Middle Fork Kaweah River and back. The easy half-mile jaunt leads past a fine display of Native American bedrock mortars and pictographs, where women of the Monache tribe ground nuts and seeds and left behind pictorial representations of their culture. During the warmer months, sandy beaches and granite slabs along the picturesque river offer swimmers and sunbathers a fine haven, where the waters of the Middle Fork glide over slabs, tumble through cataracts, and swirl through delightful pools. A wood suspension bridge over the river is of special interest to the young and young at heart, although children should be closely supervised at all times; the river can be quite treacherous when swollen with snowmelt from the mountains above.

TRAIL USE
Day Hike, Child Friendly

LENGTH
0.5 mile, ½ hour

VERTICAL FEET
+200/-200/±400

DIFFICULTY
– **1** 2 3 4 5 +

TRAIL TYPE
Loop

FEATURES
Stream
Camping
Swimming
Historical Interest

FACILITIES
Campground

Best Time

Within the foothills zone, the Potwisha Loop can be hiked year-round, although hikers will find the most pleasant conditions in spring, when temperatures are mild, the grasses are green, and the wildflowers are in bloom. Afternoon temperatures are quite hot during the summer months, when the flow of the Kaweah River is usually safe enough for a refreshing swim.

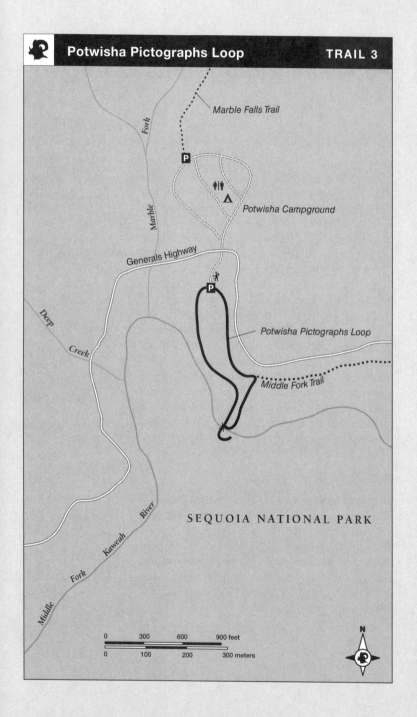

Potwisha Pictographs Loop   TRAIL 3

Marble Falls Trail

Potwisha Campground

Generals Highway

Potwisha Pictographs Loop

Middle Fork Trail

Deep

Creek

SEQUOIA NATIONAL PARK

Kaweah   *River*

Fork

Middle

| 0 | 300 | 600 | 900 feet |
| 0 | 100 | 200 | 300 meters |

N

HISTORY

Bedrock Mortars

The Monache used bedrock mortars to grind acorns from the native oak trees into meal, a staple of their diet. Since only females were involved in this activity, anthropologists assume female members of the tribe drew the nearby pictographs, the meanings of which remain a mystery.

Finding the Trail

From Visalia, follow CA 198 to Three Rivers and proceed east into Sequoia National Park, where the road becomes Generals Highway. Follow Generals Highway for 3.8 miles past the Ash Mountain Entrance to Potwisha Campground (fee, flush toilets, running water, bear boxes, and phone). Rather than turning left into the campground, turn right toward the campground dump station. Instead of continuing down the dump station loop toward the Middle Fork trailhead, follow the gravel surface to the end of a broad clearing above the river and park near some trash bins, where a path heads down toward the river.

> **The easy half-mile jaunt leads past a fine display of Native American bedrock mortars and pictographs.**

Logistics

During the summer season, the free In-park Shuttle runs between Potwisha Campground and the Giant Forest Museum via Red Route 3. In the foothills zone, hikers should be on the lookout for poison oak, ticks, and rattlesnakes.

Trail Description

▶1 Descend along a path toward Middle Fork Kaweah River, soon arriving near a series of granite slabs, site of numerous Native American bedrock

Historical Interest

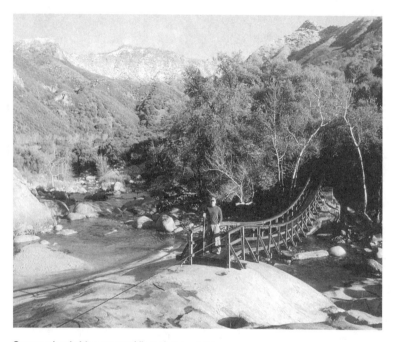

Suspension bridge *over Middle Fork Kaweah River*

mortars. An overhanging rock to the south has several pictographs on the underside surface.

Leaving the mortars and pictographs behind, continue across a slope dotted with granite boulders toward the river and a wood suspension bridge. ▶2 Cross the bridge to granite slabs on the far bank, which provide excellent views of the pools and cataracts of the Middle Fork and offer fine spots on a warm summer day for sunbathing after a refreshing dip in the water. Swimmers should exercise caution here, as the turbulent waters of the Middle Fork can be quite hazardous when the river is running swift and high. The path quickly dead-ends above the bridge near an old flume.

Swimming

Once you've enjoyed this pleasant site to the fullest, retrace your steps across the bridge and veer to the right on a path heading toward a large-diameter steel pipe. Faint tread follows the pipe on a short, steep climb up the hillside to an informal junction with the Middle Fork Trail. Turn left at the junction and follow the trail high above the level of the river through typical oak woodland back to the dump station parking area. From there, walk across the gravel parking area to your car. ▶3

🚶	**MILESTONES**

▶1	0.0	Start at trailhead
▶2	0.25	Bridge over Middle Fork Kaweah River
▶3	0.5	Return to trailhead

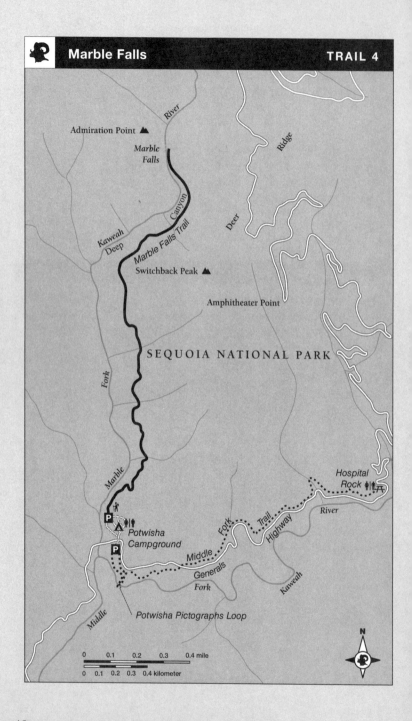

Admiration Point ▲

*Marble
Falls*

Ridge

Canyon

Deer

Kaweah Deep

Marble Falls Trail

Switchback Peak ▲

Amphitheater Point

SEQUOIA NATIONAL PARK

Fork

Marble

Hospital
Rock ♦∏♠

Fork   Trail   Highway   River

Potwisha
Campground

Middle

Generals

Fork   Kaweah

Potwisha Pictographs Loop

Middle

N

| 0 | 0.1 | 0.2 | 0.3 | 0.4 mile |

| 0 | 0.1 | 0.2 | 0.3 | 0.4 kilometer |

Marble Falls

A year-round hiking opportunity, Marble Falls is especially delightful in spring, when the Marble Fork Kaweah River tumbles down marble-filled Deep Canyon in full regalia and the High Sierra is still cloaked in winter's mantle. The waterfalls are not the only delights this trail offers in springtime; patches of verdant meadow grass and an assortment of vibrant wildflowers provide an added bonus. Hiking in the foothills zone does pose a trio of concerns uncommon in the high country, namely ticks, poison oak, and rattlesnakes, although they should be more than manageable with the proper precautions.

Best Time

For this all-year hike in the foothills zone of west Sequoia, the conditions are best from March to May when the falls are at peak glory.

TRAIL USE
Day Hike
LENGTH
6.8 miles, 3–4 hours
VERTICAL FEET
+1750/-300/±4100
DIFFICULTY
– 1 2 **3** 4 5 +
TRAIL TYPE
Out-and-back

FEATURES
Canyon
Stream
Waterfall
Wildflowers
Great Views
Secluded

FACILITIES
Campground

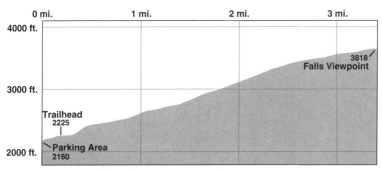

TRAIL 4   Marble Falls Elevation Profile

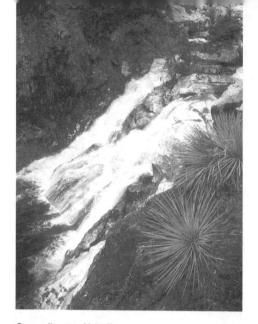

Cascading *Marble Falls*

Finding the Trail

From Visalia, follow CA 198 to Three Rivers and proceed east into Sequoia National Park, where the road becomes Generals Highway. Follow Generals Highway for 3.8 miles past the Ash Mountain Entrance to Potwisha Campground (fee, flush toilets, running water, bear boxes, and phone) and turn left into the campground. Follow the loop through the campground to the dirt access road at the northwest end; turn up this short road and park in the small parking area.

Logistics

In the foothills zone, hikers should be on the lookout for poison oak, ticks, and rattlesnakes.

Trail Description

▶1 From the parking area, walk up the continuation of the dirt road to a wood plank bridge spanning a concrete-lined flume, cross the bridge, and then continue up the road on the far side to a stream-flow gauge and a fenced control gate. The signed Marble Falls Trail begins opposite the gate. ▶2

Leave the road behind and start climbing moderately via switchbacks across a hillside dotted with typical foothill woodland trees and brilliant wildflowers in spring. Be on the alert for poison oak, which is prevalent along the initial stretch of trail. Beyond the switchbacks the trees are left behind and replaced by chaparral, as the trail climbs high above the Marble Fork around ridges and through seams on the east side of Deep Canyon. The chaparral-covered slopes allow views down the turbulent Middle Fork, which are briefly interrupted by short forays into small woodland groves lining the crossings of numerous rivulets and seasonal swales on the way up the canyon. The Marble Fork provides dramatic scenery in spring, when the swollen watercourse cascades over rock steps and swirls through churning pools, producing a raucous thunder reverberating between the walls of the deep canyon. Continue the climb up the east side of the canyon to the last stream crossing, which drains the southwest slope of Switchback Peak. Amid woodland, you wrap back around into the main canyon and climb across a hillside to meet the river, where the trail abruptly ends amid a jumble of boulders and steep slabs that inhibit further progress. ▶3

Although the name "Marble Falls" specifically applies to the uppermost fall in Deep Canyon, which is hidden from sight by the steep canyon walls, a collective series of picturesque falls visible from the end of the trail will delight visitors. Across the cleft, Admiration Point stands guard over the thunderous clamor the water creates, spilling over glistening marble precipices into wildly churning pools. The most accessible vantage point is just down from the end of the trail, where short paths

 Stream

The Marble Fork provides dramatic scenery in spring, when the swollen watercourse cascades over rock steps and swirls through churning pools.

 Waterfall

Great Views lead to impressive views from thin grassy benches above the lower falls. By scrambling over boulders, angled slabs, and steep sections of canyon wall, you could make limited progress up-canyon to more views, but the terrain becomes quite treacherous—this off-trail route should be attempted only by adventurers skilled in such travel. The terrain becomes even more difficult farther up-canyon.

MILESTONES

►1	0.0	Start at parking area
►2	0.2	Trailhead
►3	3.4	Viewpoint

Paradise Creek Trail

Paradise Creek Trail is somewhat neglected by tourists visiting the foothills area. Perhaps the half-mile-plus walk along a paved road at the start is enough to deter the easily dissuaded. For the more diligent, the short climb beyond the Buckeye Flat Campground is a peaceful journey past lovely cataracts on both the Middle Fork Kaweah River and Paradise Creek. Before the Mineral King Road was improved, a much longer trail provided the main route to Mineral King from the Middle Fork. Today, only the first couple of miles are maintained.

Best Time

As with most foothills trails, Paradise Creek Trail is a fine trip for spring, when wildflowers are blooming and temperatures are pleasant. Situated beneath shady forest for most of the journey, the trail is a good choice for summer as well, although visitors will be most comfortable with an early start during the hottest days. Autumn is also a nice time to visit, when temperatures are mild, deciduous foliage is ablaze with color, and the height of tourist season has passed.

Finding the Trail

Follow the Generals Highway to the Hospital Rock Picnic Area parking lot, 6.1 miles east of the Ash Mountain Entrance. From the parking lot, cross Generals Highway and follow the paved road toward Buckeye Flat Campground (flush toilets, running water, bear boxes). After a half mile, veer

TRAIL USE
Day Hike, Run

LENGTH
4.4 miles, 2–2½ hours

VERTICAL FEET
+975/-280/±2510

DIFFICULTY
– 1 2 **3** 4 5 +

TRAIL TYPE
Out-and-back

FEATURES
Canyon
Stream
Wildflowers
Waterfall
Secluded
Swimming

FACILITIES
Campground

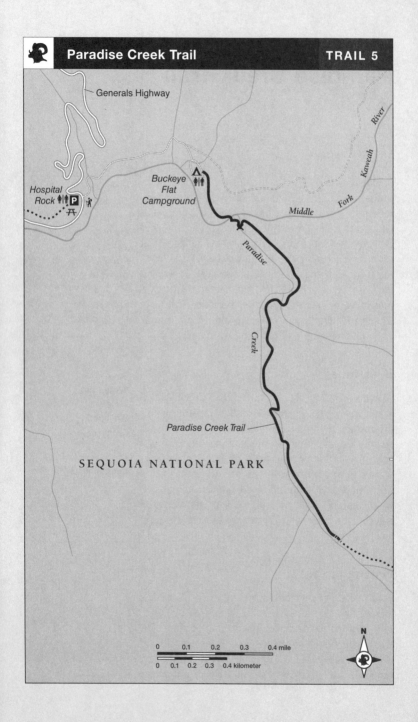

Generals Highway

Hospital
Rock

Buckeye
Flat
Campground

Kaweah

River

Middle

Fork

Paradise

Creek

Paradise Creek Trail

SEQUOIA NATIONAL PARK

| 0 | 0.1 | 0.2 | 0.3 | 0.4 mile |

| 0 | 0.1 | 0.2 | 0.3 | 0.4 kilometer |

N

right at a junction and continue downhill a short distance to the campground entrance. Proceed to the far (east) side of the campground and find the trailhead across from campsite #28.

Logistics

In the foothills zone, hikers should be on the look-out for poison oak, ticks, and rattlesnakes.

Trail Description

▶1 From the official trailhead, on gently ascending singletrack trail, you wander through oak woodland before a brief descent leads to a bridge ▶2 across Middle Fork Kaweah River. On the far side of the bridge, use trails head upstream and downstream to access the riverbank. By following the upstream path you'll soon come to a picturesque waterfall cascading into a large pool bordered by colorful rock formations. The downstream path leads to a smaller waterfall and an excellent swimming hole in Paradise Creek.

 Swimming

Waterfall

The middle trail at the far end of the bridge is the continuation of the Paradise Creek Trail, on which you ascend easily through oak woodland and lush groundcover. Climbing high above the river,

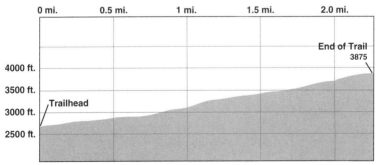

TRAIL5 Paradise Creek Trail Elevation Profile

the trees part enough to allow glimpses of the turbulent river below. Ignore a use trail on the right and continue up the main trail to a crossing of Paradise Creek, possibly a wet ford in early season. After 0.1 mile the trail crosses back over the creek and becomes steeper, as the track grows faint and brush starts to crowd the trail. Where the vegetation parts briefly, there are good views of Paradise Creek Canyon and Paradise Ridge. Perseverance pays off when, sometime later, you arrive at a pretty 15-foot-high waterfall ▶3 on the east branch of the creek. From there, retrace your steps to the parking lot.

Waterfall

🚶	**MILESTONES**		
▶1	0.0	Middle Fork Trailhead
▶2	0.2	Bridge
▶3	2.2	Waterfall

Middle Fork Trail to Panther Creek

The sunny Middle Fork Trail offers fine scenery with good views of the Great Western Divide, Moro Rock, Castle Rocks, Alta Peak, and the river canyon. After an exposed 2.8-mile hike, the shady grotto of Panther Creek is a welcome respite above a dramatic, 100-foot waterfall.

Best Times

Spring is an excellent time to use the Middle Fork Trail to Panther Creek, when the path is free of snow, mild temperatures prevail, colorful wildflowers are in bloom, and the river is full of snowmelt. The surrounding scenery is fine no matter what time of year, but summers can be unbearably hot on this virtually shadeless trail.

Finding the Trail

Follow the Generals Highway to Hospital Rock Picnic Area, 6.1 miles east of the Ash Mountain Entrance. When the road to Buckeye Flat Campground (fee, flush toilets, running water, bear boxes) is open, you can drive east from the Generals Highway a half mile to a Y-junction with the campground access road. Continue ahead from the junction on a dirt road for another 0.8 mile to the trailhead. When the road is closed, you will have to park in the Hospital Rock parking lot and walk the extra 1.3 miles to the start of the trail.

TRAIL USE
Day Hike, Backpack, Run, Horse

LENGTH
5.6 miles (8.2 miles when road closed), 3 hours (4½ hours)

VERTICAL FEET
+1325/-935/±4520

DIFFICULTY
– 1 2 **3** 4 5 +

TRAIL TYPE
Out-and-back

FEATURES
Canyon
Stream
Waterfall
Wildflowers
Great Views
Camping
Secluded

FACILITIES
Campground

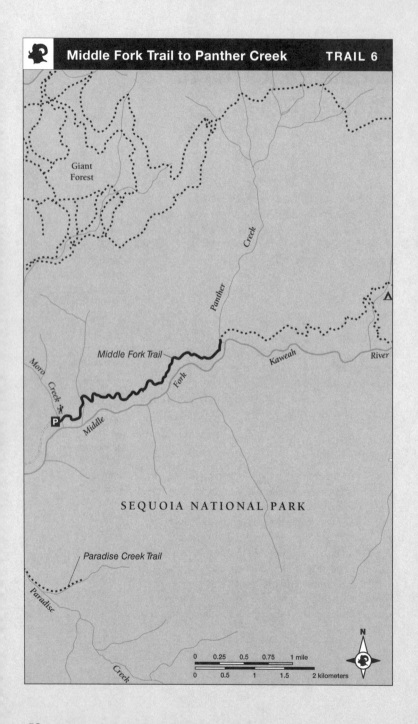

Giant
Forest

Panther Creek

Middle Fork Trail

Middle Fork

Moro Creek

Kaweah River

P

SEQUOIA NATIONAL PARK

Paradise Creek Trail

Paradise

Creek

N

| 0 | 0.25 | 0.5 | 0.75 | 1 mile |
| 0 | 0.5 | 1 | 1.5 | 2 kilometers |

Logistics

Before the Buckeye Flat Campground opens, usually in late March, you will have to walk an additional 1.3 miles on the road to access the trailhead. In the foothills zone, hikers should be on the lookout for poison oak, ticks, and rattlesnakes.

Trail Description

▶1 From the Middle Fork Trailhead, descend single-track tread shortly to a boulder-hop crossing of Moro Creek, which may be a wet ford early in the season. The stream is a picturesque setting—alders and laurels line the banks, the water dances over slanted slabs of rock, and the narrow V-shaped gorge is backdropped by the granodiorite dome of Moro Rock standing 3,000 feet above.

From the creek, a moderate climb on sandy tread slices across the canyon wall over chaparral-covered slopes. The trail soon bends into the gorge of an unnamed tributary canyon and an easy crossing of its lively but diminutive stream. From there, the trail weaves a serpentine course around the folds and creases of the river canyon. Although the vegetation blocks any view of the Middle Fork, the raucous

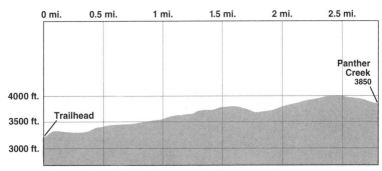

TRAIL 6 Middle Fork Trail to Panther Creek Elevation Profile

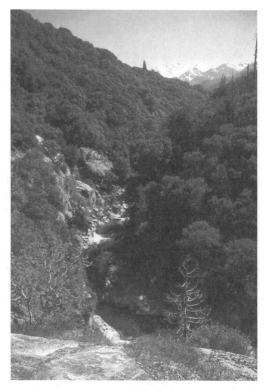

Great Western Divide *from the trail*

river is always within earshot. While the river remains mostly hidden, across the canyon are views of the spires and pinnacles of Castle Rocks, which lend a bit of ruggedness to the otherwise shrub-covered terrain. Prior to arriving at Panther Creek, three switchbacks lead up to a vista point with impressive views of the Great Western Divide, Moro Rock, Castle Rocks, and the turbulent Middle Fork Kaweah River below. Away from the viewpoint, you

Great Views

climb moderately until a steep ascent leads to the west bank of Panther Creek. ▶2

Middle Fork Trail continues for several more miles to connections with other trails near Redwood Meadow. If you wish to continue past Panther Creek, you'll have to negotiate the crossing of the shallow but fast-moving creek. Well-placed boulders usually provide a straightforward crossing, provided you're not intimidated by the presence of a precipitous waterfall just downstream, where water hurtles through a narrow chute of rock before plummeting 100 feet straight down toward the river. Whether you decide to make this crossing or swim in the inviting pools above, be extra cautious. Backpackers may find good campsites with fine views of the Great Western Divide on a bench above the far side of the creek, near some slabs toward the lip of the canyon.

 Waterfall

 Camping

🚶	**MILESTONES**

▶1   0.0   Start at Middle Fork Trailhead
▶2   2.8   Panther Creek

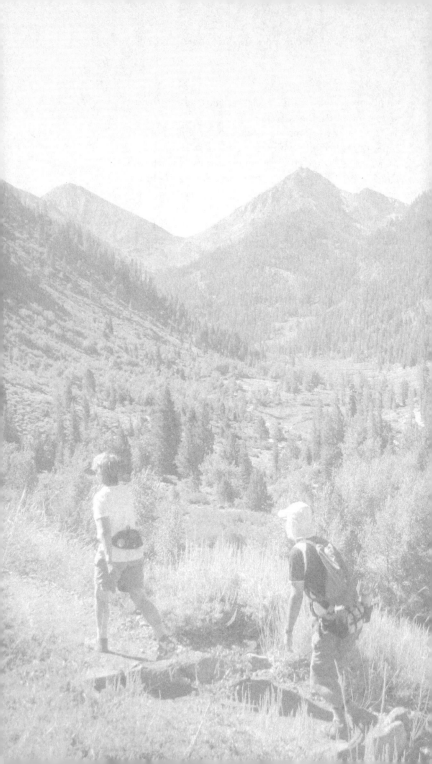

Mineral King

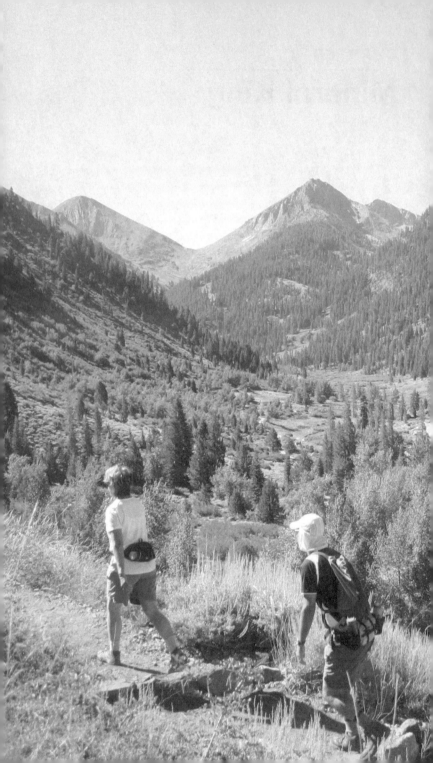

Mineral King

Access to the lovely valley of Mineral King, bordered by high, impressive-looking peaks, is via a narrow and twisting road requiring a sometimes-white-knuckle, one-hour-plus drive from the town of Three Rivers. However, the rewards are more than satisfactory upon reaching this picturesque vale bordered by alpine-looking peaks. At one time, the Disney Corporation slated Mineral King for development, with plans for a destination ski resort, which would have necessitated improving the road but at the high cost of irrevocable devastation to the wilderness ambience. Access is limited to the warmer months of the year because the National Park Service closes the road about 2.5 miles before Atwell Mill from the first of November to late May.

The first two trails in this chapter begin at a trailhead inside Atwell Mill Campground. The stiff climb to Paradise Peak offers excellent views, while the initial segment of the Atwell-Hockett Trail leads down to East Fork Kaweah River and to a lovely grove of giant sequoias. Beginning in Mineral King, all but one of the remaining trips climb stiffly out of the valley to the beautiful high country beyond. The lone exception, Cold Springs Trail, is a short and easy stroll along the river with an interpretive loop.

Permits

Permits are not required for day hikes. Backpackers must obtain a wilderness permit for all overnight trips. Between late May and late September, a quota system is in place, with a $15 fee per group. Outside the quota period, permits are free, self-issue, and available 24 hours a day. Advance reservations are available for approximately 75% of the quota, with the remainder set aside for walk-in permits. All permits must be picked up from

Overleaf and opposite: *Mineral King Valley*

the Mineral King Ranger Station between 8 a.m. and 3:45 p.m. Applications for advance reservations are accepted only by fax or mail, no earlier than midnight March 1 and no later than two weeks prior to the start of the trip. Visit the park website to download a permit application and to check on quota availability.

Maps

For the Mineral King area, the U.S. Geological Survey 7.5-minute (1:24,000 scale) topographic maps are listed below, corresponding to the trails described in this section. Sequoia Natural History Association publishes *Mineral King,* a handy foldout map for this area. Trail users may also want to consider using some of the Tom Harrison maps of this area, including *Sequoia & Kings Canyon National Parks* (1:125,000) and *Mineral King* (1:63,360).

Trail 7: *Silver City*

Trail 8: *Silver City*

Trail 9: *Mineral King*

Trail 10: *Mineral King*

Trail 11: *Mineral King*

Trail 12: *Mineral King*

Trail 13: *Mineral King*

Trail 14: *Mineral King*

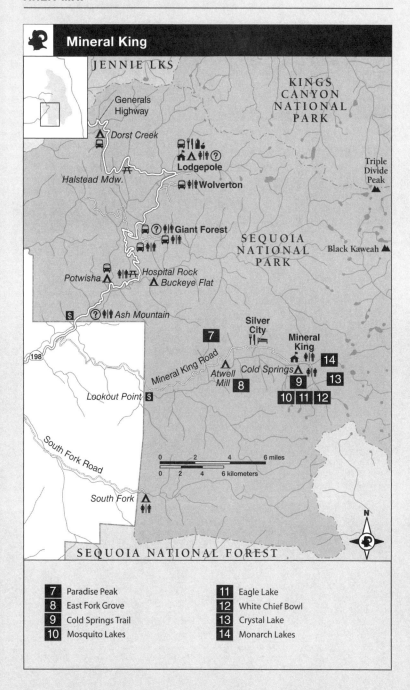

Mineral King

JENNIE LKS

KINGS CANYON NATIONAL PARK

Generals Highway

Dorst Creek

Triple Divide Peak

Lodgepole

Halstead Mdw.

Wolverton

Giant Forest

SEQUOIA NATIONAL PARK

Black Kaweah

Potwisha

Hospital Rock

Buckeye Flat

Ash Mountain

198

Mineral King Road

Silver City

Mineral King

7

14

Atwell Mill

Cold Springs

9

13

8

10 11 12

Lookout Point

South Fork Road

0   2   4   6 miles
0 2 4 6 kilometers

South Fork

N

SEQUOIA NATIONAL FOREST

7 Paradise Peak
8 East Fork Grove
9 Cold Springs Trail
10 Mosquito Lakes

11 Eagle Lake
12 White Chief Bowl
13 Crystal Lake
14 Monarch Lakes

TRAIL FEATURES TABLE

Mineral King

TRAIL	DIFFICULTY	LENGTH	TYPE	USES & ACCESS	TERRAIN	FLORA & FAUNA	OTHER
7	4	9.6	⟋	🚶🏃🐎	⛰△	❋🌲	⋔🛏⬮
8	3	5.0	⟋	🚶🏃🐎	🏞🌊	❋🌲	🛏🏠
9	1	1.2	⟍	🚶👫	🌊	❋	➤⚓🏠
10	4	7.6	⟋	🚶🎒🏃🐎	⛰🌊		△➤⚓
11	4	6.5	⟋	🚶🎒🏃	⛰🌊🌊	❋	⋔△➤⚓
12	5	7.5	⟋	🚶🎒	🏞⛰🌊🌊	❋	⋔△
13	4	7.6	⟋	🚶🎒🏃🐎	⛰🌊🌊	❋	⋔△➤
14	4	6.5	⟋	🚶🎒🏃🐎	🌊🌊	❋	⋔△➤⬮

USES & ACCESS	TYPE	TERRAIN	FLORA & FAUNA	OTHER
🚶 Day Hiking	⟲ Loop	🏞 Canyon	❋ Fall Colors	⋔ Great Views
🎒 Backpacking	⟋ Out-and-back	⛰ Mountain	❋ Wildflowers	△ Camping
🏃 Running	⟍ Point-to-point	△ Summit	🌲 Giant Sequoias	➤ Swimming
🐎 Horses		🌊 Lake		🛏 Secluded
🐕 Dogs Allowed	DIFFICULTY - 1 2 3 4 5 + less more	🌊 Stream		⬮ Steep
👫 Child Friendly		🌊 Waterfall		⚓ Fishing
♿ Wheelchair-Access				🏠 Historical Interest

Mineral King

Paradise Peak 71
A rugged climb to the top of a 9,362-foot mountain is rewarded by great views. Giant sequoias in the Atwell Grove along the way provide an added bonus. Bring along plenty of water for the south-facing ascent.

TRAIL 7

Day Hike, Run, Horse
9.6 miles, Out-and-back
Difficulty: 1 2 3 **4** 5

East Fork Grove 76
Follow the initial section of the Atwell-Hockett Trail from Atwell Mill down to East Fork Kaweah River and to the giant sequoias of the East Fork Grove.

TRAIL 8

Day Hike, Run, Horse
5 miles, Out-and-back
Difficulty: 1 2 **3** 4 5

Cold Springs Trail 80
Interpretive signs on this easy route following a short stretch of the East Fork Kaweah River provide information about the ecology and history of the Mineral King area.

TRAIL 9

Day Hike, Child Friendly
1.2 miles, Point-to-point
Difficulty: **1** 2 3 4 5

Mosquito Lakes. 84
The six Mosquito Lakes offer a variety of beautiful mountain scenery. Along with the usual recreationists, swimmers and anglers will find the lakes to be attractive destinations as well. The trail is maintained only as far as Mosquito Lake #1, but a distinct use trail can be followed to Lake #3. Straightforward cross-country travel from there is necessary to reach the upper lakes.

TRAIL 10

Day Hike, Backpack, Run, Horse
7.6 miles, Out-and-back
Difficulty: 1 2 3 **4** 5

TRAIL 11

Day Hike, Backpack,
Run, Horse

6.5 miles, Out-and-back

Difficulty: 1 2 3 **4** 5

Eagle Lake.................... 89

Perhaps the most popular hike in the Mineral King area, attractive Eagle Lake is a fine destination for those who have the stamina and are well acclimatized.

TRAIL 12

Day Hike, Backpack,
Run, Horse

7.5 miles, Out-and-back

Difficulty: 1 2 3 4 **5**

White Chief Bowl................ 95

Grand views will hopefully take your mind off the steep ascent on the way up White Chief Canyon, where you'll discover wildflower-filled meadows, old mining relics, caves, and lots of beautiful scenery.

TRAIL 13

Day Hike, Backpack,
Run, Horse

7.6 miles, Out-and-back

Difficulty: 1 2 3 **4** 5

Crystal Lake 100

Starting out on the popular Sawtooth Pass Trail, the path to Crystal Lake veers away after a couple of miles and then climbs across a scenic bowl up to a beautiful lake ringed by peaks.

TRAIL 14

Day Hike, Backpack,
Run, Horse

6.6 miles, Out-and-back

Difficulty: 1 2 3 **4** 5

Monarch Lakes 104

Just about every trail out of Mineral King requires a stiff climb, and this trail to the Monarch Lakes is no exception. En route to the spectacularly scenic lakes, you have splendid views of Mineral King valley bordered by dramatic-looking peaks.

Paradise Peak

You can avoid the crowds on this nearly 10-mile out-and-back hike to the top of Paradise Peak, as most recreationists willing to drive the long and winding Mineral King Road are headed farther up the road to trailheads in Mineral King valley. Additionally, the climb to the former lookout is relatively stiff, which deters even more hikers from taking this trail. However, only the first 3.2 miles are moderately steep up a south-facing slope before you gain gentler terrain along Paradise Ridge. Along the way, the Atwell Grove boasts some of the largest giant sequoias in existence. Your effort to reach the summit is well rewarded with fine views of the Great Western Divide and the surrounding foothills.

Best Time

Mineral King Road is usually open by Memorial Day weekend, but the trail to the top of Paradise Peak remains snowbound until mid-June and then closes with the first major storm of the season, generally in late October or early November.

Finding the Trail

Drive eastbound from Visalia on CA 198 to the east edge of Three Rivers and turn onto Mineral King Road. Follow the narrow and sometimes winding road to the Lookout Point Entrance Station (fee), past the entrance to Atwell Mill Campground (fee, vault toilets, running water, bear boxes, and phone), and then 0.2 mile farther to the signed trailhead parking area near the east edge of the campground,

TRAIL USE
Day Hike, Run, Horse
LENGTH
9.6 miles, 4–5 hours
VERTICAL FEET
+2990/-185/±6350
DIFFICULTY
– 1 2 3 **4 5** +
TRAIL TYPE
Out-and-back

FEATURES
Mountain
Summit
Wildflowers
Giant Sequoias
Great Views
Secluded
Steep

FACILITIES
Campground
Bear Box

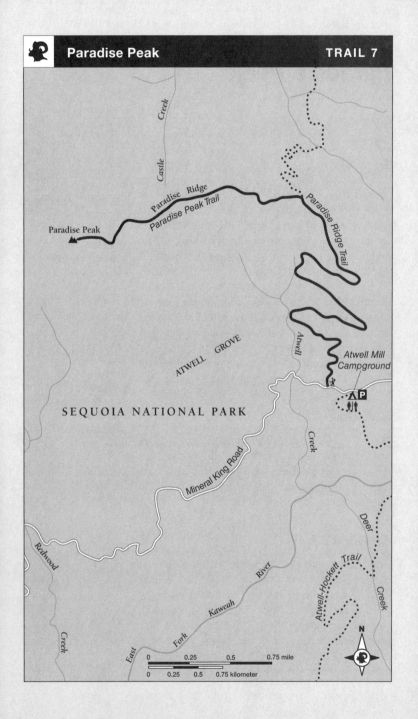

Paradise Peak

TRAIL 7

Creek

Castle

Paradise Ridge

Paradise Peak Trail

Paradise Peak

Paradise Ridge Trail

ATWELL GROVE

Atwell

Atwell Mill
Campground

SEQUOIA NATIONAL PARK

Creek

Mineral King Road

Deer

Redwood

River

Kaweah

Atwell-Hockett Trail

Creek

East

Fork

Creek

0   0.25   0.5   0.75 mile

0   0.25   0.5   0.75 kilometer

N

18.2 miles from CA 198. Silver City Mountain Resort is a short distance up the road, offering cabins, chalets, showers, a restaurant and bakery, and a limited selection of supplies.

Trail Description

▶1 From the parking area you must head back down the Mineral King Road for a quarter mile to the signed Paradise Ridge Trailhead, where singletrack trail begins a moderate climb through a mixed forest of white firs, ponderosa pines, sugar pines, incense cedars, and young sequoias shading an understory of mountain misery and manzanita. Soon a series of switchbacks leads far up the hillside past an opening in the forest, where medium-size giant sequoias make an appearance, just before a small fern-and-alder-lined seasonal rivulet. Larger sequoias will be seen farther up the trail, which are some of the 20 to 30 largest specimens in the Sierra.

Additional switchbacks lead steeply up the hillside and toward Atwell Creek—contrary to what is shown on the U.S. Geological Survey 7.5-minute Silver City quadrangle, the trail approaches but does not cross the creek. If you need water after the thirst-inducing climb, you'll have to thrash your way through thick brush to this stream, which

> **Your effort to reach the summit is well rewarded with fine views of the Great Western Divide and the surrounding foothills.**

 Steep

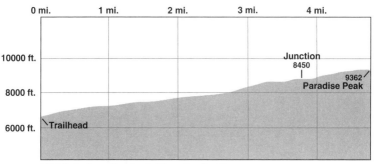

TRAIL 7 Paradise Peak Elevation Profile

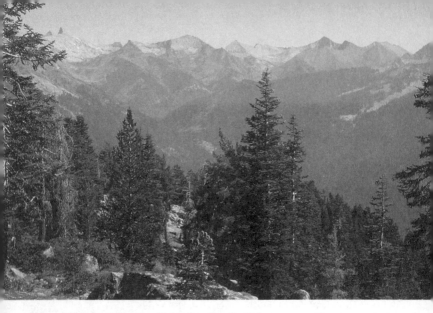

View of the Great Western Divide *from Paradise Peak*

is the only reliable water source along the entire route. Away from the stream, the switchbacking ascent continues to a junction on the crest of **Paradise Ridge.** ▶2

Turn west at the junction and proceed through a light forest of red firs and widely scattered patches of snowbush, chinquapin, and manzanita. The gentle grade of the trail along the ridge is a welcome respite following the steep climb up the south-facing hillside below. After passing to the north of Peak 8863, keen eyes may be able to spy the crown of the giant sequoia growing at the highest elevation in the Sierra (8,800 feet) downslope to the southeast. Proceed up the ridge and then wind toward the top of the peak over rocky terrain, where distinct tread falters but the way to the summit is clear. From the summit of **Paradise Peak,** ▶3 you have fine views to the east of the Great Western Divide, and to the north of Castle Rocks and the granite domes of Big and Little Baldy.

A trip to Paradise Peak is incomplete without experiencing the stunning view from the site of the

Giant Sequoias 🌲

Summit △

Paradise Peak Lookout

The lookout on top of Paradise Peak was in operation until the 1950s, when many of the fire lookouts were decommissioned in the Sierra. Today, a nearby radio repeater stands as an unwelcome reminder of more-contemporary human presence.

old lookout, directly southwest of the true summit. Work your way through brush and over boulders to the base of the rock at the end of the ridge, climb some rock steps, and then scramble up a crack to the top. You may not be able to see the Great Western Divide from this vantage, thanks to a mature stand of trees, but the impressive vista to the west includes the steep cleft of Paradise Creek running into Middle Fork Kaweah River. Also visible are Moro Rock, Alta Peak, and the Generals Highway.

MILESTONES

▶1	0.0	Start at Paradise Peak Trailhead
▶2	3.2	Turn left (west) at junction
▶3	4.8	Summit of Paradise Peak

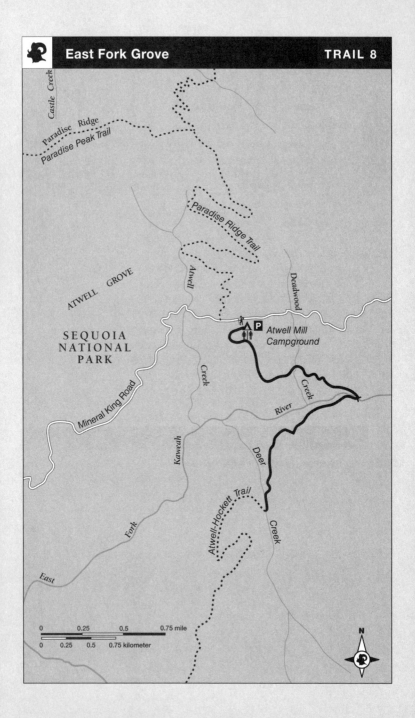

Castle Creek

Paradise Ridge
Paradise Peak Trail

Paradise Ridge Trail

ATWELL GROVE

Atwell

Deadwood

SEQUOIA
NATIONAL
PARK

Atwell Mill
Campground

P

Creek

Creek

River

Mineral King Road

Kaweah

Deer

Atwell-Hockett Trail

Creek

Fork

East

| 0 | 0.25 | 0.5 | 0.75 mile |
| 0 | 0.25 | 0.5 | 0.75 kilometer |

N

East Fork Grove

The Atwell-Hockett Trail is not as well traveled as the more popular trails leaving Mineral King, which makes even this short jaunt to the East Fork Grove of giant sequoias a usually secluded experience. After passing through the former site of Atwell Mill, where the big trees were cut down to be made into grape stakes in the late 1800s, the trail drops to a sturdy bridge spanning East Fork Kaweah River. Beyond the river, the path wanders another mile into the heart of the East Fork Grove to Deer Creek, a good turnaround point for day hikers.

Best Times

While giant sequoias are always in season, this trail is typically free of snow from late May to early November, corresponding to the time when the National Park Service opens the road. Peak flows in East Fork Kaweah River usually occur in early summer, about the same time as when wildflowers reach their zenith.

TRAIL USE
Day Hike, Run, Horse

LENGTH
5.0 miles, 2 hours

VERTICAL FEET
+525/-820/±2690

DIFFICULTY
– 1 2 **3** 4 5 +

TRAIL TYPE
Out-and-back

FEATURES
Canyon
Stream
Wildflowers
Giant Sequoias
Secluded
Historical Interest

FACILITIES
Campground

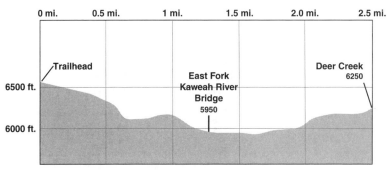

TRAIL 8 East Fork Grove Elevation Profile

77

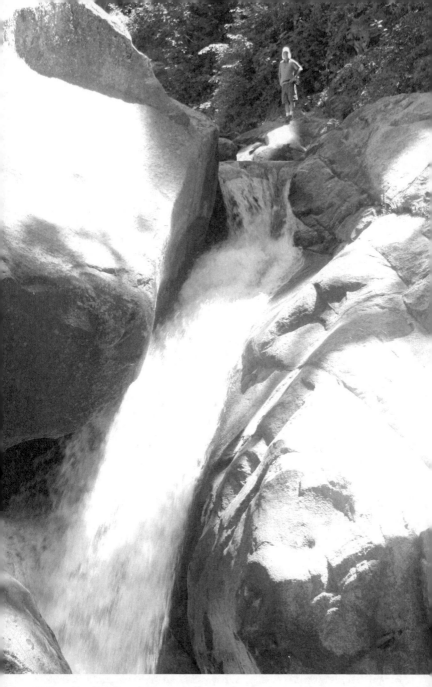

Falls *on East Fork Kaweah River*

Finding the Trail

From the east side of Three Rivers, leave CA 198 and turn onto Mineral King Road. Follow the narrow and sometimes winding road for 18.2 miles to the entrance for Atwell Mill Campground (vault toilets, running water, bear boxes), and then continue another 0.2 mile to the signed trailhead parking area at the east end of the campground.

Trail Description

▶1 Walk down a road toward the campground for about 250 yards to the signed Atwell Mill Trailhead. From there, follow the trail past redwood stumps to a small meadow with old relics left over from the long abandoned Atwell Mill. Beyond the mill site, you descend through a mixed forest of black and canyon oaks, white firs, ponderosa pines, incense cedars, and scattered sequoias to Deadwood Creek. The descent continues for another half mile to a steel-and-wood bridge across the granite cleft of East Fork Kaweah River, ▶2 1.25 miles from the parking area. From the bridge, you have a fine view of the cascading river plummeting over slabs and dancing around boulders through a narrow, sequoia-lined gorge.

A mild-to-moderate climb leads away from the bridge and through the East Fork Grove for another mile to Deer Creek, ▶3 which provides a good turnaround point for day hikers.

Giant
Sequoias

🚶	**MILESTONES**	
▶1	0.0	Start at Atwell Mill Trailhead
▶2	1.25	East Fork Kaweah River Bridge
▶3	2.5	Deer Creek

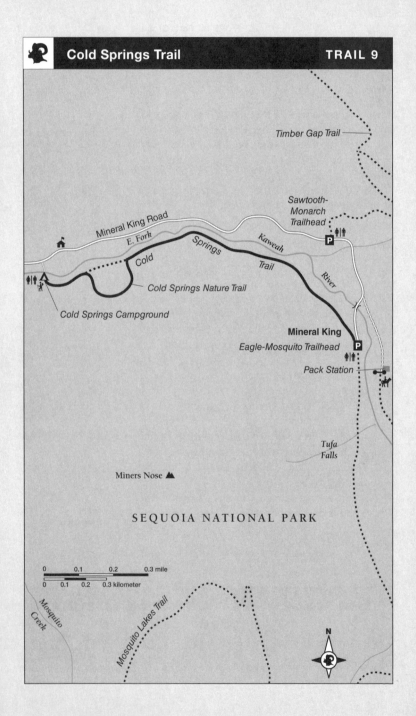

Cold Springs Trail **TRAIL 9**

Timber Gap Trail

Sawtooth-
Monarch
Trailhead

Mineral King Road

E. Fork

Kaweah

Cold

Springs

Trail

River

Cold Springs Nature Trail

Mineral King

Cold Springs Campground

Eagle-Mosquito Trailhead

Pack Station

Tufa
Falls

Miners Nose ▲▲

SEQUOIA NATIONAL PARK

| 0 | 0.1 | 0.2 | 0.3 mile |
| 0 | 0.1 | 0.2 | 0.3 kilometer |

Mosquito Lakes Trail

Mosquito
Creek

N

Cold Springs Trail

Enjoy the stunning scenery of Mineral King while learning about the human and natural history of the area on this short and easy jaunt along East Fork Kaweah River. The trail is well suited for campers at the adjacent Cold Springs Campground and for families with young children.

Best Times

Wildflowers are at their peak in early to midsummer. On the hottest days, plan on an early start because most of the trail is exposed to the sun.

Finding the Trail

START: From the east side of Three Rivers, leave CA 198 and turn onto Mineral King Road. Follow the narrow and sometimes winding road for 22 miles to the Cold Springs Campground entrance, 2.5 miles past Silver City. Just after crossing a bridge over East Fork Kaweah River, turn left at the first intersection, and drive 0.1 mile to the small parking area near campsite #6.

END: Continue on Mineral King Road past the Cold Springs Campground entrance another 1.2 miles, passing the ranger station on the way, to the Eagle-Mosquito Trailhead parking area at the end of the road.

Trail Description

►1 From the campground trailhead the trail follows the south bank of East Fork Kaweah River upstream

TRAIL USE
Day Hike, Child Friendly
LENGTH
1.2 miles, 1 hour
VERTICAL FEET
+350/-20/±370
DIFFICULTY
– **1** 2 3 4 5 +
TRAIL TYPE
Point-to-point

FEATURES
Stream
Wildflowers
Swimming
Historical Interest
Fishing

FACILITIES
Campground

Beulah

During the 1880s, the mining town springing up in Mineral King was named Beulah for the biblical land of promise, but the area never lived up to such expectations—the mines produced just enough ore to limp along but never enough to be profitable. The San Francisco earthquake of 1906 triggered a massive avalanche that put the final nail in the town's coffin.

Wildflowers

at a gentle grade, crossing grassland dotted with aspens and cottonwoods. Early summer visitors will be treated to a fine display of colorful wildflowers. Reach the west junction ▶2 of the Cold Springs Nature Trail after 0.1 mile.

Turn right and follow the loop with interpretive signs about the flora, geology, and mining history of the Mineral King area. Shortly rejoin the Cold Springs Trail again at the east junction ▶3 at the end of the loop.

From the east junction of the nature trail, the Cold Springs Trail continues upstream closer to the river, passing some dramatic cascades and lovely

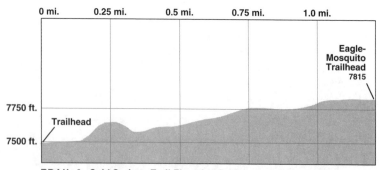

TRAIL 9 Cold Springs Trail Elevation Profile

pools. This section of the trail offers access for fishing and wading, as well as nearby picnic spots. Farther on, switchbacks lead higher up the slope into a copse of red firs. Soon breaking out of the trees, you traverse drier, sagebrush-covered slopes, crossing several small rivulets on short wood bridges on the way. A series of rock steps leads to the last stretch of trail, passing a number of old cabins on the way to the end at the Eagle-Mosquito Trailhead. ▶4

Fishing

Swimming

		MILESTONES
▶1	0.0	Start at Cold Springs Campground Trailhead
▶2	0.1	Right at Cold Springs Nature Trail West Junction
▶3	0.2	Right at Cold Springs Nature Trail East Junction
▶4	1.2	Eagle-Mosquito Trailhead

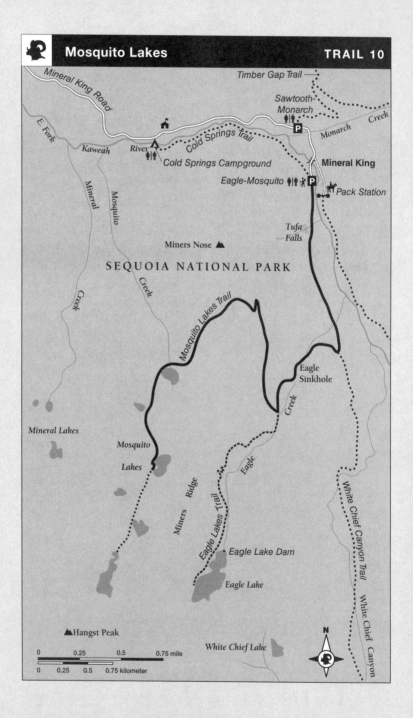

Mosquito Lakes — TRAIL 10

Timber Gap Trail

Sawtooth-Monarch

Mineral King Road

E. Fork

Kaweah

Mineral

Mosquito

Creek

Creek

Monarch Creek

Cold Springs Trail

Cold Springs Campground

River

Eagle-Mosquito

Mineral King

Pack Station

Tufa Falls

Miners Nose ▲

SEQUOIA NATIONAL PARK

Mosquito Lakes Trail

Eagle Sinkhole

Creek

Mineral Lakes

Mosquito Lakes

Miners Ridge

Eagle Lakes Trail

Eagle

Creek

White Chief Canyon Trail

Eagle Lake Dam

Eagle Lake

White Chief Canyon

▲ Hangst Peak

0   0.25   0.5   0.75 mile

0   0.25   0.5   0.75 kilometer

White Chief Lake

N

Mosquito Lakes

The diverse scenery found around the six Mosquito Lakes varies from forest-rimmed lakes to barren and rockbound. The trail is only maintained as far as Mosquito Lake #1, but a distinct use trail can be easily followed to Lake #3. Beyond there, cross-country skills will be necessary to access the upper lakes. Those who travel that far should have the area pretty much to themselves. All of the beautiful lakes are well suited for swimming and fishing. Backpackers will find the best campsites at Mosquito Lake #3.

Best Time

The Mineral King Road is usually open by Memorial Day weekend, but the trail to Mosquito Lakes is generally snowbound until early July following winters of average snowfall. Trail use is highest from mid-July through August. The weather in September can be quite enjoyable.

TRAIL USE
Day Hike, Backpack, Run, Horse

LENGTH
7.6 miles, 3½ hours

VERTICAL FEET
+2075/-300/±4750

DIFFICULTY
– 1 2 3 **4** 5 +

TRAIL TYPE
Out-and-back

FEATURES
Mountain
Lakes
Camping
Swimming
Fishing

FACILITIES
Campground
Ranger Station

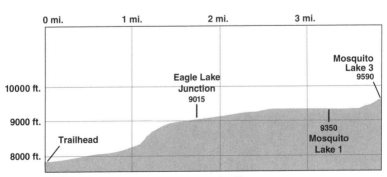

TRAIL 10 **Mosquito Lakes Elevation Profile**

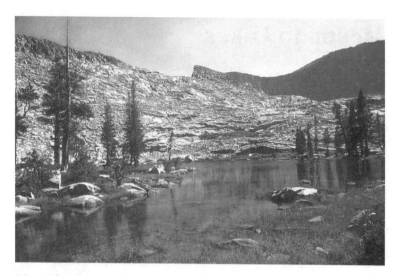

Lake #3 *from Mosquito Lakes Trail*

Finding the Trail

From the east side of Three Rivers, leave CA 198 and turn onto Mineral King Road. Continue past the Cold Springs Campground entrance and the ranger station to the Eagle-Mosquito Trailhead parking area at the end of the road.

Logistics

Backpackers must obtain a wilderness permit for all overnight visits. See pages 65–66 for more details about how to obtain one. Camping is banned at Lake #1, and campfires are prohibited.

Trail Description

►1 South of the parking area, a dirt road begins near the trailhead signboard and the restored Honeymoon Cabin. Follow this road on a mild climb up the East Fork Kaweah River canyon through open vegetation, sprinkled with red firs, mountain maples, and an occasional juniper. After a quarter mile, cross a removable wood bridge over Spring Creek and soon pass a lateral descending to the west bank of the river. Across the valley, cascading Crystal Creek can be seen plummeting down the canyon wall. A mile from the trailhead, hop across willow-lined Eagle Creek and shortly arrive at a signed junction with the White Chief Trail. ▶2

Turn right and follow the trail around a hillside to a set of steep switchbacks climbing through pockets of meadow alternating with stands of red firs and lodgepole pines. The grade eases on the approach to Eagle Sinkhole, where a stretch of Eagle Creek mysteriously disappears to adopt a temporary subterranean course. The ascent resumes past this anomaly, soon leading to a junction with the trail to Eagle Lake. ▶3

Turn right at the junction and climb through red firs to the crest of Miners Ridge, from where a 0.75-mile switchbacking descent leads to Mosquito

OPTIONS

Cross-Country to Mosquito Lakes 4–6

Above Lake #3, signs of the old trail finally disappear for good. Cairns may be of assistance as you head cross-country up the next hillside to the right of a rocky slope. The next part of the route passes well to the east of Lake #4, from where Mineral Lakes are accessible via an off-trail route over a saddle west of the lake. Proceed toward irregularly shaped Lake #5 tucked against the cliffs of Miners Ridge, where the grassy shoreline is dotted with scattered lodgepole pines.

The cross-country route to austere, treeless Lake #6, the last in the chain, continues another quarter mile up the canyon. From this lake, an off-trail route over Miners Ridge to Eagle Lake is possible.

Lake #1 ▸4 at 3.25 miles from the trailhead. The oval-shaped lake is backdropped by a talus slope and encircled by lodgepole pines. Camping has been banned here in an attempt to restore the native vegetation.

Beyond the first lake the trail is not maintained but is still discernible as far as Lake #3. Follow distinct tread around the west shore of Lake #1, and then head south up a steep hillside, where old blazes and cairns mark the route. To the east of Lake #2, another steep but short climb leads to Lake #3, ▸5 where a pair of small islands and an amphitheater of towering white cliffs enhance the scenery. Slabs near the south shore surely will entice both sunbathers and swimmers, while anglers may ply the waters in search of landing a brook trout. A sparse forest of lodgepole pines encircling the lake shades some fine campsites.

Swimming

Fishing

Camping

🚶 MILESTONES

▸1	0.0	Start at Eagle-Mosquito Trailhead
▸2	1.0	Right (south) at White Chief Canyon junction
▸3	1.75	Right (southwest) at Eagle Lake junction
▸4	3.25	Mosquito Lake #1
▸5	3.8	Mosquito Lake #3

Eagle Lake

Crystalline Eagle Lake, reposing majestically in a deep and scenic cirque, lures flocks of anglers, photographers, day hikers, and backpackers to its shores seemingly every summer day. The lake's popularity is well deserved, requiring only a 3-plus-mile journey to reach, but the stiff climb demands that visitors be in reasonable physical condition. Although camping is permitted at Eagle Lake (except between the trail and the lake on the west shore) campsites are at a premium, making this trip better suited for day hiking. Backpackers leaving cars overnight in Mineral King will need to place all food and scented items in the storage shed directly across from the ranger station because bear boxes are not available at trailheads. Especially in early season, marmots in the area have been known to nibble on radiator hoses, fan belts, brake lines, and even radiators—check with park rangers for current conditions.

Best Time

The Mineral King Road is usually open by Memorial Day weekend, but the trail to Eagle Lake is generally snowbound until early July following winters of average snowfall. Trail use is highest from mid-July through August. The weather in September can be quite enjoyable, but Eagle Lake becomes less attractive as the water level drops by late summer.

Finding the Trail

Drive eastbound from Visalia on CA 198 to the east edge of Three Rivers and turn onto Mineral King

TRAIL USE
Day Hike, Backpack, Run, Horse
LENGTH
6.5 miles, 3–4 hours
VERTICAL FEET
+2285/-55/±4680
DIFFICULTY
– 1 2 3 **4** 5 +
TRAIL TYPE
Out-and-back

FEATURES
Mountain
Lake
Stream
Wildflowers
Great Views
Camping
Swimming
Fishing

FACILITIES
Campground
Ranger Station

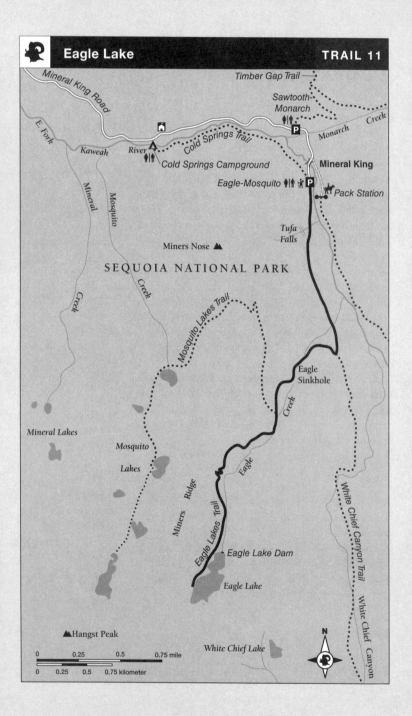

Eagle Lake — TRAIL 11

Timber Gap Trail

Mineral King Road

Sawtooth-
Monarch

P

Monarch Creek

E. Fork

Cold Springs Trail

Kaweah River

Cold Springs Campground

Mineral King

Eagle-Mosquito

P

Pack Station

Mineral

Mosquito

Tufa
Falls

Miners Nose ▲

SEQUOIA NATIONAL PARK

Creek

Mosquito Lakes Trail

Eagle
Sinkhole

Creek

Eagle Creek

Mineral Lakes

Mosquito

Lakes

Miners Ridge

Eagle

White Chief Canyon Trail

Eagle Lakes Trail

Eagle Lake Dam

Eagle Lake

White Chief Canyon

▲Hangst Peak

| 0 | 0.25 | 0.5 | 0.75 mile |

| 0 | 0.25 | 0.5 | 0.75 kilometer |

White Chief Lake

N

Road. Follow the narrow and sometimes winding road to the Lookout Point Entrance Station (fee) and proceed through the tiny resort community of Silver City. Silver City Mountain Resort offers cabins, chalets, showers, a restaurant and bakery, and a limited selection of supplies.

Continue past the entrance to Cold Springs Campground (fee, vault toilets, running water, bear boxes, and phone) and the Mineral King Ranger Station to the Mosquito-Eagle Trailhead at the end of the road, 23.5 miles from CA 198. Plan on a minimum of 1.25 hours for the drive along the Mineral King Road.

Logistics

Backpackers must obtain a wilderness permit for all overnight visits. See pages 65–66 for more details about how to obtain one.

Trail Description

▶1 South of the parking area a dirt road begins near the trailhead signboard and the restored Honeymoon Cabin. Follow this road on a mild climb up the East Fork Kaweah River canyon through open vegetation, sprinkled with red firs, mountain maples, and

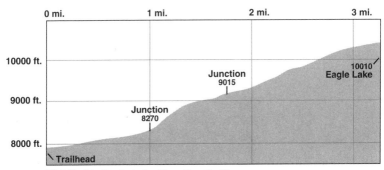

TRAIL 11 Eagle Lake Elevation Profile

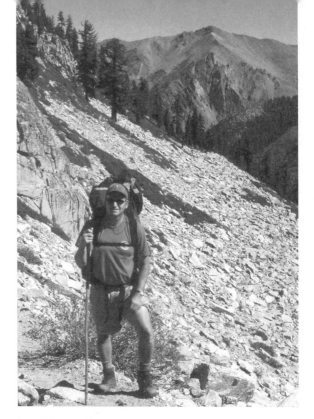

Talus slide *on the trail*

an occasional juniper. After a quarter mile, cross a removable wood bridge over Spring Creek and soon pass a lateral descending to the west bank of the river. Across the valley, cascading Crystal Creek can be seen plummeting down the far canyon wall. A mile from the trailhead, you hop across willow-lined Eagle Creek and shortly arrive at a signed junction with the White Chief Trail. ▶2

Stream ↻

Follow the trail around a hillside to a set of steep switchbacks climbing through pockets of meadow alternating with stands of red firs and lodgepole pines. The grade eases on the approach to Eagle Sinkhole, where a stretch of Eagle Creek mysteriously disappears on a temporarily subterranean course. The ascent resumes past this anomaly, soon leading to a junction with the trail to Mosquito Lakes. ▶3

From the junction, the trail climbs mildly alongside Eagle Creek to the far end of a meadow, where a steeper, switchbacking ascent leads up a forested hillside and then to the base of an expansive, talus-littered slope. A long, ascending traverse across the talus heads toward the lip of Eagle Lake's basin, with fine views of Mineral Peak, Sawtooth Peak, and the silvery thread of cascading Crystal Creek along the way. The grade eases past the talus, as you pass through pockets of grasses and shrubs, and scattered boulders and rock slabs beneath a light forest of lodgepole pines. A short section of steeper climbing leads to the concrete dam at the north end of Eagle Lake. ▶4

The stunning scenery of Eagle Lake's steep-walled cirque is complemented by the soaring summit of Eagle Crest immediately to the south. Opposite, a row of multicolored peaks rims the deep cleft of Mineral King. Just beyond the dam, a lateral heads uphill a short distance to a screened pit toilet, placed here by the National Park Service in hopes of minimizing the pollution generated at this popular destination. Camping is not allowed between the trail and the

> The stunning scenery of Eagle Lake's steep-walled cirque is complemented by the soaring summit of Eagle Crest.

 Lake

 Great Views

OPTIONS

Mosquito Lakes Cross-Country Route

Off-trail enthusiasts can ascend Miners Ridge to the west and then drop down to the Mosquito Lakes basin. The route is short but quite steep, with a particularly rocky descent on the Mosquito Lakes side. The least difficult crossing is directly upslope from the Eagle Lake Dam. Once at Mosquito Lake #4 (around 9,910 feet in elevation), you could work your way cross-country down-canyon to pick up an unmaintained path to Mosquito Lake #1, where distinct and maintained tread leads 1.5 miles back to the junction with the Eagle Lake Trail. From there, retrace your steps 1.75 miles to the Mosquito-Eagle Trailhead. Plan on an hour or two extra for this diversion.

Eagle Lake Dam

The Mt. Whitney Power and Electric Company built the dam at Eagle Lake in the early 1900s to regulate water flow for power production at a downstream generating plant in Hammond. Similar dams were constructed nearby at Crystal, Franklin, and Monarch Lakes. Today, the water in Eagle Lake is regulated by Southern California Edison Company, resulting in a dramatic drop in lake level by late season, which has a tendency to diminish the attractiveness of the lake toward the end of summer.

Camping lake, with the best sites for overnight accommodations about midway down the west shore. Anglers may enjoy fishing for small to medium brook trout.

🚶 MILESTONES

▶1	0.0	Start at Mosquito-Eagle Trailhead
▶2	1.0	Turn right (south) at White Chief Canyon junction
▶3	1.75	Proceed straight ahead (south-southwest) at Mosquito Lakes junction
▶4	3.25	Eagle Lake

White Chief Bowl

White Chief Trail climbs steeply at times into a horseshoe-shaped canyon with towering walls holding a pair of lovely meadows, historic mining ruins, and caves. Along the way are great views and delightful wildflower gardens. The naturally occurring caves and old mine shafts (some privately owned) are potentially dangerous—check with the park rangers about current conditions.

Best Time

The Mineral King Road is usually open by Memorial Day weekend, but the trail to White Chief Meadow is generally snowbound until early July following winters of average snowfall. Trail use is highest from mid-July through August. The weather in September can be quite enjoyable.

Finding the Trail

From the east side of Three Rivers, leave CA 198 and turn onto Mineral King Road. Continue on the narrow and sometimes winding road past the Cold Springs Campground entrance and the ranger station to the Eagle-Mosquito Trailhead parking area at the end of the road.

Logistics

Backpackers must obtain a wilderness permit for all overnight visits. See pages 65–66 for more details about how to obtain one. Campfires are prohibited.

TRAIL USE
Day Hike, Backpack, Run, Horse
LENGTH
7.5 miles, 4 hours
VERTICAL FEET
+2360/-150/±5020
DIFFICULTY
– 1 2 3 4 **5** +
TRAIL TYPE
Out-and-back

FEATURES
Canyon
Mountain
Lake
Stream
Wildflowers
Great Views
Camping

FACILITIES
Campground
Ranger Station

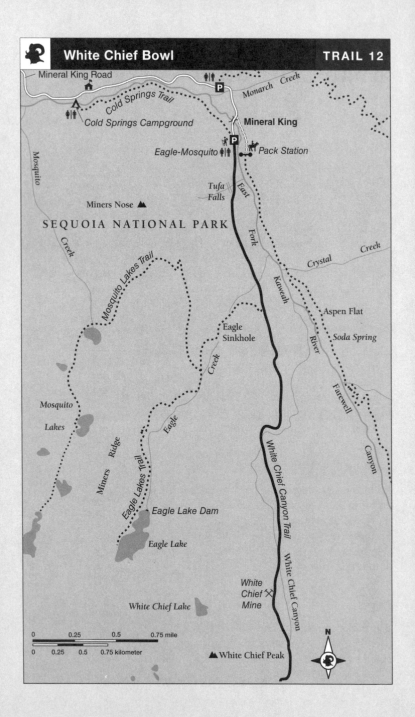

Mineral King Road

Cold Springs Trail

Monarch Creek

Cold Springs Campground

Mineral King

Eagle-Mosquito

Pack Station

Mosquito

Tufa Falls

East

Miners Nose ▲

SEQUOIA NATIONAL PARK

Creek

Fork

Crystal Creek

Mosquito Lakes Trail

Kaweah

Eagle Sinkhole

Aspen Flat

Soda Spring

Creek

River

Mosquito Lakes

Eagle

Farewell

Miners Ridge

Eagle Lakes Trail

White Chief Canyon Trail

Canyon

Eagle Lake Dam

Eagle Lake

White Chief Canyon

White Chief Lake

White Chief Mine ✕

0   0.25   0.5   0.75 mile
0   0.25   0.5   0.75 kilometer

▲ White Chief Peak

N

Trail Description

▶1 South of the parking area a dirt road begins near the trailhead signboard and the restored Honeymoon Cabin. Follow this road on a mild climb up the East Fork Kaweah River canyon through open vegetation, sprinkled with red firs, mountain maples, and an occasional juniper. After a quarter mile, cross a removable wood bridge over Spring Creek and soon pass a lateral descending to the west bank of the river. Across the valley, cascading Crystal Creek can be seen plummeting down the canyon wall. A mile from the trailhead, hop across willow-lined Eagle Creek and shortly arrive at a signed junction with the White Chief Trail. ▶2

Head south (straight ahead) from the junction and follow the White Chief Trail up the canyon. If you thought the previous mile-long climb was tough, the next stretch of trail is as steep as any maintained trail in the parks. Hopefully, the excellent view of the canyon and the peaks above will distract you from the grueling ascent. Fortunately, the grade eventually moderates, as you cross sagebrush-covered slopes dotted with junipers and pass outcrops of dark metamorphic rock. The grade eases even more on the approach to White Chief Meadow, 2 miles from the trailhead. ▶3

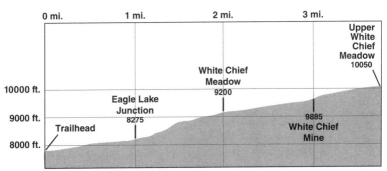

TRAIL 12 White Chief Bowl Elevation Profile

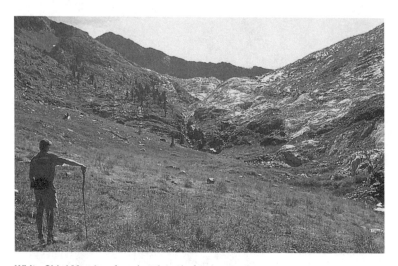

White Chief Meadow *from the White Chief Canyon Trail*

Cross the creek and follow the trail across the edge of the meadow. Over the years, numerous avalanches have swept the slopes above and deposited debris across the flat. Soon the trail climbs a rib to a bench overlooking the meadow, where campsites are nestled beneath red firs and foxtail pines. A resident herd of deer is often seen nearby around dusk.

Camping

Away from the meadow, you soon leave the trees behind and cross open, view-packed slopes carpeted with wildflowers, including gentian, yarrow, and bluebell. The stream plays a game of cat and mouse in the canyon below, frequently disappearing and then reappearing; this seemingly erratic behavior is actually quite common for creeks in areas of marble and limestone. Cross the main

Wildflowers

White Chief Mine

HISTORY

Claiming they were guided by an Indian spirit on an all-night vision quest, John Crabtree and two companions discovered this deposit and then built the mine, which sparked the Mineral King gold rush. The mines never produced a single bar of gold or silver.

Crabtree Cabin

The ruins of Crabtree Cabin, a hump of debris on a low rise just west of the lower end of the meadow, are all that remain of the cabin built by John Crabtree, who bunked miners here working at the White Chief Mine nearby.

branch of the creek, ascend the far hillside, and pass through tailings directly below White Chief Mine, ▶4 which was blasted out of a huge vein of marble. Do not explore the privately owned mine without permission from the owners.

Past the mine, ascend rocky slopes across the west wall of the canyon. Where the tread becomes hard to follow, cairns should help keep you on track. Continue up the canyon past numerous mine shafts, sinkholes, and caves to another crossing of the creek. The trail moves away from the creek temporarily on the east side of the drainage, climbs a grassy slope, and then returns. From there, follow the creek to a meadow-rimmed tarn at the head of the canyon, where you may find ruins from old mining cabins and natural marble caverns.

Reaching White Chief Lake from the upper meadow is possible by heading cross-country on a rising traverse of the talus-filled slope below White Chief Peak. ▶5

⚑ MILESTONES

▶1	0.0	Start at Eagle-Mosquito Trailhead
▶2	1.0	Straight at the Eagle Lake Trail junction
▶3	2.0	White Chief Meadow
▶4	3.0	White Chief Mine
▶5	3.75	Upper White Chief Meadow

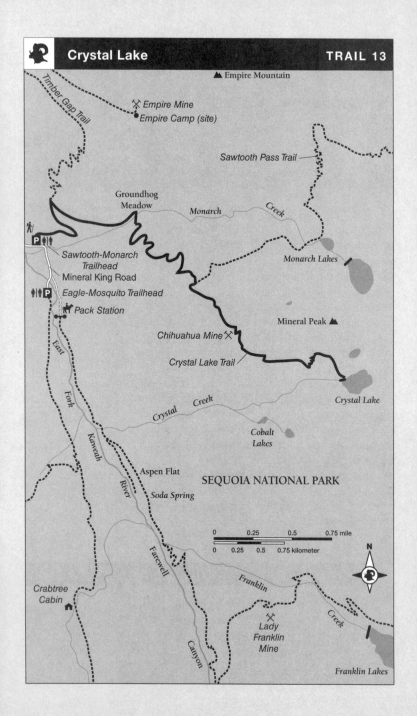

▲ Empire Mountain

⚒ Empire Mine
● Empire Camp (site)

Sawtooth Pass Trail

Timber Gap Trail

Groundhog Meadow

Monarch   Creek

Monarch Lakes

Sawtooth-Monarch Trailhead

Mineral King Road

Eagle-Mosquito Trailhead

🐎 Pack Station

P

Mineral Peak ▲

Chihuahua Mine ⚒

Crystal Lake Trail

Crystal Lake

East

Fork

Kaweah

Crystal   Creek

Cobalt Lakes

Aspen Flat   SEQUOIA NATIONAL PARK

River

Soda Spring

0   0.25   0.5   0.75 mile
0   0.25   0.5   0.75 kilometer

N

Farewell

Franklin

Creek

Crabtree Cabin

Canyon

⚒ Lady Franklin Mine

Franklin Lakes

Crystal Lake

While the start of this route follows the popular Sawtooth Pass Trail, after 2.9 miles the trail to Crystal Lake veers away to the southeast across open, view-packed Chihuahua Bowl, crosses over an airy ridge, and then traverses above Crystal Creek before zigzagging up to the lake. Occupying a horseshoe-shaped bowl south of Mineral Peak and immediately west of the Great Western Divide, beautiful Crystal Lake is a fine destination for day hikers and overnighters.

TRAIL USE
Day Hike, Backpack, Run, Horse

LENGTH
9.6 miles, 4 hours

VERTICAL FEET
+3675/-500/±8350

DIFFICULTY
– 1 2 3 **4** 5 +

TRAIL TYPE
Out-and-back

Best Time

The Mineral King Road is usually open by Memorial Day weekend, but the trail to Crystal Lake is generally snowbound until early July following winters of average snowfall. Trail use is highest from mid-July through August. The weather in September can be quite enjoyable.

FEATURES
Mountain
Lake
Stream
Wildflowers
Great Views
Camping
Swimming

FACILITIES
Campground
Ranger Station

Finding the Trail

From the east side of Three Rivers, leave CA 198 and turn onto Mineral King Road. Continue on the narrow and sometimes winding road past the Cold Springs Campground entrance and the ranger station to the Sawtooth-Monarch Trailhead, 0.8 mile from the ranger station and 23 miles from CA 198.

Logistics

Backpackers must obtain a wilderness permit for all overnight visits. See pages 65–66 for more details about how to obtain one. Campfires are prohibited.

Trail Description

►1 Climb steeply away from the trailhead up a hillside carpeted with sagebrush, manzanita, chinquapin, and gooseberry to a junction with the Timber Gap Trail at 0.6 mile. ►2

Remaining on the Sawtooth Pass Trail, veer right and head up the hillside on more moderately graded, long-legged switchbacks. After another 0.6 mile, you reach Groundhog Meadow, cross Monarch Creek, and then follow a series of switchbacks in and out of shady red-fir forest on the way to a Y-junction with the Crystal Lake Trail, 2.9 miles from the trailhead. ►3

Veer right onto the lightly used Crystal Lake Trail and climb across the barren, avalanche-ridden slopes of Chihuahua Bowl, so dubbed for the nearby mine of the same name. The ruins of the old mine are clearly visible on the southeast side of the bowl. Beyond Chihuahua Bowl, the trail crests a ridge,

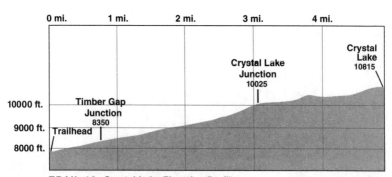

TRAIL 13 Crystal Lake Elevation Profile

from where you have good views between scattered foxtail pines. A short descent off the ridge leads to an ascending traverse across the north side of upper Crystal Creek canyon, followed by a steep, switch-backing climb up to the narrow slot of the outlet to lovely Crystal Lake. ▶4

A lack of trees around the lake's shoreline sends most overnighters to more-sheltered campsites on a terrace just below the lake, where gnarled foxtail pines offer a modicum of protection from the elements. The lake's brook trout will test the patience of anglers, and swimmers may find the water temperature to be a tad chilly at this elevation. A short scramble over low bluffs to the northeast leads to Little Crystal Lake below Mineral Peak.

Camping

Fishing

Swimming

		MILESTONES
▶1	0.0	Start at Sawtooth-Monarch Trailhead
▶2	0.6	Right at Timber Gap Trail junction
▶3	2.9	Right at Crystal Lake Trail junction
▶4	4.8	Crystal Lake

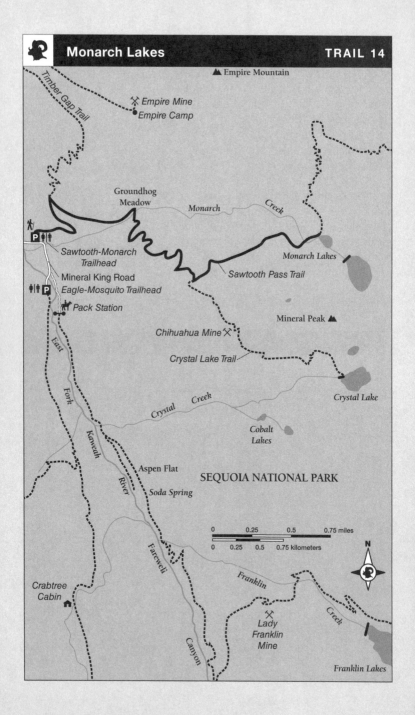

▲ Empire Mountain

Timber Gap Trail

⚒ Empire Mine
● Empire Camp

Groundhog
Meadow

Monarch   Creek

Monarch Lakes

Sawtooth-Monarch
Trailhead

Sawtooth Pass Trail

Mineral King Road
Eagle-Mosquito Trailhead

🏕 Pack Station

Mineral Peak ▲▲

Chihuahua Mine ⚒

Crystal Lake Trail

Crystal Lake

East

Crystal   Creek

Cobalt
Lakes

Fork

Kaweah

Aspen Flat

SEQUOIA NATIONAL PARK

River

Soda Spring

0   0.25   0.5   0.75 miles

0   0.25   0.5   0.75 kilometers

N

Farewell

Franklin

Crabtree
Cabin 🏠

⚒
Lady
Franklin
Mine

Canyon

Creek

Franklin Lakes

Monarch Lakes

The reward for this hike's stiff climb is a pair of picturesque subalpine lakes cradled in a dramatic cirque basin beneath multicolored peaks of metamorphic rock. Not only is the destination stunningly beautiful, but also the vistas of the Mineral King area during the ascent are equally impressive. Despite the climb—2,500 feet in 3-plus miles—the trip up the Sawtooth Pass Trail is popular with backpackers and day hikers alike.

Since the overused campsites become cramped during peak season, you may want to view this trip as a day hike only. If you insist on camping, don't expect a lot of peace and quiet. Backpackers leaving cars overnight in Mineral King need to place all food and scented items in the storage shed directly across from the ranger station because bear boxes are not available at trailheads. Especially in early season, marmots in the area have been known to nibble on radiator hoses, fan belts, brake lines, and even radiators—check with park rangers for current conditions.

Best Time

The Mineral King Road is usually open by Memorial Day weekend, but the trail to Monarch Lakes is usually snowbound until early July following winters of average snowfall. Trail use is highest from mid-July through August. The weather in September can be quite enjoyable.

TRAIL USE
Day Hike, Backpack,
Run, Horse

LENGTH
7.8 miles, 3–4 hours

VERTICAL FEET
+2740/-400/±6280

DIFFICULTY
– 1 2 3 **4** 5 +

TRAIL TYPE
Out-and-back

FEATURES
Lake
Stream
Wildflowers
Great Views
Steep
Camping
Swimming

FACILITIES
Campground
Ranger Station
Bear Box

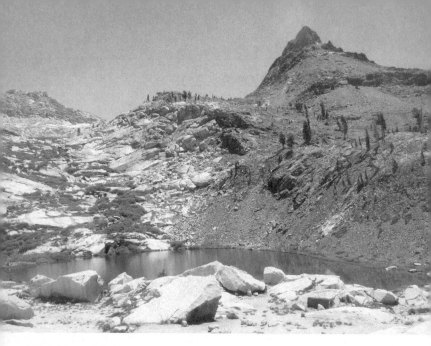

Lower Monarch Lake

Finding the Trailhead

Drive eastbound from Visalia on CA 198 to the east edge of Three Rivers and turn onto Mineral King Road. Follow the narrow and sometimes winding road to the Lookout Point Entrance Station (fee) and proceed through the tiny resort community of Silver

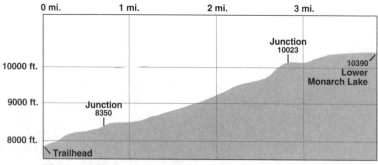

TRAIL 14 Monarch Lakes Elevation Profile

Cross-Country Route to Crystal Lakes

OPTIONS

A steep but relatively straightforward off-trail route connects the Monarch Lakes with Crystal Lake. From Upper Monarch Lake, head south and ascend a steep chute to a saddle at around 11,170 feet, descend toward the tarn below, and then proceed on a short use trail down to Crystal Lake. To return to the trailhead, follow maintained trail from Crystal Lake west and then northwest on a 1.4-mile moderately steep descent over the west ridge of Mineral Peak and across Chihuahua Bowl to the junction with the Sawtooth Pass Trail. From there, retrace your steps 2.4 miles to the trailhead. Plan on an extra hour or two for this diversion.

City. Silver City Mountain Resort offers cabins, chalets, showers, a restaurant and bakery, and a limited selection of supplies.

Continue past the entrance to Cold Springs Campground (fee, vault toilets, running water, bear boxes, and phone) and the Mineral King Ranger Station to the Sawtooth-Monarch Trailhead, 0.8 mile from the ranger station and 23 miles from CA 198.

Logistics

Backpackers must obtain a wilderness permit for all overnight visits. See pages 65–66 for more details about how to obtain one.

Trail Description

▶1 A steep climb leads away from the trailhead up a hillside covered with sagebrush, manzanita, and gooseberry for 0.6 mile to a junction with the Timber Gap Trail ▶2 heading north toward Timber Gap.

Turn right at the junction and continue southeast on the Sawtooth Pass Trail. More-reasonably graded trail follows long-legged switchbacks up the

 Steep

Upper Monarch Lake Dam

Upper Monarch Lake was dammed in the early 1900s by the
Mt. Whitney Power and Electric Company to regulate water
flow for power production at a generating plant downstream in
Hammond. Similar dams were constructed nearby at Crystal,
Franklin, and Eagle Lakes. Today, the water in these lakes is
regulated by Southern California Edison Company.

Sandwiched between multihued Sawtooth and Mineral Peaks on the Great Western Divide, the two Monarch Lakes nestle picturesquely in a scenic cirque basin.

---

hillside to Groundhog Meadow, slightly misnamed
for the ubiquitous yellow-bellied marmot, a relative
of the eastern woodchuck, that inhabits the meadows
and rocky slopes of the subalpine Sierra. Near the
meadow, you hop across sparkling Monarch Creek
and begin a series of lengthy switchbacks leading in
and out of shady red-fir forest on the way to a junction with the seldom-used Crystal Lake Trail. ▶3

Veer left (northeast) at the junction and continue climbing up the Sawtooth Pass Trail. After a
pair of switchbacks, cross a minor ridge at the edge
of expansive and rock-strewn Chihuahua Bowl and
begin a mildly ascending traverse across a barren,
austere rock slope well above the level of Monarch Creek coursing through the deep cleft below.
Eventually, the trail curves toward more-hospitable-
looking terrain again, meeting the meadow-lined
creek just below the outlet of Lower Monarch Lake
and ascending shortly to the west side of the lake.
▶4 Sandwiched between multihued Sawtooth and
Mineral Peaks on the Great Western Divide, the
two Monarch Lakes nestle picturesquely in a scenic
cirque basin. Scratched out of the rocky slopes to
the west of the lakes are exposed, overused campsites with a couple of bear boxes and a partially
screened toilet nearby.

Lake 〰

Camping

To reach the upper lake, find a use trail near the inlet amid a patch of willows and follow it up a steep hillside to larger Upper Monarch Lake. Most hikers go no farther than the lower lake, so the upper lake offers a reasonable expectation of solitude away from the well-traveled Sawtooth Pass Trail.

		MILESTONES
▶1	0.0	Start at Sawtooth-Monarch Trailhead
▶2	0.6	Turn right (southeast) at Timber Gap junction
▶3	2.9	Veer left (northeast) at Crystal Lake junction
▶4	3.9	Lower Monarch Lake

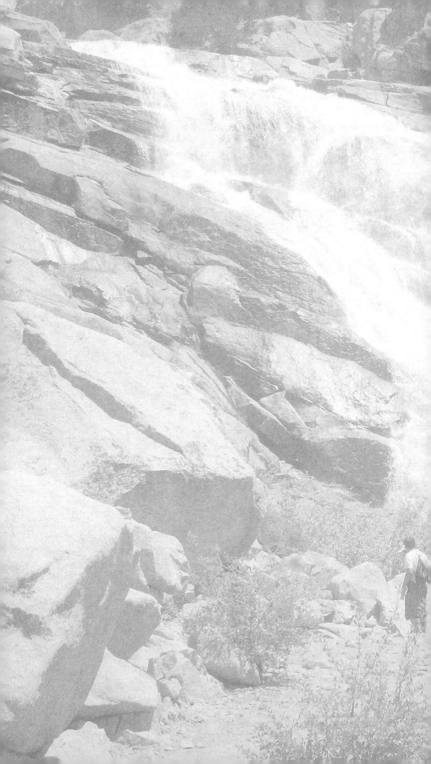

CHAPTER 3

Giant Forest and Lodgepole

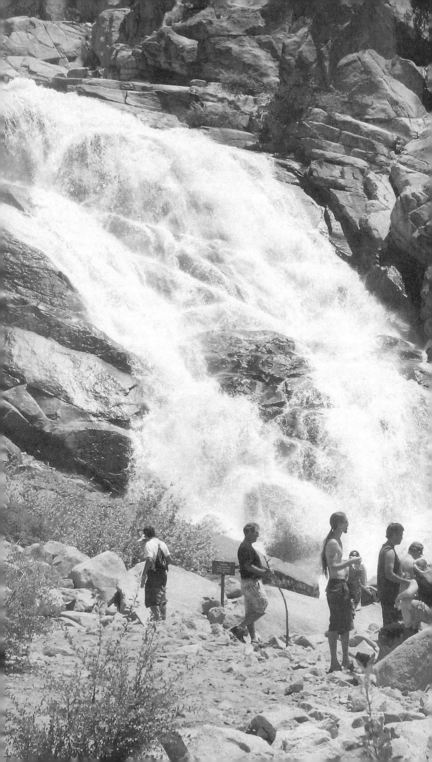

Giant Forest and Lodgepole

As well as being home to the world's largest living tree, General Sherman, the Giant Forest Plateau has the largest concentration of giant sequoias on earth. An extensive network of trails, from handicapped-accessible paths to extended loops, provides miles and miles of alternatives for visitors to experience the giant monarchs of the forest. Lovely, flower-laden meadows appear sprinkled throughout the area as well. While sequoias are the big draw in Giant Forest, there are other notable attributes, including some spectacular views from Moro Rock, Bobcat Point, and Eagle View, as described in Trails 15, 17, and 18. The remaining trails in Giant Forest, excluding the out-and-back hike to General Sherman, provide a variety of scenic loops through the heart of the area.

Lodgepole, with an array of park facilities, is the jumping-off point for a handful of excellent trails. Trail 25 offers a rigorous climb to the summit of Alta Peak, from where successful peakbaggers can take in an expansive view. A popular and scenic quartet of lakes in the next trip offers excellent destinations for both daytrippers and overnighters. An early-summer hike to Tokopah Falls reveals a dose of watery splendor when Marble Fork Kaweah River is near peak flows. Trail 28 heads north from Lodgepole through serene forests and past verdant meadows to a pair of attractive lakes nestled below Silliman Crest. Just north of Lodgepole, Trail 29 offers a short climb to a fine view from the top of the granite dome of Little Baldy, and Trail 30 travels to one of the more remote sequoia groves in either of the parks.

The Giant Forest area is accessible via public transportation from Visalia and the gateway town of Three Rivers on the Sequoia Shuttle. A round-trip ticket is $15 and includes the park entrance fee. Reservations are necessary and can be made at **sequoiashuttle.com,** or by calling 877-BUS-HIKE. From the Giant Forest Museum, free in-park shuttles provide transportation to stops at Moro Rock and Crescent Meadow, Sherman Tree, Wolverton, Lodgepole, Wuksachi Village, and Dorst Campground.

Overleaf and opposite: *Lower Tokopah Falls*

Permits

Permits are not required for day hikes. Backpackers must obtain a wilderness permit for all overnight trips. Between late May and late September, a quota system is in place, with a $15 fee per group. Outside the quota period, permits are free, self-issue, and available 24 hours a day. Advance reservations are available for approximately 75% of the quota, with the remainder set aside for walk-in permits. All permits must be picked up from the Lodgepole Visitor Center between 7 a.m. and 3:45 p.m. (closed for lunch between 11 a.m. and noon). Applications for advance reservations are accepted only by fax or mail, no earlier than midnight March 1 and no later than two weeks prior to the start of the trip. Visit the park website to download a permit application and to check on quota availability.

Maps

For the Giant Forest and Lodgepole area, the U.S. Geological Survey 7.5-minute (1:24,000 scale) topographic maps are listed below, corresponding to the trails described in this section. Sequoia Natural History Association publishes *Giant Forest* and *Lodgepole,* handy foldout maps for this area. Trail users also may want to consider using some of the Tom Harrison maps of this area, including *Sequoia & Kings Canyon National Parks* (1:125,000).

Trail 15: *Giant Forest*

Trail 16: *Giant Forest, Lodgepole*

Trail 17: *Giant Forest, Lodgepole*

Trail 18: *Giant Forest, Lodgepole*

Trail 19: *Giant Forest, Lodgepole*

Trail 20: *Giant Forest, Lodgepole*

Trail 21: *Giant Forest*

Trail 22: *Giant Forest*

Trail 23: *Giant Forest, Lodgepole*

Trail 24: *Giant Forest, Lodgepole*

Trail 25: *Lodgepole*

Trail 26: *Lodgepole*

Trail 27: *Lodgepole*

Trail 28: *Lodgepole, Mt. Silliman*

Trail 29: *Giant Forest*

Trail 30: *Muir Grove*

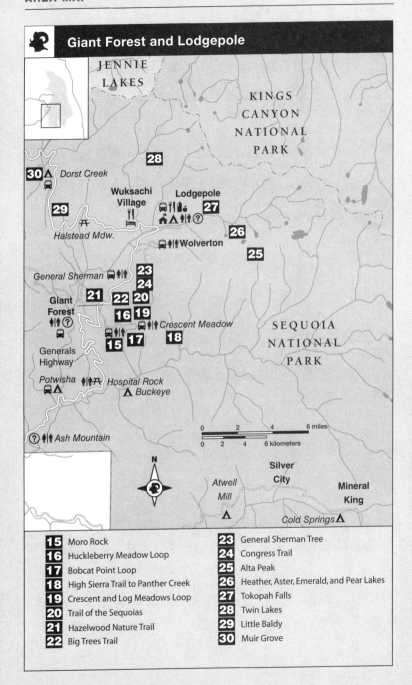

Giant Forest and Lodgepole

JENNIE
LAKES

KINGS
CANYON
NATIONAL
PARK

SEQUOIA
NATIONAL
PARK

28

30 Dorst Creek

29

Wuksachi
Village

Halstead Mdw.

Lodgepole

27

26

Wolverton

25

General Sherman

23
24
20
19

Giant
Forest

21

22
16

15 **17**

Crescent Meadow

18

Generals
Highway

Potwisha

Hospital Rock
Buckeye

Ash Mountain

| 0 | | 2 | | 4 | | 6 miles |
| 0 | 2 | | 4 | | 6 kilometers | |

N

Silver
City

Atwell
Mill

Mineral
King

Cold Springs

15	Moro Rock	**23**	General Sherman Tree
16	Huckleberry Meadow Loop	**24**	Congress Trail
17	Bobcat Point Loop	**25**	Alta Peak
18	High Sierra Trail to Panther Creek	**26**	Heather, Aster, Emerald, and Pear Lakes
19	Crescent and Log Meadows Loop	**27**	Tokopah Falls
20	Trail of the Sequoias	**28**	Twin Lakes
21	Hazelwood Nature Trail	**29**	Little Baldy
22	Big Trees Trail	**30**	Muir Grove

TRAIL FEATURES TABLE

Giant Forest and Lodgepole

TRAIL	DIFFICULTY	LENGTH	TYPE	USES & ACCESS	TERRAIN	FLORA & FAUNA	OTHER
15	2	0.6	Out-and-back	Day Hiking	Mountain		Great Views, Historical Interest
16	2	3.8	Loop	Day Hiking, Running		Wildflowers, Giant Sequoias	Historical Interest
17	1	1.25	Loop	Day Hiking, Running			Great Views, Historical Interest
18	2	5.4	Out-and-back	Day Hiking, Backpacking, Running	Waterfall	Giant Sequoias	Great Views, Camping
19	2	2.4	Loop	Day Hiking, Child Friendly		Fall Colors, Wildflowers, Giant Sequoias	Historical Interest
20	3	5.8	Loop	Day Hiking, Running		Wildflowers, Giant Sequoias	Historical Interest
21	1	1.3	Loop	Day Hiking, Child Friendly		Wildflowers, Giant Sequoias	
22	1	1.2	Loop	Day Hiking, Wheelchair-Access, Child Friendly		Wildflowers, Giant Sequoias	
23	1	0.9	Out-and-back	Day Hiking, Wheelchair-Access, Child Friendly		Giant Sequoias	
24	2	3.1	Loop	Day Hiking, Child Friendly		Fall Colors, Wildflowers, Giant Sequoias	
25	5	13.4	Out-and-back	Day Hiking, Backpacking, Horses	Mountain, Summit	Wildflowers	Great Views, Camping, Secluded
26	4	11.5	Out-and-back	Day Hiking, Backpacking, Horses	Mountain, Lake	Wildflowers	Great Views, Camping, Swimming, Fishing
27	2	4.1	Out-and-back	Day Hiking, Horses	Canyon, Waterfall	Wildflowers	Great Views
28	4	13.0	Out-and-back	Backpacking, Horses	Lake	Wildflowers	Camping, Swimming, Fishing
29	3	3.5	Out-and-back	Backpacking	Mountain, Summit		Great Views
30	3	4.2	Out-and-back			Fall Colors, Giant Sequoias	Great Views, Steep

Legend

USES & ACCESS
- Day Hiking
- Backpacking
- Running
- Horses
- Dogs Allowed
- Child Friendly
- Wheelchair-Access

TYPE
- Loop
- Out-and-back
- Point-to-point

DIFFICULTY
- 1 2 3 4 5 +
- less — more

TERRAIN
- Canyon
- Mountain
- Summit
- Lake
- Stream
- Waterfall

FLORA & FAUNA
- Fall Colors
- Wildflowers
- Giant Sequoias

OTHER
- Great Views
- Camping
- Swimming
- Secluded
- Steep
- Fishing
- Historical Interest

Giant Forest and Lodgepole

Moro Rock 121

A short climb to the top of 6,725-foot Moro Rock at the south edge of the Giant Forest plateau is rewarded by great views of two forks of the Kaweah River, the snow-capped Great Western Divide, and cars snaking their way along the Generals Highway.

TRAIL 15

Day Hike
0.6 mile, Out-and-back
Difficulty: 1 **2** 3 4 5

Huckleberry Meadow Loop 125

A less popular path through Giant Forest leading to a trio of lovely meadows—Huckleberry, Circle, and Crescent—as well as some notable giant sequoias, including the Washington Tree, formerly the second largest in the world. An old log cabin and a Native American site offer some historical interest along the way as well.

TRAIL 16

Day Hike, Run
3.8 miles, Loop
Difficulty: 1 **2** 3 4 5

Bobcat Point Loop 131

Grand views from Kaweah Vista and Bobcat Point are the main points of interest along this short loop, which also provides some bedrock mortars for historical interest.

TRAIL 17

Day Hike, Run
1.25 miles, Loop
Difficulty: **1** 2 3 4 5

High Sierra Trail to Eagle View and Panther Creek 137

Day hikers can enjoy the initial segment of the famed High Sierra Trail with fine views of the canyon of Middle Fork Kaweah River and the Great Western Divide.

TRAIL 18

Day Hike, Backpack, Run
5.4 miles, Out-and-back
Difficulty: 1 **2** 3 4 5

Congress Trail 165

TRAIL 24

Day Hike, Child Friendly
3.1 miles, Loop
Difficulty: 1 **2** 3 4 5

After visiting the world's largest giant sequoia and largest living organism on the planet, the General Sherman Tree, one of the most popular trails in Giant Forest leads to some of the more significant giant sequoias and groups of big trees in the area. Pavement makes the trail accessible to just about anyone, and the route can be shortened by a mile round-trip by riding the free park shuttle to the General Sherman Tree bus stop.

Alta Peak 171

TRAIL 25

Day Hike, Backpack, Horse
13.4 miles,
Out-and-back
Difficulty: 1 2 3 4 **5**

A rigorous hike to one of Sequoia National Park's most impressive views leads along the Alta and Alta Peak Trails to the summit of 11,204-foot Alta Peak. The total distance and elevation gain makes this a trail for hikers in good condition who are well acclimatized. The sweeping view from the summit takes in a large chunk of the Great Western Divide and most of the western part of the park.

Heather, Aster, Emerald, and Pear Lakes 179

TRAIL 26

Day Hike, Backpack, Horse
11.5 miles,
Out-and-back
Difficulty: 1 2 3 **4** 5

A popular route to classic High Sierra terrain, this trail visits four picturesque lakes in the heart of Sequoia National Park's backcountry. The lakes appeal to hikers, backpackers, equestrians, photographers, swimmers, sunbathers, and anglers. Cross-country enthusiasts can set up a basecamp at Pear Lake for off-trail forays into the granite-filled terrain known as The Tableland. Impressive views along the Watchtower Route straight down a 2,000-foot cliff to Tokopah Valley are sure to knock your socks off.

TRAIL 27

Day Hike, Horse

4.1 miles, Out-and-back

Difficulty: 1 **2** 3 4 5

Tokopah Falls 187

Tokopah Valley lies at the bottom of a steep-sided canyon with a spectacular waterfall plunging down the headwall. This 2-mile excursion leads along Middle Fork Kaweah River to a viewpoint of the falls, which reach a spectacular climax during the peak of snowmelt.

TRAIL 28

Day Hike, Backpack, Horse

13.0 miles, Out-and-back

Difficulty: 1 2 3 **4** 5

Twin Lakes. 191

After an exposed and often hot first-mile climb, hikers on the Twin Lakes Trail travel through mixed forest, past flower-laced meadows, and over gurgling streams on the way to Twin Lakes. The two lakes don't look much like twins, but they offer plenty of fine scenery, and overnighters may find pleasant campsites around the shorelines.

TRAIL 29

Day Hike

3.5 miles, Out-and-back

Difficulty: 1 2 **3** 4 5

Little Baldy. 197

One of the best western Sequoia vista points requires just a short hike to reach the site of a former fire lookout. Pack plenty of water because none is available en route to the summit.

TRAIL 30

Day Hike

4.2 miles, Out-and-back

Difficulty: 1 2 **3** 4 5

Muir Grove. 201

An opportunity to stand among giant sequoias, monarchs of the forest, in relative seclusion makes this a trip more than worthy of the name of the Sierra Nevada's foremost preservationist.

Moro Rock

Hale Tharp and his stepson were the first settlers to scale Moro Rock in 1861. In modern times, hundreds of tourists attempt to walk to the top every summer day via the 350 steps built in 1931, which were subsequently listed in the National Register of Historic Places. The view from the top of the dome of the Great Western Divide and the canyon of Middle Fork Kaweah River, although not as pristine as the days of Tharp due to the persistent smog from the San Joaquin Valley, is still remarkable.

Best Time

Once the road opens, usually sometime in May, the view from Moro Rock is always in season, provided the atmospheric conditions are cooperative—smog from the San Joaquin Valley often inhibits the vista. The first significant snowfall closes the road in the fall.

Finding the Trail

Public transportation to the Giant Forest Museum is available from Visalia and Three Rivers on the Sequoia Shuttle. The round-trip cost is $15, and reservations are required. Call 877-BUS-HIKE or visit **sequoiashuttle.com.**

From the vicinity of the Giant Forest Museum, you can ride the free In-park Shuttle on Gray Route 2 to Moro Rock.

From Visalia, private vehicles should follow CA 198 to Three Rivers and proceed east into Sequoia National Park, where the road becomes Generals

TRAIL USE
Day Hike
LENGTH
0.6 mile, ½ hour
VERTICAL FEET
+300/-0/±600
DIFFICULTY
– 1 **2** 3 4 5 +
TRAIL TYPE
Out-and-back

FEATURES
Summit
Great Views
Historical Interest

FACILITIES
Restrooms
Water

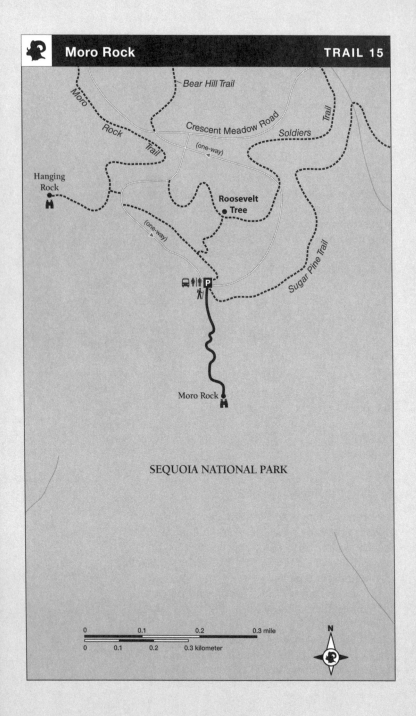

Bear Hill Trail

Moro Rock Trail

Crescent Meadow Road

(one-way)

Soldiers Trail

Hanging Rock

Roosevelt Tree

(one-way)

Sugar Pine Trail

Moro Rock

SEQUOIA NATIONAL PARK

| 0 | 0.1 | 0.2 | 0.3 mile |
| 0 | 0.1 | 0.2 | 0.3 kilometer |

N

Highway. Drive Generals Highway to the Giant Forest Museum. Either park your vehicle in the large parking lot and ride the free shuttle bus, or drive along the narrow Crescent Meadow Road 1.2 miles to the Moro Rock junction. Veer right and follow this road 0.4 mile to the parking lot.

Lodgepole is the nearest campground, about 9 miles on Generals Highway from the Giant Forest Museum (fee, flush toilets, running water, bear boxes, and phone). Wuksachi Village, a short distance north of Lodgepole, offers upscale lodging and dining. Both Lodgepole and Wuksachi Village are accessible via the free In-park Shuttle system.

Trail Description

▶1 Find the start of the Moro Rock Trail across from the parking lot. The winding, occasionally switchbacking trail climbs 300 feet to the top via rock ramps and 350 rock steps built in 1931. Interpretive displays on the way allow tourists unaccustomed to the 7,000-foot elevation the chance to catch their breath, and steel railings attempt to keep them safe. The trail eventually crests the top of the dome, from where an incredible view unfolds. ▶2 The Giant Forest plateau spreads out in the northern foreground, the crowns of giant sequoias rising above the lesser

 Great Views

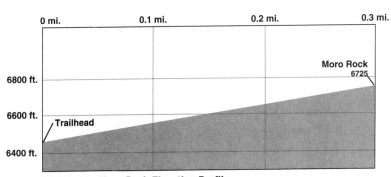

TRAIL 15 Moro Rock Elevation Profile

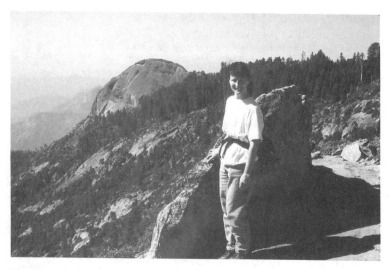

Moro Rock *from Eagle View*

conifers, while the sculpted summits of the Great Western Divide scrape the eastern sky. The deep cleft of Middle Fork Kaweah River plunges 4,000 feet below, with the multispired Castle Crags dominating the far canyon wall. Miniature-looking cars can be seen snaking up and down serpentine Generals Highway, with the community of Three Rivers visible farther down the canyon. On those extremely rare days when the air is clear, views extend westward across the San Joaquin Valley. When the time comes to return, retrace your steps to the trailhead.

🚶 MILESTONES

▶1   0.0   Start at Moro Rock Trailhead
▶2   0.3   Summit of Moro Rock

Huckleberry Meadow Loop

Sandwiched between two of the most popular trails in Giant Forest, Crescent Meadow Loop on the south and Congress Trail to the north, this pleasant, little-used loop should be much more peaceful. The circuit passes by three delightful meadows, Huckleberry, Circle, and Crescent, which are dotted with colorful wildflowers in early summer. The route visits a number of prominent giant sequoia features, including what was once the second largest (Washington Tree), the Dead Giant, and Bears Bathtub. Historical interest is found at Squatters Cabin, built by a prospector in the 1880s, and at some bedrock mortars used by Native Americans to grind nuts and seeds.

Best Time

Snow generally leaves the trails sometime in May in this part of Giant Forest, permitting snow-free hiking until the first snowfall of the season, usually in late October or early November. Late spring, when the azalea flowers are in bloom, is a particularly fine time for a visit, as is early fall, when the azalea leaves are cloaked in autumn splendor. Colorful wildflowers put on a showy display in early summer.

Finding the Trail

Public transportation to the Giant Forest Museum is available from Visalia and Three Rivers on the Sequoia Shuttle. The round-trip cost is $15, and reservations are required. Call 877-BUS-HIKE or visit **sequoiashuttle.com.**

TRAIL USE
Day Hike, Run

LENGTH
3.7 miles, 2 hours

VERTICAL FEET
+850/-850/±1700

DIFFICULTY
– 1 **2** 3 4 5 +

TRAIL TYPE
Loop

FEATURES
Wildflowers
Giant Sequoias
Historical Interest

FACILITIES
At Crescent Meadow:
Restrooms
Water
Picnic Area
Shuttle Bus Stop

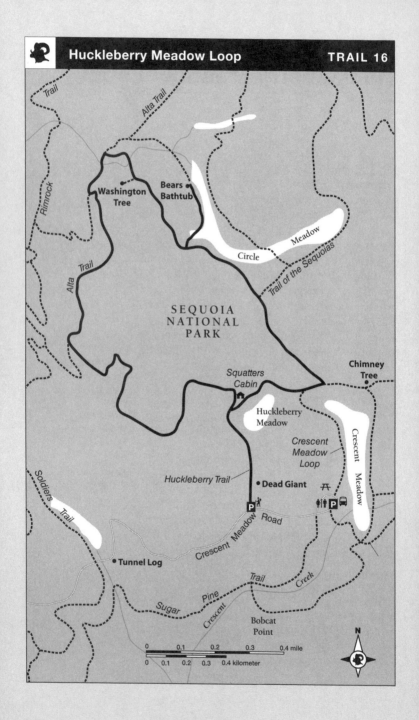

Trail

Alta Trail

Rimrock

Alta Trail

Washington Tree

Bears Bathtub

Circle Meadow

Trail of the Sequoias

SEQUOIA
NATIONAL
PARK

Chimney Tree

Squatters Cabin

Huckleberry Meadow

Crescent Meadow Loop

Crescent Meadow

Huckleberry Trail

Dead Giant

Soldiers Trail

Crescent Meadow Road

Tunnel Log

Sugar Pine Trail

Crescent Creek

Bobcat Point

0   0.1   0.2   0.3   0.4 mile
0   0.1   0.2   0.3   0.4 kilometer

N

From the vicinity of the Giant Forest Museum, you can ride the free In-park Shuttle on Gray Route 2 to Crescent Meadow. From there, walk back down the road for 0.3 mile to the Huckleberry Trailhead.

From Visalia, private vehicles should follow CA 198 to Three Rivers and proceed east into Sequoia National Park, where the road becomes Generals Highway. Drive Generals Highway to the Giant Forest Museum. Either park your vehicle in the large parking lot and ride the free shuttle bus, or drive along the narrow Crescent Meadow Road 1.2 miles to the Moro Rock junction. Veer left and follow Crescent Meadow Road for 1 mile to the small parking area for the Huckleberry Trail.

Lodgepole is the nearest campground, about 9 miles on Generals Highway from the Giant Forest Museum (fee, flush toilets, running water, bear boxes, and phone). Wuksachi Village, a short distance north of Lodgepole, offers upscale lodging and dining. Both Lodgepole and Wuksachi Village are accessible via the free In-park Shuttle system.

Trail Description

▶1 Follow the Huckleberry Trail through a mixed forest of giant sequoias, sugar pines, and dogwoods

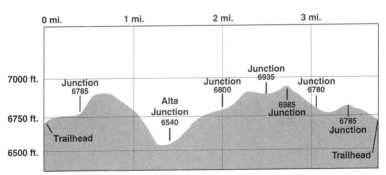

TRAIL 16 Huckleberry Meadow Loop Elevation Profile

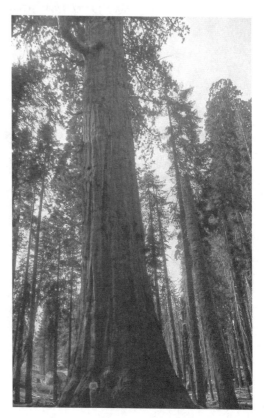

The Washington Tree

to the Dead Giant, one of the few examples of a sequoia succumbing to a forest fire. Typically, the sequoia's thick bark provides adequate protection from all but the most intense fires. A short distance farther is Huckleberry Meadow, carpeted with lush grasses and decorated with splashes of color from an assortment of wildflowers. Continue to the far end of the meadow, where towering trees shade Squatters Cabin. Just past the cabin is a junction, 0.4 mile from the trailhead. ▶2

Bearing left at the junction, make a winding ascent over a low ridge into a drier forest of Jeffrey pines with an understory of manzanita. After a

Wildflowers

Historical Interest 🏠

moderate descent from the ridgecrest, return to the damper conditions of a mixed forest, where azaleas, wildflowers, and ferns carpet the floor. Reach a well-signed junction with the Alta Trail, 1 mile from the previous junction. ►3

Turning right at the junction, you head north on the Alta Trail and make a half-mile climb past an abandoned spur trail on the left. A short distance later, a sign points the way to some bedrock mortars, where Native Americans once ground nuts and seeds. Cross Little Deer Creek, a reliable water source until late summer, and continue to the next junction, 2.0 miles from the trailhead. ►4

Historical Interest

Leave the Alta Trail and follow signed directions toward the Washington Tree on a gently rising ascent. The azalea-lined trail leads back across Little Deer Creek, lined with a narrow strip of lush foliage. Beyond the creek is an area of young sequoias, beneficiaries of a controlled burn back in the late 1970s. Nearby, a signed, short lateral heads to the base of the Washington Tree, with a volume of 47,850 cubic feet, this behemoth was at one time second in size only to General Sherman. A forest fire in 2003 reduced the size of the tree, which today no longer ranks within the top 30 sequoias.

Giant Sequoias

From the lateral to the Washington Tree, a moderate ascent leads over a low rise and down to a junction near the edge of Circle Meadow, 2.4 miles from the trailhead. ►5 Before continuing on the right-hand trail, follow the left-hand trail shortly for a look at Bears Bathtub.

Heading southeast along the fringe of Circle Meadow, you climb over a low hill to the next junction, 0.25 mile from the previous one. ►6 Continue southeast on a 0.3-mile descent to the north side of Crescent Meadow and a junction of the Crescent Meadow Loop at 3.0 miles. ►7 (Shuttle bus riders may elect to head south from here on the Crescent Meadow Loop Trail around the west side of the meadow to the bus stop at the Crescent Meadow parking lot.)

To return to the Huckleberry Trailhead, turn right (west) and proceed on a nearly level course, eventually passing around the north edge of Huckleberry Meadow on the way to the close of the loop at the first junction near Squatters Cabin. ▶8 From there, turn left and retrace your steps back to the trailhead. ▶9

MILESTONES

▶1	0.0	Start at Huckleberry Trailhead
▶2	0.4	Left at junction
▶3	1.4	Right at Alta Trail junction
▶4	2.0	Right at junction
▶5	2.4	Right at junction
▶6	2.65	Right at junction
▶7	3.0	Right at Crescent Meadow Loop junction
▶8	3.3	Left at junction
▶9	3.7	End at trailhead

Bobcat Point Loop

Despite the short length of only 1.25 miles, this loop trip will take you away from the usual hubbub at Crescent Meadow to magnificent vistas of the Great Western Divide and Middle Fork Kaweah River Canyon, as well as an up-close view of the profile of Moro Rock. A couple of sites with bedrock mortars add historical interest.

Best Time

Snow generally leaves the trails sometime in May in this part of Giant Forest, permitting snow-free hiking until the first snowfall of the season, usually in late October or early November. Late spring, when the azalea flowers are in bloom, is a particularly fine time for a visit, as is early fall, when the azalea leaves are cloaked in autumn splendor. Colorful wildflowers put on a showy display in early summer.

Finding the Trail

Public transportation to the Giant Forest Museum is available from Visalia and Three Rivers on the Sequoia Shuttle. The round-trip cost is $15, and reservations are required. Call 877-BUS-HIKE or visit **sequoiashuttle.com.**

From the vicinity of the Giant Forest Museum, you can ride the free In-park Shuttle on Gray Route 2 to Crescent Meadow.

From Visalia, private vehicles should follow CA 198 to Three Rivers and proceed east into Sequoia National Park, where the road becomes Generals Highway. Drive Generals Highway to the Giant

TRAIL USE
Day Hike, Run

LENGTH
1.25 miles, 1 hour

VERTICAL FEET
+250/-250/±500

DIFFICULTY
– **1** 2 3 4 5 +

TRAIL TYPE
Loop

FEATURES
Great Views
Historical Interest

FACILITIES
Restrooms
Water
Picnic Area
Shuttle Bus Stop

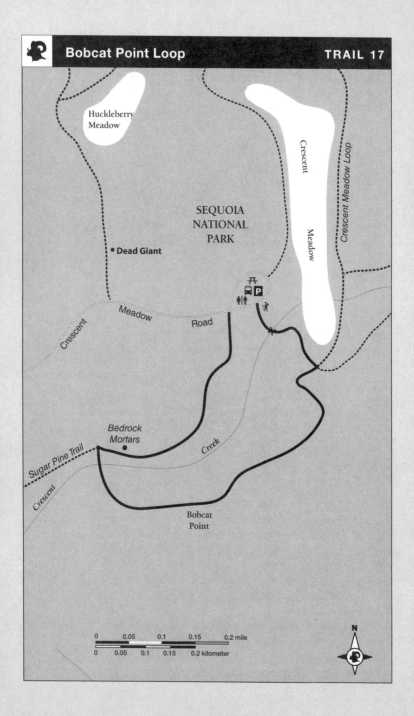

Huckleberry
Meadow

SEQUOIA
NATIONAL
PARK

Crescent

Meadow

Crescent Meadow Loop

• Dead Giant

Crescent   Meadow   Road

Bedrock
Mortars
•

Creek

Sugar Pine Trail

Crescent

Bobcat
Point

0   0.05   0.1   0.15   0.2 mile

0   0.05   0.1   0.15   0.2 kilometer

N

Forest Museum. Either park your vehicle in the large parking lot and ride the free shuttle bus, or drive along the narrow Crescent Meadow Road 1.2 miles to the Moro Rock junction. Motorists should continue on Crescent Meadow Road another 1.3 miles to the end of the road at the Crescent Meadow parking lot.

Lodgepole is the nearest campground, about 9 miles on Generals Highway from the Giant Forest Museum (fee, flush toilets, running water, bear boxes, and phone). Wuksachi Village, a short distance north of Lodgepole, offers upscale lodging and dining. Both Lodgepole and Wuksachi Village are accessible via the free In-park Shuttle system.

Trail Description

▶1 Begin the loop by following the initial section of the High Sierra Trail, which heads east from the vicinity of the restrooms at the Crescent Meadow parking lot. Cross a pair of short wood bridges over Crescent Creek and soon come to a junction with the Crescent Meadow Loop on the left. Veer right, remaining on the High Sierra Trail for about 25 yards to a second junction with your trail to Bobcat Point. ▶2

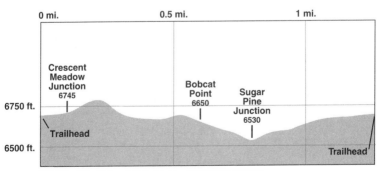

TRAIL 17 Bobcat Point Loop Elevation Profile

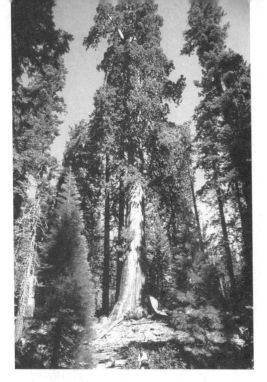

A majestic giant sequoia

Turning right at the junction, climb up a lightly forested hillside and then follow the trail as it bends west, drops into a saddle, and ascends along a ridge well above Middle Fork Kaweah River. Break out of the trees as you reach the rock outcrop known as Kaweah Vista, where a splendid view unfolds of the 3,000-foot-deep canyon below and the airy summits of the Great Western Divide to the east. A short distance farther is another vista at Bobcat Point, ▶3 where the impressive-looking granite dome of Moro Rock stands a mere 0.75 mile southwest. Across the yawning chasm of the Middle Fork are the crags and spires of Castle Rocks.

Great Views

Leaving Bobcat Point, head back into the trees and cross Crescent Creek, which flows picturesquely over a broad, sloping slab of granite. Near this scenic spot are several bedrock mortars worth inspecting. A short distance past the creek is a junction with the Sugar Pine Trail, ▶4 that offers a straightforward 0.9-mile traverse over to the base of Moro Rock (see Trail 15).

Historical Interest

To return to the Crescent Meadow Trailhead, bear right at the junction and climb steadily through a light forest to a short lateral to the bedrock mortars. Away from the lateral, a gentler ascent proceeds through mixed forest to the end of the loop at the Crescent Meadow Road. From there, walk a short distance to the parking lot. ▶5.

🚶 MILESTONES

▶1	0.0	Start at Crescent Meadow Trailhead
▶2	0.1	Right at Crescent Meadow Loop junction
		Right at Bobcat Point junction
▶3	0.6	Bobcat Point
▶4	0.8	Right at Sugar Pine Trail junction
▶5	1.25	Crescent Meadow Trailhead

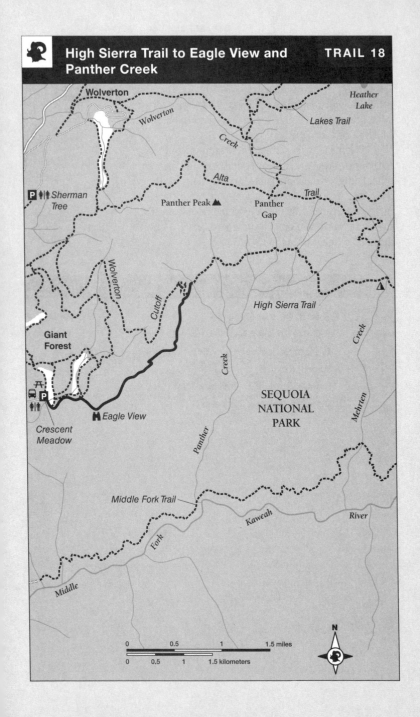

Wolverton

Heather Lake

Wolverton Creek

Lakes Trail

P ♦♦ Sherman Tree

Panther Peak ▲

Alta Trail

Panther Gap

Wolverton Cutoff

High Sierra Trail

Creek

Giant Forest

⚠

Ⓐ P ♦♦

Ⓜ Eagle View

Panther Creek

SEQUOIA NATIONAL PARK

Mehrten Creek

Crescent Meadow

Middle Fork Trail

Kaweah River

Middle Fork

Middle

N

0   0.5   1   1.5 miles

0   0.5   1   1.5 kilometers

High Sierra Trail to Eagle View and Panther Creek

Although not nearly as famous as the John Muir Trail, the High Sierra Trail is the second most noteworthy long-distance path in the High Sierra, traveling from the big trees (Giant Forest) to the big mountain (Mount Whitney).

Best Time

Snow generally leaves the trails sometime in May in this part of Giant Forest, permitting snow-free hiking until the first snowfall of the season, usually in late October or early November. Late spring, when the azalea flowers are in bloom, is a particularly fine time for a visit, as is early fall, when the azalea leaves are cloaked in autumn splendor. Colorful wildflowers put on a showy display in early summer. Much of the trail is fully exposed to the sun, so get an early start if the weather forecast calls for high afternoon temperatures.

Finding the Trail

Public transportation to the Giant Forest Museum is available from Visalia and Three Rivers on the Sequoia Shuttle. The round-trip cost is $15, and reservations are required. Call 877-BUS-HIKE or visit **sequoiashuttle.com.**

From the vicinity of the Giant Forest Museum, you can ride the free In-park Shuttle on Gray Route 2 to Crescent Meadow.

From Visalia, private vehicles should follow CA 198 to Three Rivers and proceed east into Sequoia National Park, where the road becomes Generals

TRAIL USE
Day Hike, Backpack, Run

LENGTH
5.4 miles, 2–3 hours

VERTICAL FEET
+850/-850/±1700

DIFFICULTY
– 1 **2** 3 4 5 +

TRAIL TYPE
Out-and-back

FEATURES
Stream
Giant Sequoias
Great Views
Camping

FACILITIES
Restrooms
Water
Picnic Area
Shuttle Bus Stop

Highway. Drive Generals Highway to the Giant Forest Museum. Either park your vehicle in the large parking lot and ride the free shuttle bus, or drive along the narrow Crescent Meadow Road 1.2 miles to the Moro Rock junction. Motorists should continue on Crescent Meadow Road another 1.3 miles to the end of the road at the Crescent Meadow parking lot.

Lodgepole is the nearest campground, about 9 miles on Generals Highway from the Giant Forest Museum (fee, flush toilets, running water, bear boxes, and phone). Wuksachi Village, a short distance north of Lodgepole, offers upscale lodging and dining. Both Lodgepole and Wuksachi Village are accessible via the free In-park Shuttle system.

Trail Description

▶1 Begin the loop by following the initial section of the High Sierra Trail, which heads east from the vicinity of the restrooms at the Crescent Meadow parking lot. Cross a pair of short wood bridges over Crescent Creek and soon come to a junction with the Crescent Meadow Loop on the left. Veer right, remaining on the High Sierra Trail for about 25 yards to a second junction with the trail to Bobcat Point. ▶2 From there, the dirt tread of the High

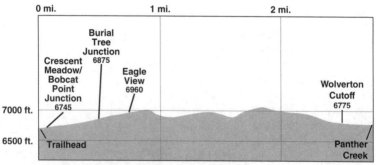

TRAIL 18 **High Sierra Trail to Eagle View and Panther Creek Elevation Profile**

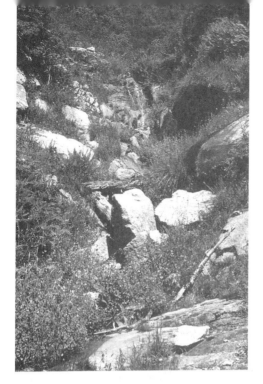

Panther Creek

Sierra Trail gently ascends across the north side of a low hill. Pass by a few more scattered sequoias on the way to a junction near the Burial Tree in a forested saddle, 0.5 mile from the trailhead. ▶3

Continue ahead from the junction, as the trail swings across an open hillside near the edge of the Giant Forest plateau and high above the canyon of Middle Fork Kaweah River. A nearly level grade leads to aptly named Eagle View at 0.75 mile. ▶4 From this aerie, 3,000 feet above the river, you have marvelous views of the canyon below, Moro Rock, Castle Rocks, and the Great Western Divide.

 Great Views

Away from Eagle View, the High Sierra Trail traverses the south-facing hillside, where open areas with sweeping views alternate with pockets of light mixed forest made up of Jeffrey pines, white firs, incense cedars, and black oaks. A set of four switchbacks interrupts the otherwise gently graded trail on the way to the high point of the route near the 2-mile mark. From there, a general descent leads through light forest and past a short rock wall to a junction with the Wolverton Cutoff, 2.5 miles from the trailhead. ▶5

From the junction you can usually hear the roar of Panther Creek ahead. An easy, 0.2-mile stroll leads to the banks of this refreshing stream, where a ribbon of water spills over moss-covered rocks and plunges down a steep chasm tangled with logs and lush vegetation. ▶6 This refreshing brook makes a good turnaround point for day hikers. Backpackers must continue another 0.8 mile farther up the trail past multiple branches of Panther Creek to the first legal campsites near Mehrten Creek.

Stream

Camping ▲

🚶	**MILESTONES**	
▶1	0.0	Start at Crescent Meadow Trailhead
▶2	0.1	Right at Crescent Meadow Loop junction
		Left at Bobcat Point junction
▶3	0.5	Straight at junction near Burial Tree
▶4	0.75	Eagle View
▶5	2.5	Straight at Wolverton Cutoff
▶6	2.7	Panther Creek

Crescent Meadow and Log Meadow Loop

The Crescent Meadow area is one of the busiest spots in Sequoia National Park. Despite the potential crowds, this short journey to two flower-filled meadows and numerous majestic giant sequoias is a must-do trip for any visitor to the Giant Forest. A stop at Tharps Log completes the quintessential experience.

Best Time

Trails in Giant Forest are generally snow-free by the first part of June and remain so usually until sometime in November. Summer is by far the busiest time, when parking spaces are at a premium—consider riding the free shuttle bus during peak season. The best time to view the verdant sedges and grasses of Crescent and Log Meadows is midsummer, when they're complemented by a palette of color from a copious variety of wildflowers. Autumn can be a fine time for a visit as well, especially when crowds are small and the dogwoods are ablaze with fall color.

Finding the Trail

Public transportation to the Giant Forest Museum is available from Visalia and Three Rivers on the Sequoia Shuttle. The round-trip cost is $15, and reservations are required. Call 877-BUS-HIKE or visit **sequoiashuttle.com.**

From the vicinity of the Giant Forest Museum, you can ride the free In-park Shuttle on Gray Route 2 to Crescent Meadow.

TRAIL USE
Day Hike, Child Friendly

LENGTH
2.4 miles, 1½ hours

VERTICAL FEET
+450/-450/±900

DIFFICULTY
– 1 **2** 3 4 5 +

TRAIL TYPE
Loop

FEATURES
Fall Colors
Wildflowers
Giant Sequoias
Historical Interest

FACILITIES
Restrooms
Water
Picnic Area
Shuttle Bus Stop

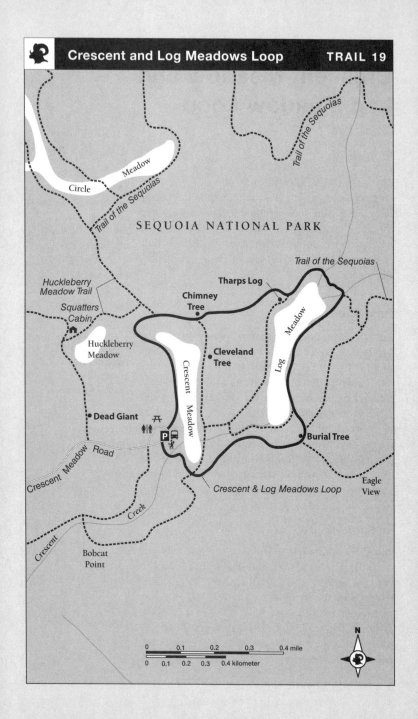

SEQUOIA NATIONAL PARK

Circle Meadow

Trail of the Sequoias

Trail of the Sequoias

Huckleberry Meadow Trail

Squatters Cabin

Tharps Log

Chimney Tree

Huckleberry Meadow

Cleveland Tree

Crescent Meadow

Log Meadow

Dead Giant

Burial Tree

Crescent Meadow Road

Crescent & Log Meadows Loop

Eagle View

Creek

Crescent

Bobcat Point

0   0.1   0.2   0.3   0.4 mile
0   0.1   0.2   0.3   0.4 kilometer

N

From Visalia, private vehicles should follow CA 198 to Three Rivers and proceed east into Sequoia National Park, where the road becomes Generals Highway. Drive Generals Highway to the Giant Forest Museum. Either park your vehicle in the large parking lot and ride the free shuttle bus, or drive along the narrow Crescent Meadow Road 1.2 miles to the Moro Rock junction. Motorists should continue on Crescent Meadow Road another 1.3 miles to the end of the road at the Crescent Meadow parking lot.

Lodgepole is the nearest campground, about 9 miles on Generals Highway from the Giant Forest Museum (fee, flush toilets, running water, bear boxes, and phone). Wuksachi Village, a short distance north of Lodgepole, offers upscale lodging and dining. Both Lodgepole and Wuksachi Village are accessible via the free In-park Shuttle system.

Trail Description

▶1 Begin your journey by following the famed High Sierra Trail, a 60-plus-mile path connecting the big trees (giant sequoias) with the big mountain (Mount Whitney). This fabled path begins as a paved trail that crosses a pair of short wood bridges over Crescent Creek and then passes junctions with the Crescent Creek and Bobcat Point Trails. ▶2 Beyond the second

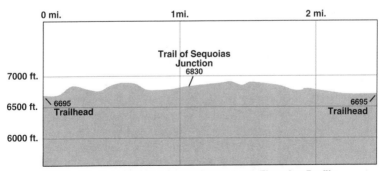

TRAIL 19 Crescent and Log Meadows Loop Elevation Profile

Hiker *at Tharps Log*

Tharps Log

HISTORY

Gaining an accurate sense of the magnitude of a mature giant sequoia is often difficult when the tree is still standing. When one of the old giants topples and stretches across the forest floor, a better perspective is gained on the true immensity of these big trees. Tharps Log is just such an example, large enough for the fire-hollowed interior to have been used for a summer cabin in the late 1800s. Modern-day visitors can view the restored cabin, complete with rock fireplace, bed, table, and rough-hewn benches and chairs. Interpretive signs provide some history associated with the tree, as well as a warning for visitors to respect the historical nature of the structure by remaining outside.

Hale D. Tharp, a Michigan native, settled near Three Rivers in 1856, where he quickly befriended the native Yokuts, who told their new friend of the giant trees. Two years later, Tharp was taken by the Yokuts to the Giant Forest and was later credited as being the first white man to see the big trees. Tharp later home-steaded Log Meadow, where he ran cattle. He used the log as a summer cabin from 1861 to 1890. Tharps Log remains the oldest human-made edifice in the park.

junction, the trail turns to dirt and makes a mild ascent across the north side of a low hill. Pass a few scattered sequoias on the way to a fork in the trail in a forested saddle near the Burial Tree. ▶3

Descend northwest from the junction, soon dropping to another junction near the southeast edge of Log Meadow, ▶4 a grass-and-flower-filled glade ringed by giant sequoias and lesser conifers.

 Wildflowers

Head north from the junction and walk along the east side of Log Meadow through an understory of azaleas and ferns beneath mixed forest cover. Near the north end of this lovely dell, you reach a signed T-junction with the Trail of the Sequoias. ▶5

 Fall Colors

Proceed ahead from the junction, step over a sliver of a stream to a forested flat, and then come almost immediately to a second stream crossing on a wood plank bridge. Nearby, a number of stately sequoias line the drainage. Heading west around the northern fringe of Log Meadow, you soon reach Tharps Log, lying in a pastoral clearing, and a junction with the designated Crescent and Log Meadows Loop. ▶6

 Historical Interest

Turn north and follow signed directions toward the Chimney Tree on the shared course of the Trail of the Sequoias and Crescent and Log Meadows Loop, climbing away from Log Meadow and soon ascending a set of stairs hewn out of a fallen sequoia. At the top of the climb, the trail crosses a low divide separating Log and Crescent meadows. Drop off the divide on a mild descent to a pair of junctions. At the first, a very short lateral leads to the base of the Chimney Tree, where hikers can stand inside the fire-hollowed snag of a dead sequoia. This giant apparently met its doom at the hands of a fire set by a careless camper in 1919. About 25 feet farther is a second junction, ▶7 where a quick detour on the left-hand trail leads shortly to the Cleveland Tree, one of the larger sequoias in the Giant Forest.

 Giant Sequoias

Veer right at the second junction and skirt around the north side of Crescent Meadow on a

Crystal Cave

Many consider a trip to Sequoia National Park incomplete without a visit to magnificent Crystal Cave, where sweater- or jacket-clad visitors take guided tours from early May to late September to such notable features as stalactites and curtains, large cathedral-like rooms, and areas of elaborately polished marble. After purchasing advance tickets at either the Foothills or Lodgepole Visitor Centers (tickets are not available at the cave), a 6-plus-mile scenic drive from Generals Highway is followed by a half-mile stroll down to the cave entrance. From there, paid ticket holders are guided on the Family Tour (50 minutes; 50-person limit; $16 adults, $8 youth ages 5–12, and $5 children under 5) or the Discovery Tour (1½ hours, 18-person limit, $18). Spelunkers have the added opportunity to make arrangements for a 6-hour tour off the beaten path on the Wild Cave Tour ($135, 16 years or older). For tour times or more information, visit **explorecrystalcave.com.**

short stroll through the forest to a Y-junction, where the Trail of the Sequoias heads northwest. ►8 Turn left (southwest) and follow the west side of picturesque Crescent Meadow a half mile back to the parking lot. ►9

🚶 MILESTONES

►1	0.0	Start at High Sierra Trailhead
►2	0.15	Straight at Crescent Creek and Bobcat Point junctions
►3	0.5	Turn left (northwest) at junction near Burial Tree
►4	0.6	Veer right (north) at junction near Log Meadow
►5	1.1	Straight at Trail of the Sequoias
►6	1.2	Turn right (north) at Tharps Log junction
►7	1.5	Veer right (northwest) at second junction near Chimney Tree
►8	1.7	Turn left (southwest) at junction of Trail of the Sequoias
►9	2.4	Return to trailhead

Trail of the Sequoias Loop

This nearly 6-mile excursion through the heart of Giant Forest allows visitors the opportunity to stand among the giant sequoias in silence and serenity, away from most of the crowds on the more popular trails in the area. Plenty of notable sequoias are passed along the way, some named and many unnamed. In addition to the Big Trees, the circuit visits three flower-laden meadows—Crescent, Log, and Circle. For those wishing to see some of Giant Forest's more popular trees, access to the southern part of the Congress Trail loop is straightforward.

Best Time

Snow generally leaves the trails sometime in May in this part of Giant Forest, permitting snow-free hiking until the first snowfall of the season, usually in late October or early November. Late spring, when the azalea flowers are in bloom, is a particularly fine time for a visit, as is early fall, when the azalea leaves are cloaked in autumn splendor. Colorful wildflowers put on a showy display in early summer.

Finding the Trail

Public transportation to the Giant Forest Museum is available from Visalia and Three Rivers on the Sequoia Shuttle. The round-trip cost is $15, and reservations are required. Call 877-BUS-HIKE or visit **sequoiashuttle.com.**

From the vicinity of the Giant Forest Museum, you can ride the free In-park Shuttle on Gray Route 2 to Crescent Meadow.

TRAIL USE
Day Hike, Run

LENGTH
5.8 miles, 3 hours

VERTICAL FEET
+1050/-1050/±2100

DIFFICULTY
– 1 2 **3** 4 5 +

TRAIL TYPE
Loop

FEATURES
Wildflowers
Giant Sequoias
Historical Interest

FACILITIES
Restrooms
Water
Picnic Area
Shuttle Bus Stop

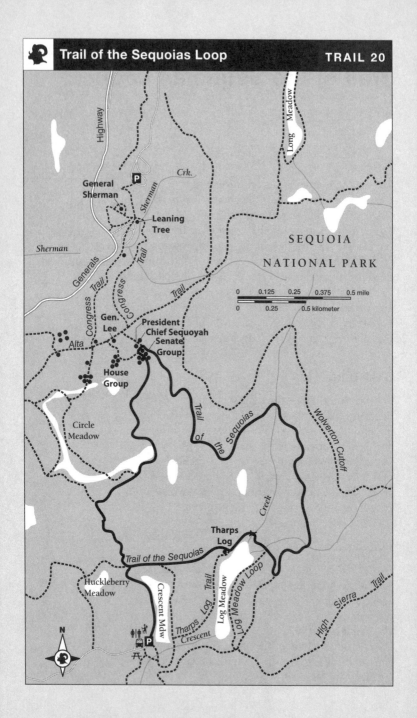

Highway

Crk.

General
Sherman

Leaning
Tree

Sherman

Sherman

SEQUOIA

NATIONAL PARK

Generals

Congress

Trail

Trail

0   0.125   0.25   0.375   0.5 mile
0   0.25   0.5 kilometer

Gen.
Lee

President
Chief Sequoyah
Senate
Group

Alta

House
Group

Congress Trail

Trail

of

the

Sequoias

Wolverton Cutoff

Circle
Meadow

Creek

Tharps
Log

Trail of the Sequoias

Huckleberry
Meadow

Crescent Mdw

Tharps Log Trail

Log Meadow

Log Meadow Loop

High Sierra

Trail

Crescent

N

From Visalia, private vehicles should follow CA 198 to Three Rivers and proceed east into Sequoia National Park, where the road becomes Generals Highway. Drive Generals Highway to the Giant Forest Museum. Either park your vehicle in the large parking lot and ride the free shuttle bus, or drive along the narrow Crescent Meadow Road 1.2 miles to the Moro Rock junction. Motorists should continue on Crescent Meadow Road another 1.3 miles to the end of the road at the Crescent Meadow parking lot.

Lodgepole is the nearest campground, about 9 miles on Generals Highway from the Giant Forest Museum (fee, flush toilets, running water, bear boxes, and phone). Wuksachi Village, a short distance north of Lodgepole, offers upscale lodging and dining. Both Lodgepole and Wuksachi Village are accessible via the free In-park Shuttle system.

Trail Description

▶1 Begin your adventure into the heart of Giant Forest by heading north on the Crescent Meadow Loop along the west edge of the lovely flower-laden meadow for a half mile to a Y-junction near the north edge. ▶2

Turn right (east) and pass above the fringe of the meadow for 0.2 mile to a pair of junctions about 10

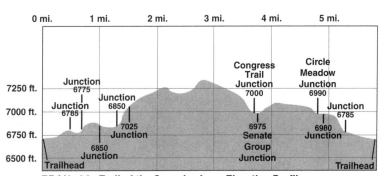

TRAIL 20   Trail of the Sequoias Loop Elevation Profile

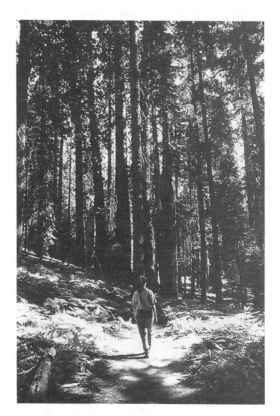

Giant Forest, *Trail of the Sequoias*

yards apart. ▶3 The Chimney Tree, a fire-hollowed giant sequoia, is just a short walk to the north. Following signed directions to Tharps Log, you continue eastbound on a short, winding ascent over a low ridge and then descend briefly to Tharps Log near the north end of Log Meadow.

Historical Interest 🏠

Near Tharps Log is a T-junction ▶4 between the Tharps Log Trail on the right and the Trail of the Sequoias on the left.

Continue east from the junction around the north tip of Log Meadow, cross Crescent Creek on a wood plank bridge, and soon step across a smaller tributary on the way to the junction with the Log Meadow Loop on the right. ▶5 Climb up

a fern-covered hillside and reach the next junction
▶6 after 0.2 mile with a little-used connector trail
headed south to the High Sierra Trail.

Remaining on the Trail of the Sequoias, veer
left and follow a lengthy traverse across a hillside,
hopping over a pair of small rivulets along the
way and encountering a number of notable giant
sequoias, including passing through a break in
the trunk of a fallen giant. The trail arcs across the
drainage of Crescent Creek and then climbs to the
top of a ridge, from where there are filtered views
of the surrounding woodland. Gazing across the
mixed forest, you may notice the characteristic
sequoia crowns overshadowing the lesser conifers.
A half-mile descent from the ridge leads past more
sequoias on the way to a junction with the Congress
Trail near the President Tree. ▶7

 Giant Sequoias

Turn left at the junction and very soon reach a
junction near the Senate Group. ▶8 Because several
notable giant sequoias are in the general vicinity, you may elect to follow a short section of the
southern loop of the Congress Trail to such trees as
General Lee, McKinley, and the House Group.

From the junction near the Senate Group, the
Trail of the Sequoias heads south and follows a general descent past a couple of scorched giants that at
first glance appear to have died but, upon further
inspection, are amazingly still alive. Cross a tiny
rivulet trickling into the southeast fringe of Circle
Meadow, and then follow the path across the slope
above this verdant, flower-dotted clearing. After passing an unsigned fork, where a use trail wanders out
into the meadow, you reach a signed junction a short
way farther with the Circle Meadow Trail. ▶9

 Wildflowers

Veer left at the junction to remain on the Trail
of the Sequoias for another 0.1 mile to the next
junction. ▶10 Turn left and head south–southeast
on a descent through moderate forest cover for 0.4
mile to a pair of Y-junctions, ▶11 approximately 25

yards apart. Turn left at the first junction and reach the close of the loop at the second junction. From there, turn right and retrace your steps 0.5 mile to the Crescent Meadow Trailhead. ▶12

🚶 MILESTONES

▶1	0.0	Start at Crescent Meadow Loop Trailhead
▶2	0.5	Right at junction
▶3	0.7	Straight at Chimney Tree junction
▶4	1.0	Left at Trail of the Sequoias junction
▶5	1.3	Straight at Log Meadow Loop junction
▶6	1.5	Left at connector junction
▶7	3.7	Left at Congress Trail junction
▶8	3.75	Left at junction near Senate Group
▶9	4.8	Left at Circle Meadow Trail junction
▶10	4.9	Left at junction
▶11	5.3	Left at first junction; right at second junction
▶12	5.8	Crescent Meadow Trailhead

Hazelwood Nature Trail

The Hazelwood Nature Trail is a short and easy stroll through a verdant forest dell, where visitors can see a fine assortment of young and old giant sequoias.

Best Time

Snow generally leaves the trails sometime in May in this part of Giant Forest, permitting snow-free hiking until the first snowfall of the season, usually in late October or early November. Late spring, when the azalea flowers are in bloom, is a particularly fine time for a visit, as is early fall, when the azalea leaves are cloaked in autumn splendor. Colorful wildflowers put on a showy display in early summer.

Finding the Trail

Public transportation to the Giant Forest Museum is available from Visalia and Three Rivers on the Sequoia Shuttle. The round-trip cost is $15, and reservations are required. Call 877-BUS-HIKE or visit **sequoiashuttle.com.**

Private vehicles should follow CA 198 to Three Rivers and proceed east into Sequoia National Park, where the road becomes Generals Highway. Drive Generals Highway to the vicinity of the Giant Forest Museum and park in the main parking lot across from the museum.

Lodgepole is the nearest campground, about 4.5 miles on Generals Highway from the Giant

TRAIL USE
Day Hike, Child Friendly
LENGTH
1.3 miles, 3/4 hour
VERTICAL FEET
Negligible
DIFFICULTY
– **1** 2 3 4 5 +
TRAIL TYPE
Loop

FEATURES
Wildflowers
Giant Sequoias

FACILITIES
Museum
Restrooms
Water
Shuttle Bus Stop

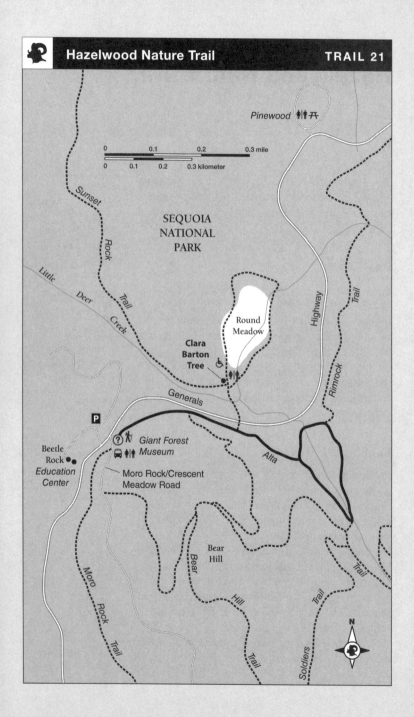

Hazelwood Nature Trail

TRAIL 21

Pinewood

0   0.1   0.2   0.3 mile
0   0.1   0.2   0.3 kilometer

Sunset

SEQUOIA
NATIONAL
PARK

Rock

Trail

Little

Deer

Creek

Round
Meadow

Clara
Barton
Tree

Highway

Rimrock

Trail

Generals

P

Giant Forest
Museum

Alta

Beetle
Rock
Education
Center

Moro Rock/Crescent
Meadow Road

Bear
Hill

Moro

Rock

Trail

Bear

Hill

Trail

Trail

Soldiers

N

Forest Museum (fee, flush toilets, running water, bear boxes, and phone). Wuksachi Village, a short distance north of Lodgepole, offers upscale lodging and dining. Both Lodgepole and Wuksachi Village are accessible via the free In-park Shuttle system.

Logistics

This trail can easily be combined with the Big Trees Trail (see Trail 22).

Trail Description

▶1 From the Giant Forest Museum, follow a paved section of the Alta Trail eastward, passing through junctions on the right with the Bear Hill Trail and on the left with a lateral across Generals Highway to connect with the Big Trees Trail. After 0.4 mile, you come to the Hazelwood Nature Trail loop. ▶2

Turn right at the junction to begin a counterclockwise circuit through mixed forest, where massive sequoias dwarf the other conifers. A smattering of dogwoods adds creamy white flowers in early summer and a blaze of orange leaves in autumn. The verdant groundcover consists of an assortment of plants, including azaleas, thimbleberries, ferns, and colorful wildflowers in season. Reach a signed junction, ▶3 where the Alta Trail veers uphill to the right but you bend to the left, cross a nascent branch of Little Deer Creek, and then head north.

The loop continues through the lovely forested dell, reaching the next junction, where the Rimrock Trail continues to the north. ▶4

Veer left at the junction and proceed to a crossing of the Little Deer Creek tributary on a short wood bridge. Reach the close of the loop ▶5 and then retrace your steps back to the museum. ▶6

Giant Sequoias

Wildflowers

🚶	**MILESTONES**		
▶1	0.0	Start at Giant Forest Museum
▶2	0.4	Right at loop junction
▶3	0.6	Left at Alta Trail junction
▶4	0.8	Left at Rimrock Trail junction
▶5	0.9	Right at loop junction
▶6	1.3	Giant Forest Museum

Big Trees Trail

Big Trees Trail is a short and easy wheelchair-accessible path around lush Round Meadow filled with seasonal wildflowers and bordered by giant sequoias. Interpretive signs along the trail offer information about the ecology of the forest.

Best Time

Snow generally leaves the trails sometime in May in this part of Giant Forest, permitting snow-free hiking until the first snowfall of the season, usually in late October or early November. Late spring, when the azalea flowers are in bloom, is a particularly fine time for a visit, as is early fall, when the azalea leaves are cloaked in autumn splendor. Colorful wildflowers put on a showy display in early summer.

Finding the Trail

Public transportation to the Giant Forest Museum is available from Visalia and Three Rivers on the Sequoia Shuttle. The round-trip cost is $15, and reservations are required. Call 877-BUS-HIKE or visit **sequoiashuttle.com.**

Private vehicles should follow CA 198 to Three Rivers and proceed east into Sequoia National Park, where the road becomes Generals Highway. Drive Generals Highway to the vicinity of the Giant Forest Museum and park in the main parking lot across from the museum.

Lodgepole is the nearest campground, about 4.5 miles on Generals Highway from the Giant Forest Museum (fee, flush toilets, running water,

TRAIL USE
Day Hike, Child Friendly, Handicapped Accessible

LENGTH
1.2 miles, 1/2 hour

VERTICAL FEET
Negligible

DIFFICULTY
– **1** 2 3 4 5 +

TRAIL TYPE
Loop

FEATURES
Wildflowers
Giant Sequoias

FACILITIES
Museum
Restrooms
Water
Shuttle Bus Stop

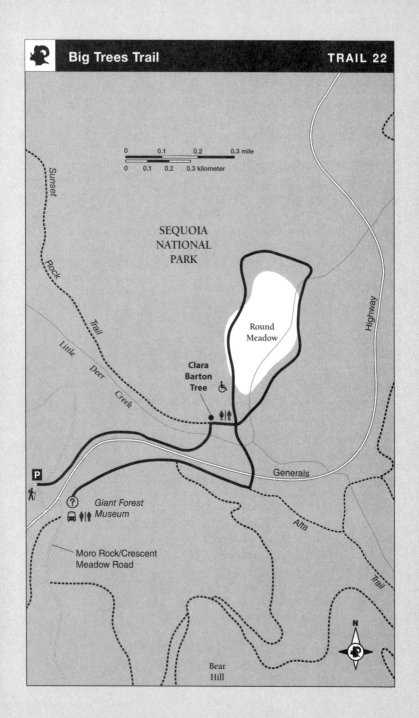

SEQUOIA
NATIONAL
PARK

Sunset

Rock

Trail

Little

Deer

Creek

Round
Meadow

**Clara
Barton
Tree**

Highway

Generals

Alta

Trail

P

Giant Forest
Museum

Moro Rock/Crescent
Meadow Road

N

Bear
Hill

0   0.1   0.2   0.3 mile
0   0.1   0.2   0.3 kilometer

bear boxes, and phone). Wuksachi Village, a short distance north of Lodgepole, offers upscale lodging and dining. Both Lodgepole and Wuksachi Village are accessible via the free In-park Shuttle system.

Logistics

This trail can easily be combined with the Hazel-wood Nature Trail (see Trail 21).

Trail Description

►1 From the Giant Forest parking lot, follow paved trail alongside Generals Highway through a junction at the Sunset Rock Trail to a second junction near the Clara Barton Tree, named for the founder of the Red Cross. Continue ahead a short distance to the beginning of the loop. ►2 Alternately, if you arrived by shuttle bus, follow the paved start of the Alta Trail on the south side of Generals Highway to a junction with a lateral on the left that crosses the highway to connect with the loop around Round Meadow.

Giant Sequoias

Turn left and begin a clockwise loop around lovely Round Meadow, crossing a tributary of Little Deer Creek twice on the way to the close of the loop near the restrooms. ►3 From there, retrace your steps back to the parking lot, or the Giant Forest Museum. ►4

Wildflowers

🚶	**MILESTONES**	
►1	0.0	Start at Giant Forest Museum
►2	0.3	Left at loop junction
►3	0.9	Left at loop junction
►4	1.2	Giant Forest Museum

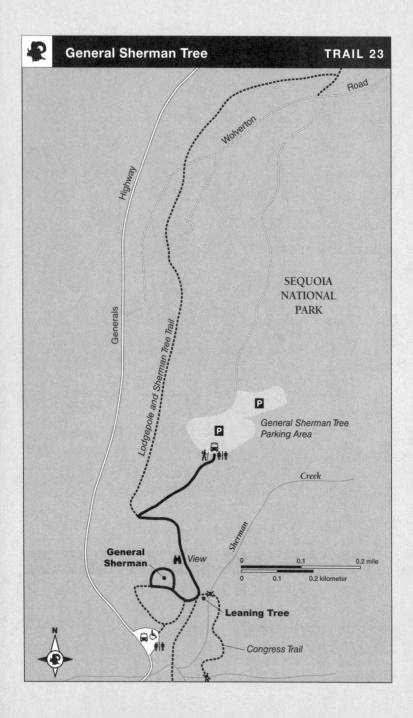

Road

Wolverton

Highway

Generals

Lodgepole and Sherman Tree Trail

SEQUOIA
NATIONAL
PARK

P

P
General Sherman Tree
Parking Area

Creek

Sherman

**General
Sherman**

View

0   0.1   0.2 mile

0   0.1   0.2 kilometer

Leaning Tree

N

Congress Trail

General Sherman Tree

The General Sherman Tree is truly one of the world's great wonders, reaching heights near 275 feet and a volume of more than 52,500 feet, and achieving a circumference at its base of more than 100 feet. In the 1800s, a skeptical public refused to believe the existence of such massive conifers. Two relatively easy routes allow visitors to admire General Sherman: a very short, handicapped-accessible trail from a shuttle bus stop off Generals Highway and a half-mile, paved path from the General Sherman parking lot (also accessible by shuttle bus). Interpretive signs and a cross section of the tree's base along the half-mile route offer interesting information and a graphic way to appreciate the tree's tremendous size. Although the area is understandably highly popular with tourists, experiencing General Sherman close up is a must-do activity for all visitors to Sequoia National Park.

TRAIL USE
Day Hike, Handicapped Accessible, Child Friendly

LENGTH
0.9 miles, 1/4 hour

VERTICAL FEET
+250/-250/±500

DIFFICULTY
– **1** 2 3 4 5 +

TRAIL TYPE
Out-and-back

FEATURES
Giant Sequoias

FACILITIES
Museum
Restrooms
Water
Shuttle Bus Stop

Best Time

Snow generally leaves the trails sometime in May in this part of the Giant Forest, permitting snow-free hiking until the first winter storm, usually in late October or early November. Late spring, when the azalea flowers are in bloom, is a particularly fine time for a visit, as is early fall, when the azalea leaves are cloaked in autumn splendor. Colorful wildflowers put on a showy display in early summer.

Finding the Trail

Public transportation to the Giant Forest Museum is available from Visalia and Three Rivers on the Sequoia Shuttle. The round-trip cost is $15, and

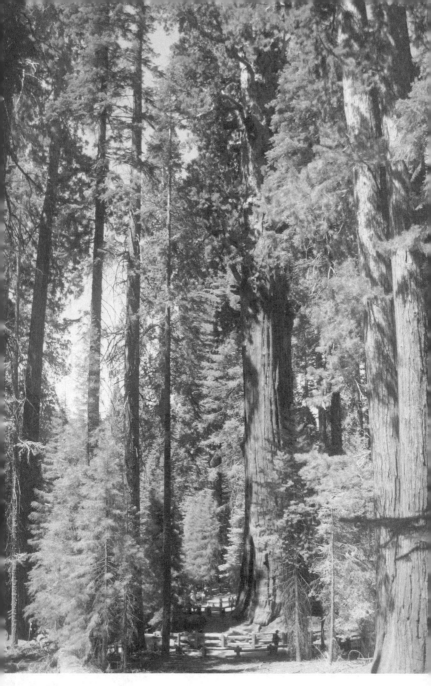

General Sherman Tree

reservations are required. Call 877-BUS-HIKE or visit **sequoiashuttle.com**. From the vicinity of the Giant Forest Museum, passengers can ride the free In-park Shuttle on Green Route 1 to either the General Sherman Tree bus stop off Generals Highway or the General Sherman parking lot off Wolverton Road.

From Visalia, private vehicles should follow CA 198 to Three Rivers and proceed east into Sequoia National Park, where the road becomes Generals Highway. Drive Generals Highway to Giant Forest and park your vehicle in the large parking lot opposite the museum if you plan on utilizing the shuttle bus. (The parking area for the General Sherman Tree was relocated in 2005 to provide a less environmentally sensitive site than the previous one just off Generals Highway).

To continue driving a vehicle to the General Sherman Trailhead, proceed on Generals Highway to the junction with Wolverton Road, 2.8 miles north of the museum and 1.75 miles south of Lodgepole. Motorists should follow Wolverton Road 0.5 mile to a three-way stop, and then turn right to follow a spur road another half mile to the General Sherman parking area at the end of the road. Lodgepole is the nearest campground (fee, flush toilets, running water, bear boxes, and phone). Wuksachi Village, just north of Lodgepole, offers upscale lodging and dining.

> The diameter of the tree's largest branch is an amazing 7 feet, larger than the diameter of the trunk on most mature conifers.

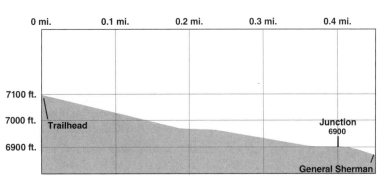

TRAIL 23 General Sherman Tree Elevation Profile

Logistics

Crowds can be avoided by making an early-morning or late-afternoon visit.

Trail Description

►1 From the parking lot, pass through an elaborate wood archway lined with informational placards and descend along a well-graded, paved trail with periodic stairs toward the General Sherman Tree. Several park benches along the way offer tourists convenient resting spots, primarily for the uphill return. Where the path makes a sharp bend, a set of stairs marks the beginning of the lightly used Lodgepole and Sherman Tree Trail that connects these two areas. Farther on, a wide spot in the trail is imprinted with a cross section of the Sherman Tree's base, a graphic picture of this truly massive giant sequoia. This spot also offers an unobstructed view of the world's largest tree, distant enough for photographers to squeeze the big tree into their camera frames. A short walk beyond the vista leads to a junction ►2 of the nature trail to General Sherman on the right and the signed Congress Trail on the left.

Giant Sequoias

Turn right and follow the path around the largest tree by volume (52,500 cubic feet) in the world. Not only is General Sherman the world's largest tree, it's also the world's largest living organism. After completing the circuit, retrace your steps from the junction ►3 uphill back to the parking lot. ►4

🚶	**MILESTONES**	
►1	0.0	Start at General Sherman parking area
►2	0.4	Right at junction
►3	0.5	Left at junction
►4	0.9	General Sherman parking area

Congress Trail

Not surprisingly, the largest tree in the world is an attraction guaranteed to lure throngs of tourists, both domestic and international, throughout the course of a Sierra summer. With the General Sherman Tree as the first stop, this 3-plus-mile, paved loop also visits the third, fourth, and 26th largest giant sequoias, and two of the most impressive clusters of the big trees, the Senate and House groups. Short side trips offer even more possibilities for viewing other notable Giant Forest landmarks. While you shouldn't expect to stand alone in reverent solitude before these awe-inspiring monarchs of the forest, the numbers of tourists drops dramatically the farther you travel away from the General Sherman Tree.

Best Times

Snow generally leaves the trails sometime in May in this part of the Giant Forest, permitting snow-free hiking until the first winter storm, usually in late October or early November. Late spring, when the azalea flowers are in bloom, is a particularly fine time for a visit, as is early fall, when the azalea leaves are cloaked in autumn splendor. Colorful wildflowers put on a showy display in early summer.

Finding the Trail

Public transportation to the Giant Forest Museum is available from Visalia and Three Rivers on the Sequoia Shuttle. The round-trip cost is $15, and reservations are required. Call 877-BUS-HIKE or visit

TRAIL USE
Day Hike, Child Friendly
LENGTH
3.1 miles, 1½–2 hours
VERTICAL FEET
+550/-550/±1100
DIFFICULTY
– 1 **2** 3 4 5 +
TRAIL TYPE
Loop

FEATURES
Fall Colors
Wildflowers
Giant Sequoias

FACILITIES
Restrooms
Water
Shuttle Bus Stop

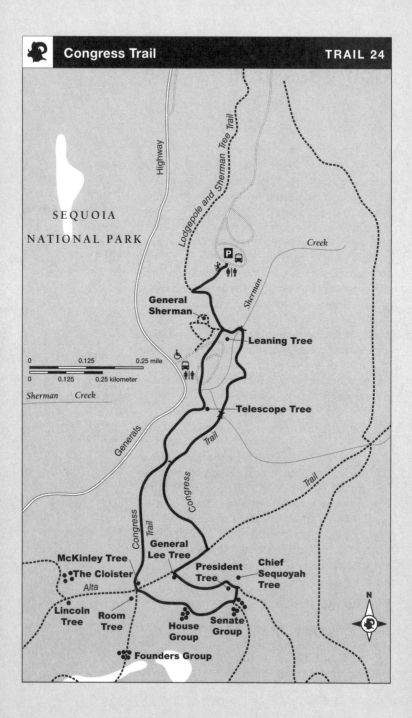

SEQUOIA

NATIONAL PARK

Highway

Lodgepole and Sherman Tree Trail

Creek

P

Sherman

General Sherman

Leaning Tree

| 0 | 0.125 | 0.25 mile |
| 0 | 0.125 | 0.25 kilometer |

Sherman   Creek

Telescope Tree

Generals

Congress   Trail

Trail

Congress   Trail

McKinley Tree
The Cloister

Alta

General Lee Tree

President Tree

Chief Sequoyah Tree

Lincoln Tree

Room Tree

House Group

Senate Group

N

Founders Group

sequoiashuttle.com. From the vicinity of the Giant Forest Museum, passengers can ride the free In-park Shuttle on Green Route 1 to either the General Sherman Tree bus stop off Generals Highway or the General Sherman parking lot off Wolverton Road.

From Visalia, private vehicles should follow CA 198 to Three Rivers and proceed east into Sequoia National Park, where the road becomes Generals Highway. Drive Generals Highway to the Giant Forest. The parking area for the General Sherman Tree (and start of the Congress Trail) was relocated in 2005 to provide a less environmentally sensitive site than the previous one just off Generals Highway. To continue driving a vehicle to the General Sherman Trailhead, proceed on Generals Highway to the junction with Wolverton Road, 1.75 miles south of Lodgepole and 2.8 miles north of the museum. Motorists should follow Wolverton Road 0.5 mile to a three-way stop and then turn right to follow a spur road another half mile to the General Sherman parking area at the end of the road. Lodgepole is the nearest campground (fee, flush toilets, running water, bear boxes, and phone). Wuksachi Village, a short distance north of Lodgepole, offers upscale lodging and dining.

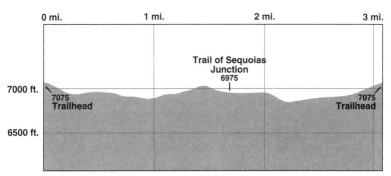

TRAIL 24 Congress Trail Elevation Profile

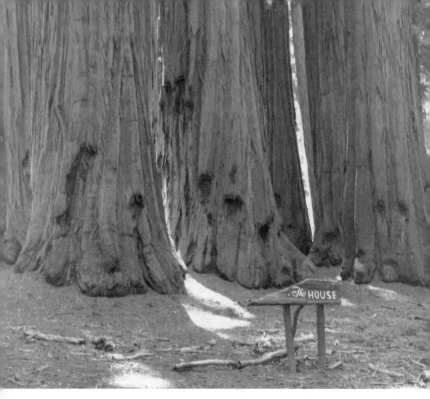

House Group *on the Congress Trail*

Logistics

Crowds can be avoided by making an early-morning or late-afternoon visit.

Trail Description

►1 From the parking lot, pass through an elaborate wood archway lined with informational placards and descend along a well-graded, paved trail with periodic stairs toward the General Sherman Tree. Several park benches along the way offer tourists convenient resting spots for the uphill return. Where the path makes a sharp bend, a set of stairs marks the beginning of the lightly used Lodgepole and Sherman Tree Trail that connects these two areas. Farther on, a wide spot in the trail is imprinted with a cross section of the Sherman Tree's base, a graphic picture of this truly massive giant sequoia. This spot also offers an unobstructed view of the world's largest tree, distant enough for photographers to squeeze the big tree into their camera frames. A short walk beyond the vista leads to a junction of the nature trail to General Sherman on the right and the signed Congress Trail on the left.

Giant Sequoias

Whether you arrive via the shuttle bus or by way of the half-mile trail from the parking area, find the signed trailhead for the Congress Trail nearby ►2 and proceed downhill to the Leaning Tree. From there, the path continues over a pair of footbridges over branches of Sherman Creek, passing a number of stately sequoias along the way. Springtime hikers will notice the lovely white blooms of dogwoods scattered throughout the Giant Forest, while autumn hikers will be blessed by the fall colors from the turning leaves. Beyond the second bridge, a lateral on the right ►3 offers a shortcut back to the trailhead for those unaccustomed to hiking at 7,000 feet.

Fall Colors

From the lateral, a winding, quarter-mile ascent leads to a four-way junction with the Alta Trail. ►4 Beyond the junction, nearing the south end of the loop, are many notable sequoias, including Chief Sequoyah (26th largest) and the President (third largest), the Senate and House groups, and General Lee and McKinley trees. Amid the staid Senate Group, the Trail of the Sequoias branches south. ►5 After 0.3 mile, reach a five-way junction with the Alta and Circle Meadows Trails near the McKinley Tree. ►6 With extra time, you can visit additional sequoia landmarks on easy side trips from this junction. The Cloister Tree and Lincoln Tree (fourth largest) are just a short jaunt southwest on the Alta Trail. A longer, 0.9-mile excursion farther southwest on the Alta Trail leads to the Huckleberry Meadow Trail, and a

General Sherman Tree

Any visit to the Giant Forest would be incomplete without taking the short stroll around this immense monarch of the forest. At 275 feet high, 103 feet around the base, and with a volume of 52,508 cubic feet, this giant sequoia has been declared not only the world's biggest tree but also the largest living organism in existence. The diameter of the tree's largest branch is an amazing 7 feet, larger than the diameter of the trunk on most mature conifers. James Wolverton, a pioneer cattleman who served under the general during the Civil War, named the tree in 1879 for General William Tecumseh Sherman, whose most remembered act during the war was the dubious March to the Sea, a campaign across Georgia from Atlanta.

short walk generally south to the Washington Tree (formerly the second largest). Southbound, the Circle Meadow Trail takes you shortly to the Room Tree, the Founders Group, and Cattle Cabin.

From the five-way junction, head north to descend mildly on the Congress Trail, weaving through the forest back to the lateral shortcut. ▶7 From there, continue north to the vicinity of the General Sherman Tree ▶8, and either pick up the shuttle bus or retrace your steps uphill to the parking area. ▶9

		MILESTONES
▶1	0.0	Start at General Sherman parking area
▶2	0.4	General Sherman Nature Trail and trailhead for Congress Trail
▶3	0.8	Straight at lateral junction
▶4	1.2	Straight at Alta Trail junction
▶5	1.7	Veer right at Trail of the Sequoias junction
▶6	2.0	Turn right (north) at five-way junction with Alta and Circle Meadow Trails
▶7	2.4	Straight at lateral junction
▶8	2.7	General Sherman Tree and trailhead for Congress Trail
▶9	3.1	Parking area

Alta Peak

Alta Peak's airy summit offers one of the best views available on the western side of Sequoia via a maintained trail. While arduous, a one-day ascent is a viable option for strong hikers who are well acclimatized. Lesser mortals have the option of a 2–3 day backpack trip, with a basecamp at either Alta Meadow or Mehrten Meadow Camp. However many days are needed, the supreme vista from Alta Peak is a just reward for the effort involved in getting there.

Best Time

The trail to Alta Peak, with a summit elevation of more than 11,000 feet, is usually snowbound through early July. The most popular time to climb the peak is midsummer, when there is the bonus of a fine wildflower display along the way. Early autumn is still a good time for an ascent, although hikers must be prepared for chilly temperatures. Once the first significant snowfall hits the southern Sierra, generally by the end of October, the trail holds onto snow until next summer.

Finding the Trail

Public transportation to the Giant Forest Museum is available from Visalia and Three Rivers on the Sequoia Shuttle. The round-trip cost is $15, and reservations are required. Call 877-BUS-HIKE or visit **sequoiashuttle.com.** From the vicinity of the Giant Forest Museum, passengers can ride the free In-park Shuttle on Orange Route 4 to the parking lot at the end of Wolverton Road.

TRAIL USE
Day Hike, Backpack, Horse
LENGTH
13.4 miles, 7–8 hours
VERTICAL FEET
+4275/-350/±9250
DIFFICULTY
– 1 2 3 4 **5** +
TRAIL TYPE
Out-and-back

FEATURES
Mountain
Summit
Wildflowers
Great Views
Camping
Steep

FACILITIES
Restrooms
Water
Bear Boxes

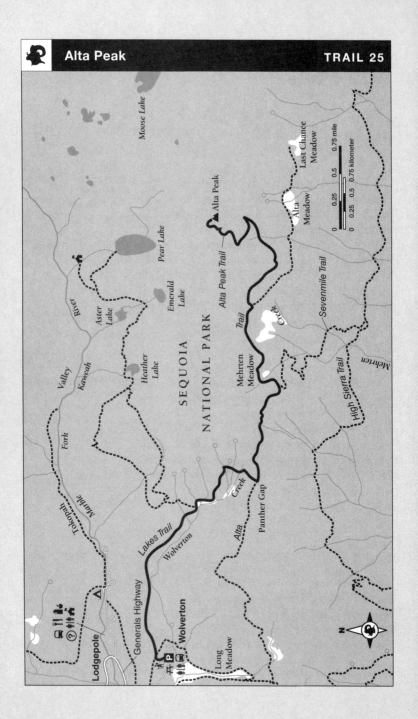

From Visalia, private vehicles should follow CA 198 to Three Rivers and proceed east into Sequoia National Park, where the road becomes Generals Highway. Follow Generals Highway to Wolverton Road, 1.75 miles southeast of Lodgepole. Head east 1.5 miles on Wolverton Road to the large trailhead parking area. Lodgepole is the nearest campground (fee, flush toilets, running water, bear boxes, and phone). Wuksachi Village, a short distance north of Lodgepole, offers upscale lodging and dining.

Logistics

Backpackers must obtain a wilderness permit for all overnight visits. See page 114 for more details about how to obtain one. Campfires are not allowed except at Panther Gap and Mehrten Meadow.

Trail Description

▶1 A barrage of trail signs with numerous destinations and mileages marks the start of the trail. Follow a series of concrete steps shortly to a wide, singletrack dirt trail that ascends a hillside to a junction at the crest with a path accessing the Lodgepole area and the old Wolverton corrals. ▶2 Turn right and follow the Lakes Trail, soon passing another

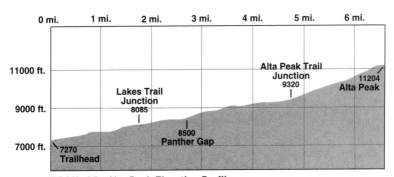

TRAIL 25 Alta Peak Elevation Profile

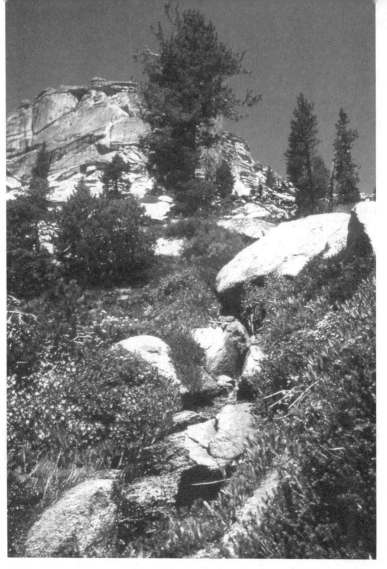

Brook *below Alta Peak*

junction with a trail on the right to Long Meadow. ►3 After the initial ascent, the grade eases to more of a mild to moderate climb along the course of Wolverton Creek. Hop across a spring-fed tributary of the creek and proceed to a junction with the trail to Panther Gap. ►4

OPTIONS

Alta Meadow

Overnighters may find favorable campsites near Alta Meadow. From the junction of Alta and Alta Peak Trails, follow mildly ascending trail around the forested base of Tharps Rock, eventually breaking out of the trees to a wide-ranging view of Middle Fork Kaweah River canyon. Beyond a stream crossing, the trail reaches the northwestern fringe of the verdant and flower-covered meadowlands of Alta Meadow, the beauty of which is complemented exquisitely by views of Tharps Rock, Alta Peak, and the Kings-Kaweah and Great Western divides. Fine campsites are nestled beneath red firs on a low ridge just south of the trail. An unmaintained path continues a short distance east over vales and rivulets to Last Chance Meadow and additional campsites.

Turn right and follow well-maintained tread through moderate forest cover on a course that roughly parallels Wolverton Creek, stepping across numerous little tributary streams along the way. Eventually, these delightful brooks lined with lush foliage are left behind, as the trail climbs out of the canyon to a T-junction with the Alta Trail at Panther Gap. ►5

Heading east on the Alta Trail, the trail soon veers onto the open, south-facing slope above Middle Fork Kaweah River, where views across this deep cleft are quite impressive. After a half mile, you hop across a nascent tributary of Panther Creek and then follow a series of switchbacks to a junction with the Sevenmile Trail. ►6 Remaining on the Alta Trail, proceed into forest cover and down to a ford of Mehrten Creek. Nearby is Mehrten Meadow Camp, ►7 where a few campsites with a bear box are sheltered by red firs. The narrow glade of Mehrten Meadow lies well below the trail. Leaving Mehrten Creek behind, the trail follows a mildly ascending,

 Great Views

 Camping

0.75-mile traverse across the north wall of the canyon to a junction with the Alta Peak Trail. ►8

Turn left and zigzag up the hillside beneath the intermittent shade from a grove of red firs, before the trees are soon left behind on an ascent to a refreshing, spring-fed, willow- and wildflower-lined stream. Ford the stream, pass a small campsite near the east bank, and begin a long ascending traverse across the face of Tharps Rock through scattered red firs and patches of chinquapin. Excellent views abound across the deep canyon of Middle Fork Kaweah River to the terrain in the southwestern part of Sequoia National Park, as well as the verdant swath of Alta Meadow below, and Tharps Rock and Alta Peak above. Nearing the end of the traverse, you reach the last reliable water source at a pretty arroyo filled with heather and wildflowers.

Following a switchback, the trail climbs stiffly on a zigzagging course above Tharps Rock. A few stunted foxtail pines herald the arrival into the alpine zone, where scattered tufts of ground-hugging flowers and plants cling to the nearly barren slopes. Over decomposed granite and around boulders, the unrelenting ascent continues just below the southwest ridge to the crest of the summit ridge. A short climb from there leads to the summit block and a final scramble to the top of Alta Peak. ►9

To describe the view from the summit as spectacular is an understatement. The body of water directly north of the peak is Pear Lake, backdropped by a sea of granite rising northeast to the Tableland and the Kings-Kaweah Divide. Numerous park landmarks are clearly visible, including the Sierra Crest stretching across the eastern horizon. With the aid of a big enough map, you'll be able to identify scads of peaks. When the ubiquitous San Joaquin Valley haze is absent, usually only after a rare, cleansing summer rainstorm, you'll be blessed with a western view across the valley's farmland to the Coast Range.

To describe the view from the summit as spectacular is an understatement.

Wildflowers

Summit

Great Views

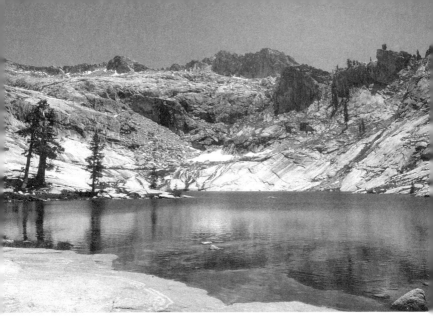

The Great Western Divide *from the Lakes Trail*

<table>
<tr><td>👣</td><td colspan="3">MILESTONES</td></tr>
<tr><td>▶1</td><td>0.0</td><td>Start at trailhead</td></tr>
<tr><td>▶2</td><td>0.1</td><td>Turn right (east) at junction</td></tr>
<tr><td>▶3</td><td>0.15</td><td>Straight at junction to Long Meadow</td></tr>
<tr><td>▶4</td><td>1.8</td><td>Turn right (south) at junction to Panther Gap</td></tr>
<tr><td>▶5</td><td>2.7</td><td>Turn left at Alta Trail junction</td></tr>
<tr><td>▶6</td><td>3.7</td><td>Straight at Sevenmile Trail junction</td></tr>
<tr><td>▶7</td><td>4.0</td><td>Mehrten Meadow Camp</td></tr>
<tr><td>▶8</td><td>4.75</td><td>Turn left (north) at Alta Peak Trail junction</td></tr>
<tr><td>▶9</td><td>6.7</td><td>Alta Peak</td></tr>
</table>

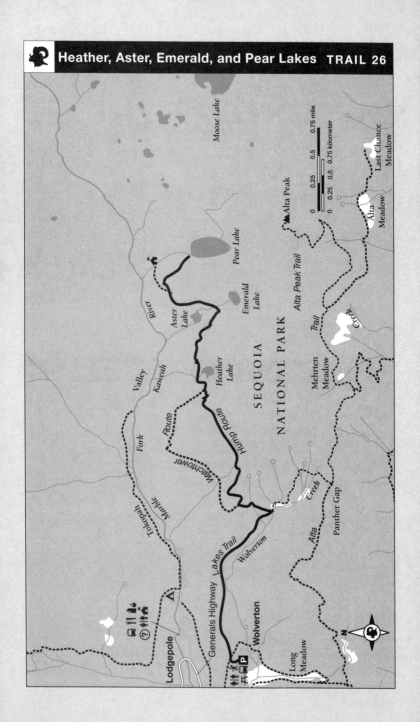

Moose Lake

Pear Lake

Aster Lake

River

Emerald Lake

Alta Peak

0   0.25   0.5   0.75 mile

0   0.25   0.5   0.75 kilometer

Last Chance Meadow

Alta Meadow

Heather Lake

Alta Peak Trail

Valley

Kaweah

SEQUOIA   NATIONAL PARK

Mehrten Meadow

Creek

Fork

Route

Hump Route

Watchtower

Marble

Creek

Panther Gap

Tokopah

Lakes Trail

Wolverton

Alta

Generals Highway

Wolverton

Lodgepole

Long Meadow

N

Heather, Aster, Emerald, and Pear Lakes

The Lakes Trail to Heather, Aster, Emerald, and Pear lakes is one of the busiest trails in Sequoia National Park, thanks to a combination of spectacular scenery and easy access. All four lakes are quite picturesque and provide fine opportunities for sunbathing on granite slabs around the shore or taking a refreshing afternoon dip in the chilly waters. Anglers can try their luck on the resident trout as well. In addition to the lovely lakes, plenty of dramatic vistas can be had along the way, including an incredible view of Tokopah Valley and the tumbling Marble Fork Kaweah River from the Watchtower Route, which follows a narrow ledge across a sheer face dynamited out of the rock some 2,000 feet above the valley floor. An early start should allow hikers in good condition to complete the trip in about 6–7 hours.

Due to the lakes' popularity, the National Park Service has instituted camping bans at Heather and Aster Lakes and limited camping to designated sites near Emerald and Pear Lakes. In addition, visitors are encouraged to use the backcountry pit toilets placed in the vicinity of the lakes. With a basecamp at Pear Lake, the open granite terrain to the east is well suited for cross-country travel to Moose Lake and the Tableland. Equestrians are limited to day-use trips.

Best Time

The Lakes Trail usually sheds its snow by mid-June, with wildflower season beginning in earnest by early July. The trail is busy with day hikers from then

TRAIL USE
Day Hike, Backpack, Horse
LENGTH
11.5 miles, 6–7 hours
VERTICAL FEET
+2800/-550/±6700
DIFFICULTY
– 1 2 3 **4** 5 +
TRAIL TYPE
Out-and-back

FEATURES
Mountain
Lake
Wildflowers
Great Views
Camping
Swimming
Fishing

FACILITIES
Restrooms
Water
Bear Boxes

179

Emerald Lake, backdropped by steep cliffs on three sides, is picturesquely set below Alta Peak.

through Labor Day weekend, when backcountry permits are also at a premium. The crowds disperse considerably after Labor Day, making September a fine time for either a day hike or backpack.

Finding the Trail

Public transportation to the Giant Forest Museum is available from Visalia and Three Rivers on the Sequoia Shuttle. The round-trip cost is $15, and reservations are required. Call 877-BUS-HIKE or visit **sequoiashuttle.com.** From the vicinity of the Giant Forest Museum, passengers can ride the free In-park Shuttle on Orange Route 4 to the parking lot at the end of Wolverton Road.

From Visalia, private vehicles should follow CA 198 to Three Rivers and proceed east into Sequoia National Park, where the road becomes Generals Highway. Follow Generals Highway to Wolverton Road, 1.75 miles southeast of Lodgepole. Head east 1.5 miles on Wolverton Road to the large trailhead parking area. Lodgepole is the nearest campground (fee, flush toilets, running water, bear boxes, and phone). Wuksachi Village, a short distance north of Lodgepole, offers upscale lodging and dining.

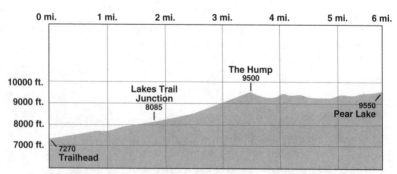

TRAIL 26 Heather, Aster, Emerald, and Pear Lakes Elevation Profile

Cross-Country Options

OPTIONS

Even though the maintained trail ends at Pear Lake, experienced cross-country enthusiasts can venture farther afield on off-trail excursions to remote Moose Lake and the Tableland.

Logistics

Backpackers must obtain a wilderness permit for all overnight visits. See page 114 for more details about how to obtain one. Camping is not allowed at Heather and Aster Lakes and is limited to designated sites at Emerald and Pear Lakes. No campfires.

Trail Description

►1 A barrage of trail signs with numerous destinations and mileages marks the start of the trail. Follow a series of concrete steps shortly to a wide, singletrack dirt trail that ascends a hillside to a junction at the crest with a path accessing the Lodgepole area and the old Wolverton corrals. ►2 Turn right and follow the Lakes Trail, soon passing another junction with a trail on the right to Long Meadow. ►3 After the initial ascent, the grade eases to more of a mild to moderate climb along the course of Wolverton Creek. Hop across a spring-fed tributary of the creek and proceed to a junction with the trail to Panther Gap. ►4

Remaining on the Lakes Trail, turn left at the junction, weave up a hillside, and then drop briefly to the crossing of a flower- and fern-lined tributary of Wolverton Creek. A moderate climb ensues on the way to a junction ►5 between the Watchtower Route on the left and the Hump Route on the right.

Turn right and follow switchbacks on a moderate to moderately steep climb through red-fir forest, crossing a tiny stream lined with pockets of

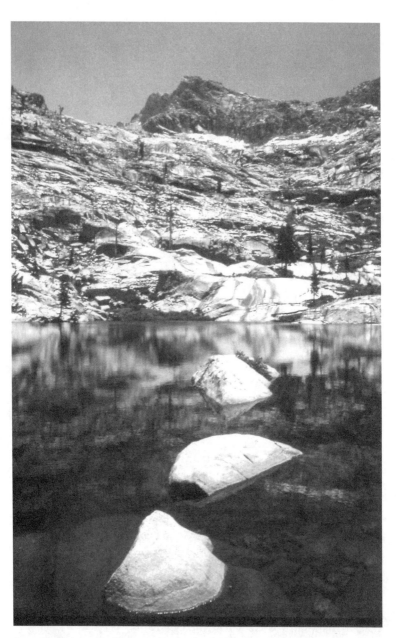

Emerald Lake

flower-dotted meadow along the way. At the apex of the climb, you gain the crest of the Hump, ▶6 where a splendid vista of the Tableland and Silliman Crest can be had by stepping off the trail toward an open stretch of hillside beyond scattered conifers.

 Wildflowers

A steep descent leads down to a small flat, carpeted with pockets of heather and dotted with a smattering of lodgepole pines, where the two routes merge at a signed junction. ▶7 From the junction, a brief, mild descent offers a glimpse of Heather Lake below, near where a lateral leads shortly to a pit toilet; the facility is screened on three sides, which allows for a splendid view. Just beyond the lateral, you reach the heather-laced shore of aptly named Heather Lake, ▶8 where a few pines formerly sheltered a number of campsites around the cliff-rimmed shoreline, but the area has been closed to camping for several years due to overuse.

 Lake

Proceed on rocky tread around boulders and scattered pines on a climb out of the Heather Lake basin. Once out of the basin, the trail leads across open granite terrain on a gentler grade, with fine views across the canyon of Marble Fork Kaweah River and up to Alta Peak. Wrap around a hillside and then drop to the floor of a basin cradling Aster Lake, 0.2 mile downhill to the left, and Emerald Lake, a shorter distance uphill to the right. ▶9 Although camping is banned at Aster Lake, granite slabs around the mostly open shoreline afford fine spots for sunbathing. Anglers can test their skills on the resident rainbow trout. Between the trail and Emerald Lake, designated campsites with bear boxes offer backpackers the first opportunity for legal camping between here and the trailhead. Scattered pines shelter the campsites, and thin strips of verdant meadow border the nearby outlet. Emerald Lake, backdropped by steep cliffs on three sides, is picturesquely set below Alta Peak. Above the far shore, the inlet cascades dramatically down

 Lake

 Fishing

 Camping

Return via the Watchtower

OPTIONS

For a scenic variation on your return to the trailhead, retrace your steps back to the junction ►7 between the Watchtower and the Hump Routes, 0.2 mile west of Heather Lake. Bear right at the junction and follow the Watchtower Route on a gentle descent. Soon the trail starts clinging to the side of a near-vertical cliff that plunges 2,000 feet straight down to Tokopah Valley. Not surprisingly, the exposed view down to the churning and careening Marble Fork is quite staggering (severe acrophobes will be best served by avoiding this route altogether and returning to the trailhead via the Hump Route). The thunderous sound of the river reverberates all the way up to the level of the trail. With all of the drama below, don't forget to turn around and experience the vista of the Silliman Crest.

Proceed down the trail on a moderate descent that leads to a wedge of rock protruding into the canyon, shown as Point 8973T on the U.S. Geological Survey 7.5-minute Lodgepole quadrangle. An unofficial scramble route leads bold adventurers to extraordinary views from the top of this feature. Beyond the wedge of rock, switchbacks head down less-precipitous slopes and into light forest cover. Hop over a vigorous creek lined with lush foliage and continue descending moderately to the junction where the Hump and Watchtower Routes come together again. ►5 From there, retrace your steps 2.1 miles to the trailhead. ►1

cliffs before gracefully pouring across granite slabs on the way into the lake. Brook trout will tempt anglers at Emerald Lake. Between the two lakes is a solar toilet.

Great Views

A mildly ascending trail leads away from the Emerald and Aster Lakes basin around a spur ridge and into the Pear Lake basin, where small pockets of wildflowers soften the otherwise rocky terrain. Fine views into the deep cleft of Marble Fork Kaweah River and Tokopah Valley capture your attention as you follow the trail around the spur. Pass a junction with a trail on the left to the Pear Lake ranger station and continue on ascending tread for another half mile to rockbound **Pear Lake**. ►10 Rimmed by craggy ridges and towered over by Alta Peak, the lake is quite scenic, with widely scattered pines and small tufts of grass finding tenuous footholds in the stony basin. Campers will find 12 designated campsites spread around the outlet, with a solar toilet nearby. Anglers can fish for brook trout.

 Camping

🚶	**MILESTONES**

►1	0.0	Start at trailhead
►2	0.1	Turn right (east) at junction
►3	0.15	Straight at junction to Long Meadow
►4	1.8	Turn left (south) at junction to Panther Gap
►5	2.1	Turn right (east) at first Watchtower/Hump junction
►6	3.4	The Hump
►7	3.6	Straight at second Watchtower/Hump junction
►8	3.8	Heather Lake
►9	4.7	Aster and Emerald Lakes
►10	5.75	Pear Lake

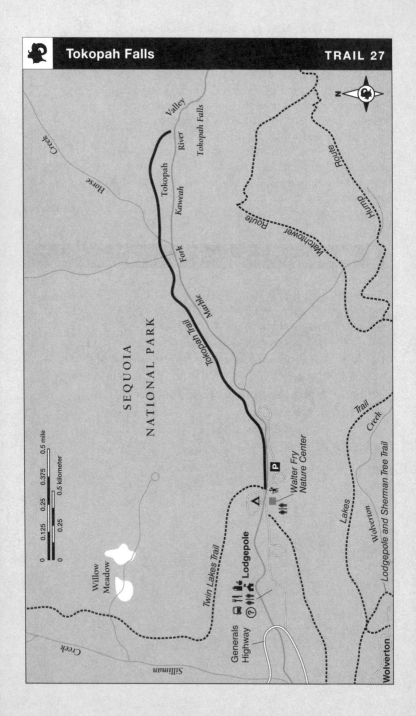

SEQUOIA

NATIONAL PARK

Horse Creek

Tokopah Valley

Tokopah Falls

Kaweah River

Fork

Tokopah

Marble Fork

Tokopah Trail

Hump Route

Watchtower Route

Willow Meadow

Twin Lakes Trail

Lakes Creek Trail

Wolverton

Lodgepole and Sherman Tree Trail

Walter Fry Nature Center

P

Lodgepole

Generals Highway

Silliman Creek

Wolverton

0   0.125   0.25   0.375   0.5 mile

0   0.25   0.5 kilometer

N

Tokopah Falls

An easy 2-mile hike leads to a viewpoint of Tokopah Falls, where the waters from Marble Fork Kaweah River plunge down a steep headwall at the upper end of Tokopah Valley. While the falls are best viewed in late spring, the straightforward hike is also quite pleasant in summer and fall. The nearby amenities at Lodgepole Village offer plenty of extra diversions.

Best Time

Tokopah Valley is usually snow-free from April to November. However, the falls are in full glory when snowmelt in the higher elevations turns Marble Fork Kaweah River into a raging torrent during late spring and early summer.

Finding the Trail

Public transportation to the Giant Forest Museum is available from Visalia and Three Rivers on the Sequoia Shuttle. The round-trip cost is $15, and reservations are required. Call 877-BUS-HIKE or visit **sequoiashuttle.com.** From the vicinity of the Giant Forest Museum, passengers can ride the free In-park Shuttle on Green Route 1 to the Lodgepole area.

From Visalia, private vehicles should follow CA 198 to Three Rivers and proceed east into Sequoia National Park, where the road becomes Generals Highway. Drive on Generals Highway to the Lodgepole junction and turn east. Proceed to the entrance station for Lodgepole Campground (fee, flush toilets, running water, bear boxes, and phone) to secure a free parking permit, and then continue

TRAIL USE
Day Hike, Horse

LENGTH
4.1 miles, 2 hours

VERTICAL FEET
+700/±1400

DIFFICULTY
– 1 **2** 3 4 5 +

TRAIL TYPE
Out-and-back

FEATURES
Canyon
Waterfall
Wildflowers
Great Views

FACILITIES
Store
Visitor Center
Nature Center
Post Office
Campground
Picnic Area
Restrooms
Laundromat
Showers
Phone
Water
Bear Boxes
Shuttle Bus Stop

to the hiker and backpacker parking area. Wuksachi Village, a short distance north of Lodgepole, offers upscale lodging and dining.

Trail Description

▶1 From the parking area, walk along the campground access road past the Walter Fry Nature Center and restrooms to a fork in the road ▶2 and veer left. Cross a log bridge over the Marble Fork and locate the beginning of the **Tokopah Trail** on the far side. ▶3 Head upstream from the trailhead on singletrack trail on a mild climb through a mixed forest of red and white firs, incense cedars, and ponderosa and Jeffrey pines, with the river lined by willows, aspens, and chokecherries. Proceed up the north bank, sometimes right alongside the churning river and sometimes a fair distance away. Low granite outcrops and small pockets of grassy meadow sprinkled with early-season wildflowers break up the otherwise continuous band of trees. Several short bridges span seasonal swales on the way up Tokopah Valley.

Depending on the time of year, you may hear Tokopah Falls well before you actually see the sometimes-mighty cascade. Early in the year the roar of the falls can be quite deafening, as a

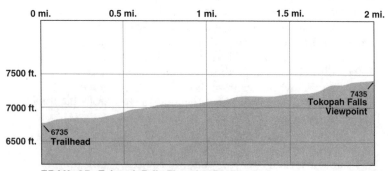

TRAIL 27 Tokopah Falls Elevation Profile

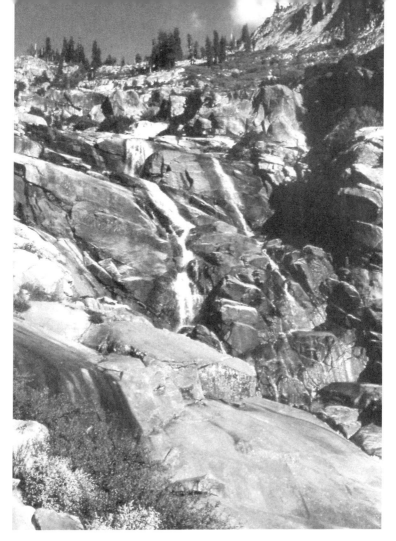

Tokopah Falls *in early summer*

snowmelt-filled torrent catapults over the lip of the canyon headwall. Eventually, the forest gives way to shrubs of elderberry, oak, and manzanita growing between piles of boulders and large blocks of granite, finally allowing views of the falls and the steep-walled canyon. Across the canyon looms the mighty wall of rock known as the Watchtower, which soars 2,000 feet above the valley floor.

 Canyon

The trail continues ascending through a sea of boulders and slabs, increasing in grade on the approach to the base of the falls. The trail abruptly terminates ►4 at a boulder-rimmed bench near the base of some steep cliffs, where a sign advises against the idea of attempting further progress up the canyon onto slippery and unstable slopes (some fatalities have occurred here over the years). Ahead, **Waterfall** silvery Tokopah Falls creates a majestic scene, plummeting down the steep headwall of the upper canyon. Once you've fully enjoyed the falls, retrace your steps to the trailhead.

🚶 MILESTONES

►1	0.0	Start at parking area
►2	0.1	Veer left at fork in the road
►3	0.15	Start of Tokopah Trail
►4	2.05	End of trail

Twin Lakes

This fine day or overnight hike passes through mixed forest, around flower-laden meadows, and over gurgling streams to a pair of scenic and popular lakes. Although dubbed Twin Lakes, these two bodies of water share little in common, other than their proximity to one another. Nonetheless, they are both quite attractive and provide fine places to pitch a tent for a night or two. Wilderness permits are often at a premium for campsites at the lakes, so you may need to make this a day hike. The first mile or so is in full sun, so an early start is best before temperatures start to climb. For those who don't wish to go the full distance to Twin Lakes, the 2.6-mile one-way journey to Cahoon Meadow should be a satisfying alternative.

Best Time

Snow-free hiking to the lakes usually begins in early July following an average winter. Wildflowers typically grace the meadows through midsummer. The hiking season ends after the first snowfall, generally by late October.

Finding the Trail

Public transportation to the Giant Forest Museum is available from Visalia and Three Rivers on the Sequoia Shuttle. The round-trip cost is $15, and reservations are required. Call 877-BUS-HIKE or visit **sequoiashuttle.com.** From the vicinity of the Giant Forest Museum, passengers can ride the free In-park Shuttle on Green Route 1 to the Lodgepole area.

TRAIL USE
Day Hike, Backpack, Horse

LENGTH
13.0 miles, 5–7 hours

VERTICAL FEET
+3030/-285/±6630

DIFFICULTY
– 1 2 3 **4** 5 +

TRAIL TYPE
Out-and-back

FEATURES
Lake
Wildflowers
Camping
Swimming
Fishing

FACILITIES
Store
Visitor Center
Nature Center
Post Office
Campground
Picnic Area
Restrooms
Laundromat
Showers
Phone
Water
Bear Boxes
Shuttle Bus Stop

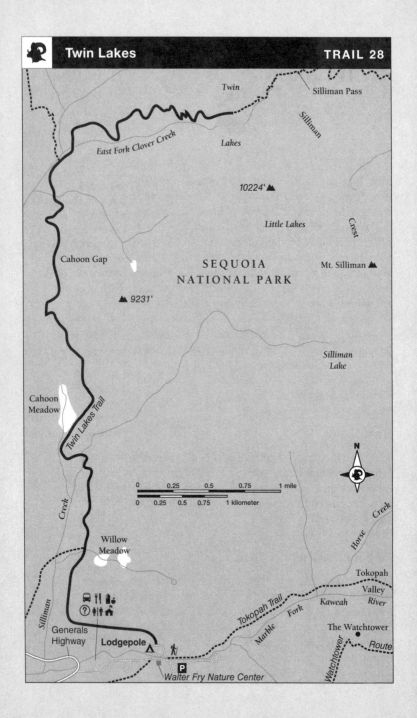

Twin

Silliman Pass

Silliman

East Fork Clover Creek

Lakes

10224' ▲▲

Little Lakes

Crest

Cahoon Gap

SEQUOIA
NATIONAL PARK

Mt. Silliman ▲▲

▲ 9231'

Silliman
Lake

Cahoon
Meadow

Twin Lakes Trail

N

0   0.25   0.5   0.75   1 mile

0   0.25   0.5   0.75   1 kilometer

Creek

Willow
Meadow

Horse
Creek

Tokopah

Valley

Tokopah Trail

Marble

Fork

Kaweah

River

The Watchtower
•

Silliman

Generals
Highway

Lodgepole

Watchtower

Route

Walter Fry Nature Center

From Visalia, private vehicles should follow CA 198 to Three Rivers and proceed east into Sequoia National Park, where the road becomes Generals Highway. Drive on Generals Highway to the Lodgepole junction and turn east. Proceed to the entrance station for Lodgepole Campground (fee, flush toilets, running water, bear boxes, and phone) to secure a free parking permit, and then continue to the hiker and backpacker parking area. Wuksachi Village, a short distance north of Lodgepole, offers upscale dining and lodging.

Logistics

Backpackers must obtain a wilderness permit for all overnight visits. See page 114 for more details about how to obtain one. No campfires.

Trail Description

▶1 From the trailhead, pass through Lodgepole Campground on a nearly level, rock-lined trail amid mixed forest. Soon, the grade increases as the trail attacks the open hillside above the campground. After about a mile, you proceed through dense red-fir and lodgepole-pine forest, as the trail veers north into the Silliman Creek drainage. Hop across a tiny,

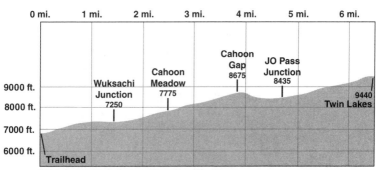

TRAIL 28 Twin Lakes Elevation Profile

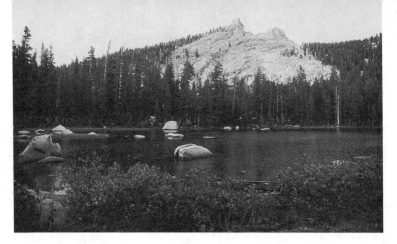

The larger Twin Lake

spring-fed brook to a T-junction with the Wuksachi Trail at 1.5 miles, which is a lateral used primarily by guests staying at Wuksachi Village. ▶2

Cross a usually dry, rock-filled wash, the former bed of Silliman Creek, which these days flows just over a low ridge on the left. A moderate climb on rocky switchbacks leads to the crossing of the main branch of Silliman Creek (possibly a difficult ford in early season), 0.75 mile from the Wuksachi junction. Because the creek is the domestic water supply for Lodgepole, camping, swimming, fishing, and picnicking are not allowed.

Head away from the creek, climb around the nose of a south-facing spur, and then head northeast to Cahoon Meadow, 2.6 miles from the trailhead. ▶3 This pleasant glade, a favorite haunt of the resident deer population, is carpeted with tall

Wildflowers

Camping

grasses and sprinkled with colorful wildflowers. A few campsites may be found beneath tall firs along the fringe of the meadow. This delightful parkland makes a good turnaround point for day hikers or backpackers who wish not to go all the way to Twin Lakes.

The stiff climb continues to a lushly lined, spring-fed stream, where lupines, tiger lilies, monkeyflowers, and asters add splashes of color to the verdant plants bordering the stream. From there, ascend to a clearing with fine views across Cahoon Meadow and then continue climbing, jumping across several tiny rivulets adorned with colorful swaths of wildflowers. The uppermost brook drains a good-size, sloping meadow you pass on the way to viewless Cahoon Gap, 4 miles from the trailhead. ▶4

 Wildflowers

A mild to moderate, half-mile-plus descent from Cahoon Gap leads alongside East Fork Clover Creek to a usually easy boulder hop of a tributary stream, with campsites with bear boxes on the far bank. Proceed upstream under the cover of fir forest to a junction with a trail to JO Pass, 4.9 miles from the trailhead, where a few fir-sheltered campsites may tempt overnighters. ▶5

 Camping

Veer right at the junction and continue a mild to moderate ascent along East Fork Clover Creek to a ford, where shooting stars, leopard lilies, and asters line the banks. Beyond the creek, the grade increases on the way up a hillside through stands of conifers alternating with small clearings. Farther on, wildflowers, including leopard lilies, shooting stars, asters, lupines, corn lilies, larkspurs, cinquefoils, wallflowers, golden senecios, and Mariposa lilies blanket an expansive slope. Beyond a series of switchbacks, the grade eventually eases. You pass an informational sign and soon get a glimpse of the larger Twin Lake through the trees. A very short, easy stroll leads to the shoreline. ▶6

 Wildflowers

The southern lake is obviously the larger of the two, bearing little resemblance to its smaller neighbor. While the smaller lake is entirely ringed by dense lodgepole and red-fir forest, the south shore of the larger lake has an open slope of talus beneath cliffs rising 600 feet above the water. The rugged towers of Twin Peaks are visible from spots along the shoreline of the larger lake as well. Backpackers will find heavily used campsites (bear boxes) beneath a strip of forest between the two lakes and

Fishing

Swimming

less-used sites scattered around both shorelines. A pit toilet is located west of the smaller lake. Anglers can ply the waters for brook trout. Swimmers will find the shallow lakes to be quite refreshing on hot afternoons.

MILESTONES

►1	0.0	Start at Twin Lakes Trailhead
►2	1.5	Straight at Wuksachi Trail junction
►3	2.6	Cahoon Meadow
►4	4.0	Cahoon Gap
►5	4.9	Right at JO Pass junction
►6	6.5	Twin Lakes

Little Baldy

An excellent vista gained by a less than 2-mile hike should tempt just about any self-respecting hiker. A moderate climb of 700-plus feet leads to arguably one of the western Sierra's supreme views from the top of Little Baldy, a vista so expansive that the National Park Service used to maintain a fire lookout there. Reach the trailhead with plenty of water because none is readily available en route or anywhere nearby. Despite the lack of water, a few parties each year spend a night on the summit, undoubtedly drawn by the incomparable sunsets and excellent stargazing.

Best Time

The absolute best time to enjoy the view from the top of Little Baldy is following a rare cleansing storm, when the rains have washed the ubiquitous haze from the skies above the San Joaquin Valley. Thankfully, the eastward view of the Great Western Divide and other notable features in the park is not as dependent on the air quality above the valley, making a snow-free hike anytime from June to mid-October a rewarding experience.

Finding the Trail

From Visalia, follow CA 198 to Three Rivers and proceed east into Sequoia National Park, where the road becomes Generals Highway. Follow Generals Highway to Little Baldy Saddle, 6.6 miles north of the Lodgepole turnoff (18 miles south of the Y-junction with CA 180). Park your vehicle along

TRAIL USE
Day Hike

LENGTH
3.5 miles, 2 hours

VERTICAL FEET
+750/-75/±1650

DIFFICULTY
– 1 2 **3** 4 5 +

TRAIL TYPE
Out-and-back

FEATURES
Mountain
Summit
Great Views

FACILITIES
None

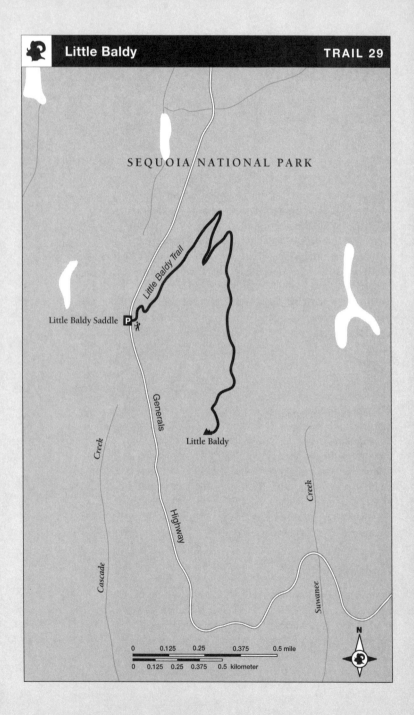

Little Baldy

TRAIL 29

SEQUOIA NATIONAL PARK

Little Baldy Trail

Little Baldy Saddle

Generals

Creek

Highway

Little Baldy

Cascade

Creek

Suwanee

| 0 | 0.125 | 0.25 | 0.375 | 0.5 mile |

| 0 | 0.125 | 0.25 | 0.375 | 0.5 kilometer |

N

the shoulder as space allows. Dorst Campground (fee, flush toilets, running water, bear boxes, and phone) is the nearest campground. Wuksachi Village, a short distance north of Lodgepole, offers upscale lodging and dining. Stony Creek Village and Montecito Lake Resort offer slightly less expensive lodging options.

Trail Description

▶1 From the roadside trail sign, head up the trail on a climb of a hillside covered with red firs and a smattering of Jeffrey pines. Beyond a pair of switchbacks, the trail makes a steady, moderate climb northeast across a steep hillside, roughly paralleling the highway below. Sporadic gaps in the forest allow brief views of Big Baldy to the northwest, while the craggy spires of Chimney Rock can be seen directly ahead. After a trio of switchbacks, the grade eases along the ridge north of Little Baldy, as you proceed toward the summit through pockets of forest, manzanita, and oak. A final short and rocky climb leads to the top and the extraordinary view. ▶2

From the summit, the view encompasses a large part of the Great Western Divide, as well as features closer at hand, such as Castle Rocks and Mineral

 Summit

 Great Views

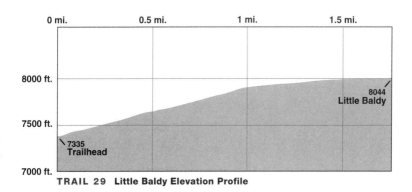

TRAIL 29 Little Baldy Elevation Profile

King valley to the southeast. To the southwest is a rugged and remote section of Sequoia National Park, where a once-prominent network of trails has mostly disappeared over the years, lost to encroaching vegetation from a combination of lack of use and no trail maintenance.

 MILESTONES

▶1   0.0   Start at trailhead
▶2   1.75 Little Baldy summit

Muir Grove

Off the beaten path and tucked away from hordes of tourists who frequent the more popular groves of giant sequoias, Muir Grove is a rare gem. The nearly 1-mile drive from the Generals Highway, when combined with the 2-mile hike to the grove, seems enough of a deterrent to keep the crowds at bay and allows hikers the opportunity to stand among the Big Trees with a strong possibility for peace and serenity. John Muir should be pleased to have his name attached to this quiet grove of stately trees.

TRAIL USE
Day Hike
LENGTH
4.2 miles, 2 hours
VERTICAL FEET
+535/-515/±2100
DIFFICULTY
– 1 2 **3** 4 5 +
TRAIL TYPE
Out-and-back

FEATURES
Fall Colors
Giant Sequoias
Great Views
Secluded

FACILITIES
Campground
Restrooms

Best Time

Since the trailhead is located nearly a mile inside Dorst Campground, the best time to hike this trail is between Memorial Day and Labor Day weekends, when the campground is open. The dogwood flowers are usually showy in late spring, followed by the wildflower bloom in early summer. If you don't mind adding an extra 1.8 miles round-trip to walk the road, autumn can be a fine time for this hike, when the campground is closed. Virtually no one is on the trail, and the dogwood leaves are ablaze with color—a fine complement to the red bark of the sequoias.

Finding the Trail

From Visalia, follow CA 198 to Three Rivers and proceed east into Sequoia National Park, where the road becomes Generals Highway. Drive on Generals Highway to the entrance into Dorst Campground (fee, flush toilets, running water, bear boxes, and

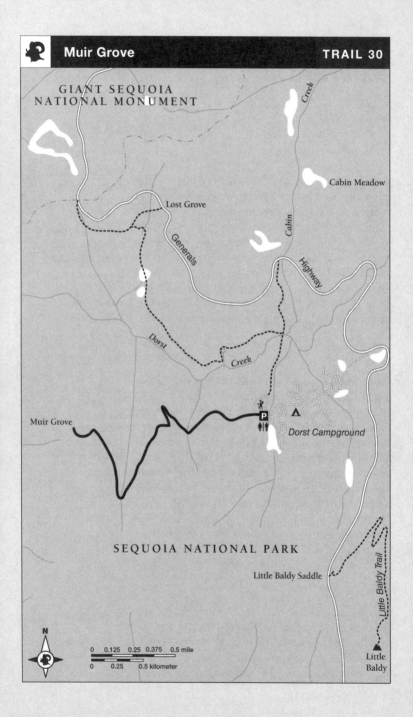

GIANT SEQUOIA
NATIONAL MONUMENT

Creek

Cabin Meadow

Lost Grove

Generals

Cabin

Highway

Dorst

Creek

Muir Grove

P

Dorst Campground

SEQUOIA NATIONAL PARK

Little Baldy Saddle

Little Baldy Trail

N

| 0 | 0.125 | 0.25 | 0.375 | 0.5 mile |

| 0 | 0.25 | 0.5 kilometer |

Little
Baldy

phone), 8 miles northwest of the Lodgepole turnoff (16.4 miles southeast of the Y-junction with CA 180). Proceed on the main access road through the campground 0.9 mile to the signed trailhead, and then continue to the parking lot near the campground amphitheater. Wuksachi Village, a short distance north of Lodgepole, offers upscale lodging and dining. Stony Creek Village and Montecito Lake Resort are slightly less expensive lodging options.

Trail Description

▶1 Begin the hike by walking back down the road from the parking lot to the start of the trail near a small metal sign marked MUIR GROVE TRAIL. Immediately cross a log bridge over a delightful tributary of Dorst Creek, and then make a mild descent through mixed forest to a junction. ▶2

Turn sharply left at the junction and traverse a hillside well above the main channel of the creek to the crossing of another tributary. A moderate ascent follows, aided by a couple of switchbacks, leading to the crest of a ridge and an exposed granite hump, where the trees part enough to allow a fine view of Chimney Rock, Big Baldy, and the densely forested drainages of Stony and Dorst Creeks. The confluence of these two streams,

Off the beaten path and tucked away from hordes of tourists who frequent the more popular groves of giant sequoias, Muir Grove is a rare gem.

 Great Views

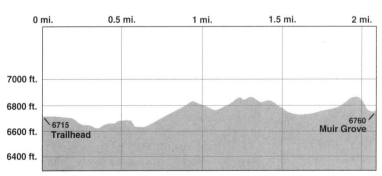

TRAIL 30 Muir Grove Elevation Profile

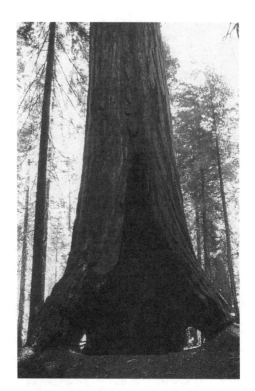

Cave Tree *in Muir Grove*

within rugged and virtually inaccessible terrain, is the birthplace of the North Fork Kaweah River. Careful observation from this vantage across the canyon will reveal the crowns of giant sequoias extending above the lesser conifers.

Leaving the granite hump behind, you proceed in and out of a mixed forest of firs, pines, and cedars on a mildly undulating traverse to the crossing of a flower-lined tributary of Dorst Creek. From there, the mildly ascending trail leads to the top of a ridge, passing azaleas and dogwoods—which provide striking colors in fall—along the way. Just beyond, you reach the first of the sequoias—a pair of burned remnants and a massive giant just off the trail. A short distance farther is perhaps the highlight of

Fall Colors

Muir Grove, ▶3 a circle of a dozen or more giant sequoias arranged in a nearly symmetrical pattern. Standing among this ring of Goliaths stirs a feeling of reverential awe fitting for such a grand cathedral. Short, faint paths lead away from this magical spot to additional sequoias scattered about, but the old trail that once continued on to Skagway Grove, Hidden Spring, and North Fork Kaweah River is overgrown and very hard, if not impossible, to follow.

 Giant Sequoias

🚶	**MILESTONES**

▶1   0.0   Start at trailhead
▶2   0.2   Turn left at junction
▶3   2.1   Muir Grove

CHAPTER 4

Grant Grove and Redwood Mountain

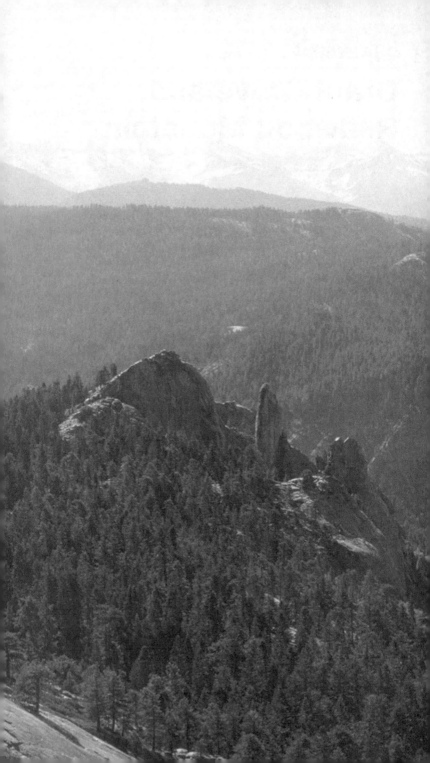

Grant Grove and Redwood Mountain

G rant Grove received federal protection in 1890, when four sections of land were set aside as General Grant National Park, in the same bill that created Yosemite and Sequoia National Parks. The remaining area we know of today as Kings Canyon National Park, including the Redwood Mountain area, was a late arrival into the national park system in 1940. The General Grant Tree, second in size only to General Sherman in Sequoia, has always been the principal attraction in Grant Grove. Although there are no backpacking trails in Grant Grove, numerous day-hiking opportunities exist on a fine network of trails. Not only do the trails lead to numerous sequoia landmarks, but to meadows, waterfalls, streams, and vistas as well. Three campgrounds (Azalea, Crystal Springs, and Sunset); Grant Grove Cabins; and John Muir Lodge offer fine options for base camps for those who wish to explore the area for more than one day.

A stop at Grant Grove Market is accessible via public transportation from stops of the Fresno/Sanger Route in Fresno at the Amtrak railroad station, Greyhound bus station, and Fresno Yosemite International Airport. The shuttle also can be caught at city hall in Sanger and at Squaw Valley/ Clingan's Junction. A round-trip ticket is $15 and includes the park entrance fee. Reservations are necessary and can be made at **sequoiashuttle. com** or by calling 800-325-RIDE (7433).

Redwood Mountain holds the distinction of harboring the largest intact sequoia grove on the planet. In spite of this notoriety, the area receives fewer tourists than one might imagine, thanks in part perhaps to a lack of signs pointing the way and access via a narrow dirt road. Unlike some of the more popular trails in Grant Grove, visitors to Redwood Mountain can experience numerous sequoia monarchs in a quiet and secluded setting. Also unlike Grant Grove, backpackers have the possibility of using campsites along Redwood Creek downstream from the grove.

Overleaf and opposite: *View from the top of Big Baldy*

Near Redwood Mountain and with trailheads next to Generals Highway are two of the park's granite domes, Big Baldy and Buena Vista Peak, both offering short day hikes to excellent viewpoints from their summits. Farther afield, on the border between Kings Canyon National Park and Jennie Lakes Wilderness, is Mitchell Peak, which also commands a spectacular view.

Permits

Permits are not required for day hikes. Backpackers must obtain a wilderness permit for all overnight trips. Between late May and late September, a quota system is in place, with a $15 fee per group. Outside the quota period, permits are free, self-issue, and available 24 hours a day. Advance reservations are available for approximately 75% of the quota, with the remainder set aside for walk-in permits. All permits must be picked up from the Kings Canyon Visitor Center in Grant Grove between 8 a.m. and 4:30 p.m. Applications for advance reservations are accepted only by fax or mail, no earlier than midnight March 1 and no later than two weeks prior to the start of the trip. Visit the park website to download a permit application and to check on quota availability.

Maps

For the Grant Grove and Redwood Mountain area, the U.S. Geological Survey 7.5-minute (1:24,000 scale) topographic maps are listed below, corresponding to the trails described in this section. Sequoia Natural History Association publishes *General Grant Grove,* a handy foldout map for the trails in the Grant Grove area (Redwood Mountain is not included). Trail users also may want to consider using Tom Harrison's map, *Sequoia & Kings Canyon National Parks* (1:125,000).

> Trails 31–39: *General Grant Grove*
>
> Trail 40: *Mt. Silliman*

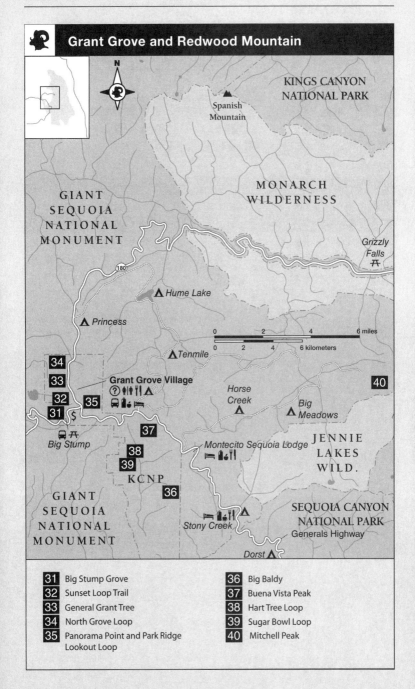

Grant Grove and Redwood Mountain

KINGS CANYON
NATIONAL PARK

Spanish
Mountain

MONARCH
WILDERNESS

GIANT
SEQUOIA
NATIONAL
MONUMENT

Grizzly
Falls

180

Hume Lake

Princess

Tenmile

Grant Grove Village

Horse
Creek

Big
Meadows

40

34
33
32
35
31 $

Big Stump

37

JENNIE
LAKES
WILD.

Montecito Sequoia Lodge

38
39
KCNP

36

GIANT
SEQUOIA
NATIONAL
MONUMENT

SEQUOIA CANYON
NATIONAL PARK
Generals Highway

Stony Creek

Dorst

| 0 | 2 | 4 | 6 miles |
| 0 | 2 | 4 | 6 kilometers |

31	Big Stump Grove		36	Big Baldy
32	Sunset Loop Trail		37	Buena Vista Peak
33	General Grant Tree		38	Hart Tree Loop
34	North Grove Loop		39	Sugar Bowl Loop
35	Panorama Point and Park Ridge Lookout Loop		40	Mitchell Peak

Grant Grove and Redwood Mountain

TRAIL	DIFFICULTY	LENGTH	TYPE	USES & ACCESS	TERRAIN	FLORA & FAUNA	OTHER
31	1	2.0	↺	🚶👫		🍁❋🌲	⌂
32	3	6.4	↺	🏃	⤵🏔	❋🌲	⋒
33	1	0.5	↺	🚶♿👫		🌲	
34	2	1.5	↺	🚶🏃		🌲	⬇
35	3	5.6	↺	🚶🏃			⋒
36	3	4.4	↗	🚶🏃	🏔		⋒
37	2	2.0	↗	🚶🏃	🏔		⋒
38	3	7.25	↺	🚶🐎🏃		🍁❋🌲	⋒△⬇
39	3	6.6	↺	🚶🐎🏃		🍁❋🌲	⋒△⬇
40	4	6.6	↗	🚶🏃	⛰△	❋	⋒⬇

USES & ACCESS	TYPE	TERRAIN	FLORA & FAUNA	OTHER
🚶 Day Hiking	↺ Loop	🟦 Canyon	🍁 Fall Colors	⋒ Great Views
🎒 Backpacking	↗ Out-and-back	🔺 Mountain	❋ Wildflowers	△ Camping
🏃 Running	↘ Point-to-point	△ Summit	🌲 Giant Sequoias	➟ Swimming
🐎 Horses		🌊 Lake		⬇ Secluded
🐕 Dogs Allowed	DIFFICULTY - 1 2 3 4 5 + less more	⤵ Stream		⬇ Steep
👫 Child Friendly		▮▮ Waterfall		🎣 Fishing
♿ Wheelchair-Access				⌂ Historical Interest

Grant Grove and Redwood Mountain

Big Stump Grove 215
This 2-mile loop is a walk through man's early history in the sequoia groves, where nearly every tree in this grove was sacrificed.

TRAIL 31

Day Hike, Child Friendly
2.0 miles, Loop
Difficulty: **1** 2 3 4 5

Sunset Loop Trail 221
This loop through part of Grant Grove combines the characteristic big trees with Viola and Ella Falls and a splendid vista from Sequoia Lake Overlook.

TRAIL 32

Day Hike, Run
6.4 miles, Loop
Difficulty: 1 2 **3** 4 5

General Grant Tree 229
General Grant Tree is the second-largest giant sequoia in the world and the most-visited feature in Kings Canyon National Park. A short, paved nature trail leads to an unobstructed view of this majestic monarch and loops past several other noteworthy trees.

TRAIL 33

Day Hike, Child Friendly,
Handicapped Access
0.5 mile, Loop
Difficulty: **1** 2 3 4 5

North Grove Loop 233
A reasonably short trail leads hikers away from the usual hubbub surrounding the General Grant Tree down into a secluded grove of giant sequoias.

TRAIL 34

Day Hike, Run
1.5 miles, Loop
Difficulty: 1 **2** 3 4 5

**Panoramic Point and
Park Ridge Lookout** 237
Gently graded segments of singletrack trail and fire road lead hikers from one fantastic vista at Panoramic Point to another one at Park Ridge Lookout. Still operational, Park Ridge is one of the few remaining fire lookouts from a former network that once spanned the length and breadth of the Sierra.

TRAIL 35

Day Hike, Run
5.6 miles, Loop
Difficulty: 1 2 **3** 4 5

TRAIL 36

Day Hike, Run
4.4 miles, Out-and-back
Difficulty: 1 2 **3** 4 5

Big Baldy 242

A short climb to the top of a granite dome leads to fine views of the Kings-Kaweah and Great Western Divides, as well as the surrounding terrain.

TRAIL 37

Day Hike, Run
2.0 miles, Out-and-back
Difficulty: 1 **2** 3 4 5

Buena Vista Peak 247

This short hike leads to the top of Buena Vista Peak and a fine view of the western part of Kings Canyon National Park.

TRAIL 38

Day Hike, Backpack, Run
7.25 miles, Loop
Difficulty: 1 2 **3** 4 5

Hart Tree Loop 251

A visit to the largest intact grove of giant sequoias in the world on a relatively lightly used trail will delight even the most discriminating hiker.

TRAIL 39

Day Hike, Backpack, Run
6.6 miles, Loop
Difficulty: 1 2 **3** 4 5

Sugar Bowl Loop. 257

Hikers and backpackers alike will find plenty of interesting sequoia terrain on the western loop through the Redwood Mountain Grove.

TRAIL 40

Day Hike, Run
6.6 miles, Out-and-back
Difficulty: 1 2 3 **4** 5

Mitchell Peak. 262

Straddling the border between Kings Canyon National Park and Jennie Lakes Wilderness, the trail to Mitchell Peak offers one of the most lightly used routes to one of the finest viewpoints on the west side of the range.

Big Stump Grove

Experience a bit of history on this 2-mile loop, which provides a glimpse into the misguided ethic of the bygone era of the late 1800s, when resources in the western forests seemed inexhaustible. Loggers and timber companies were drawn to the immense trees in the sequoia groves with the lure of jobs and big-time profits. Although the wood from the sequoias would eventually prove to be too brittle for most commercial applications, nearly every tree in the Big Stump Grove was sacrificed. Modern-day visitors will bear witness to the results: Countless giant stumps are a vivid reminder of an era's shortsightedness. Unfortunately, what would have been one of the region's most impressive giant sequoia groves is instead a graveyard of fallen monarchs.

Best Time

Trails in this area are usually free of snow from late May until the first major snowfall in autumn, usually by November. Wildflowers reach the peak of bloom in late spring and early summer; watch for the crescendo of autumn color in mid- to late October.

Finding the Trail

Public transportation to Grant Grove Market is available from stops in Fresno, Sanger, and Squaw Valley/Clingan's Junction on the Fresno/Sanger Shuttle. The round-trip cost is $15, and reservations are required. Call 800-325-RIDE (7433). From the vicinity of the Grant Grove Market, passengers can

TRAIL USE
Day Hike, Child Friendly
LENGTH
2.0 miles, 1 hour
VERTICAL FEET
+300/-300/±600
DIFFICULTY
– **1** 2 3 4 5 +
TRAIL TYPE
Loop

FEATURES
Fall Colors
Wildflowers
Giant Sequoias
Historical Interest

FACILITIES
Restrooms
Picnic Tables
Shuttle Bus Stop

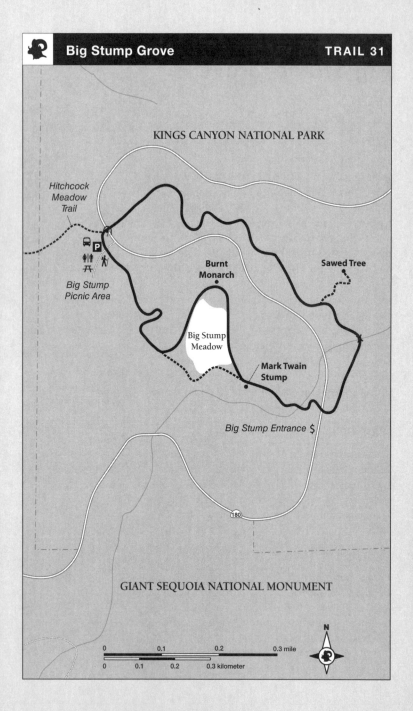

Big Stump Grove

TRAIL 31

KINGS CANYON NATIONAL PARK

Hitchcock Meadow Trail

Big Stump Picnic Area

Burnt Monarch

Sawed Tree

Big Stump Meadow

Mark Twain Stump

Big Stump Entrance $

180

GIANT SEQUOIA NATIONAL MONUMENT

N

| 0 | 0.1 | 0.2 | 0.3 mile |

| 0 | 0.1 | 0.2 | 0.3 kilometer |

ride the park's free Big Tree Shuttle to the Big Stump Picnic Area and Trailhead.

Private vehicles should follow CA 180 east from Fresno to the Big Stump Picnic Area a short way past the Big Stump Entrance.

Trail Description

▶1 Find the start of the trail near the restroom building on the south side of the parking area and head downhill on a wide, well-graded path through pockets of manzanita and stands of a mixed forest of incense cedars, Jeffrey pines, sugar pines, and firs. You soon come to the first notable giant sequoia, the Resurrection Tree, a topless sequoia still thriving despite having been struck by lightning. The winding descent continues down to the west junction ▶2 with the loop around Big Stump Meadow, 0.3 mile from the parking lot.

Giant Sequoias

Veer left at the junction on a clockwise circuit around the meadow, site of the long-abandoned Smith Comstock Mill, which occupied the clearing in the late 1800s. A number of large sequoia stumps and piles of redwood sawdust litter the otherwise pristine clearing. Partway around the meadow is the Burnt Monarch, a huge sequoia that succumbed to fire but remains erect. Just beyond are two young

Wildflowers

Historical Interest

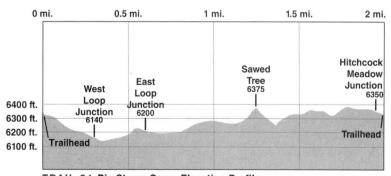

TRAIL 31 Big Stump Grove Elevation Profile

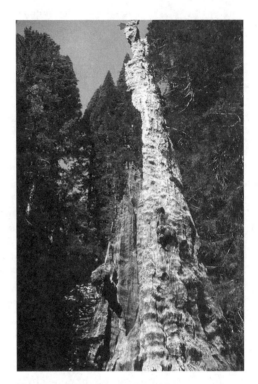

The Burnt Monarch *in Big Stump Grove*

sequoias, planted in 1888 by Jesse Pattee, a lumberjack who lived in a nearby cabin. A cursory glance at this pair of sequoias reveals their limited stature in comparison to the massive stumps nearby. Just past a short lateral to the Feather Bed is the east junction. ▶3

BEGIN SIDE TRIP: Before continuing the loop, turn right (west) at the junction and walk around the south side of Big Stump Meadow to a small brook and the Shattered Giant. Rather than using the standard practice of the day, loggers dropped this particular sequoia down-slope and watched it fragment into hundreds of useless pieces, which remain in the streambed. After marveling at the results of this mishap, retrace your steps back to the east junction. **END SIDE TRIP**

From the east junction, turn left, head across a short bridge, and soon reach the Mark Twain Stump.

Away from the stump, the trail leads through a narrow swath of meadow to CA 180, a mile from the trailhead. Follow an angling crosswalk over the highway to the resumption of trail on the far side, where a moderate climb ensues through mixed forest. Follow the trail as it roughly parallels the highway to a bridge across a tiny brook and a junction with a short but steep lateral to the Sawed Tree. It's an easy walk worth the side trip. ▶4 Loggers attempted to cut down this massive sequoia but eventually gave up, most likely exhausted from the prolonged labor. Since the bark wasn't completely severed, life-giving nutrients continued to travel up the tree.

From the Sawed Tree lateral, continue climbing, passing by more sequoia stumps on the way. Soon, the grade eases and the trail veers southwest back toward the highway, where a tunnel safely leads hikers to the far side and a junction with the Hitchcock Meadow Trail. ▶5

Turn left at the junction and ascend a hill to the close of the loop at the Big Stump parking lot. ▶6

Mark Twain Stump

HISTORY

Rather than being chopped down for lumber, in 1891 this tree was meticulously disassembled and transported for exhibition at the American Museum of Natural History and the British Museum in London. Thirteen days of chopping, sawing, and wedging were necessary to drop the tree. Today, a set of stairs takes visitors to the top of the stump to gain a better appreciation of the immensity of this giant sequoia.

Feather Beds

Since the brittle sequoias tend to burst into pieces when felled, loggers would dig a trench and line it with boughs to cushion the blow and keep the Big Tree intact. The feather beds of Big Stump Meadow are now overgrown with a tangle of willows and other shrubs, a jumble of vegetation that belies the former purpose.

MILESTONES

►1	0.0	Start at Big Stump Picnic Area Trailhead
►2	0.3	Left at west junction with loop around Big Stump Meadow
►3	0.6	Left at east junction with loop around Big Stump Meadow
►4	1.25	Lateral to Sawed Tree
►5	1.95	Left at Hitchcock Meadow Trail junction
►6	2.0	Big Stump Picnic Area Trailhead

Sunset Loop Trail

Waterfalls, vistas, and big trees are the prime attractions for this trip through a section of Grant Grove, an area with far fewer visitors than around General Grant Tree. Ella and Viola Falls put on a showy display in late spring and early summer, when Sequoia Creek is running high from snowmelt. Added treats include an overlook offering a grand view of Sequoia Lake and, of course, the opportunity to see some notable giant sequoias.

Best Time

Hikers will usually find the trails in Grant Grove to be free of snow from late May to mid-October.

Finding the Trail

Public transportation to Grant Grove Market is available from stops in Fresno, Sanger, and Squaw Valley/Clingan's Junction on the Fresno/Sanger Shuttle. The round-trip cost is $15, and reservations are required. Call 800-325-RIDE (7433). From the vicinity of the Grant Grove Market, simply walk a short distance to the Kings Canyon Visitor Center.

Private vehicles should follow CA 180 east from Fresno into Kings Canyon National Park and continue to Grant Grove Village. Park your vehicle in the visitor center parking lot. Grant Grove has three campgrounds—Azalea, Crystal Springs, and Sunset (fee, flush toilets, and bear boxes). John Muir Lodge and Grant Grove Cabins offer accommodations, and the village has a restaurant, general store, gift shop, and showers.

TRAIL USE
Day Hike, Run

LENGTH
6.4 miles, 3 hours

VERTICAL FEET
+1885/-1885/±3770

DIFFICULTY
– 1 2 **3** 4 5 +

TRAIL TYPE
Loop

FEATURES
Streams
Waterfalls
Wildflowers
Giant Sequoias
Great Views

FACILITIES
Lodging
Store
Café
Visitor Center
Post Office
Restrooms
Water
Picnic Area
Campgrounds
Stables
Shuttle Bus Stop

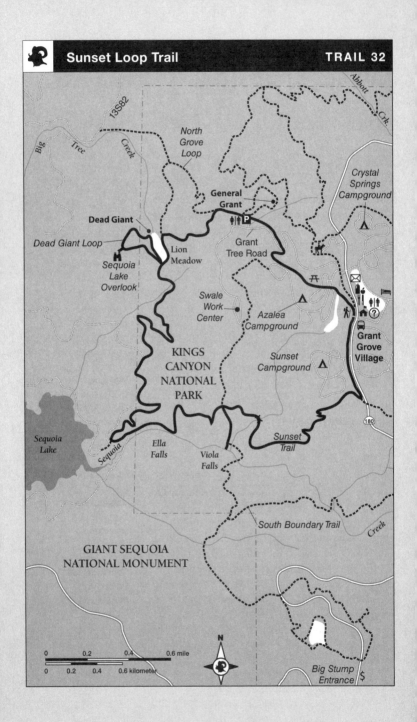

Big Tree Creek

13S82

North Grove Loop

Abbott Crk.

Crystal Springs Campground

General Grant

Dead Giant

Dead Giant Loop

Lion Meadow

Grant Tree Road

Sequoia Lake Overlook

Swale Work Center

Azalea Campground

Grant Grove Village

KINGS CANYON NATIONAL PARK

Sunset Campground

Sequoia Lake

Sequoia

Ella Falls

Viola Falls

Sunset Trail

180

South Boundary Trail

Creek

GIANT SEQUOIA NATIONAL MONUMENT

0   0.2   0.4   0.6 mile

0   0.2   0.4   0.6 kilometer

N

Big Stump Entrance

Trail Description

▶1 To locate the start of the Sunset and Azalea Trails, follow the crosswalk directly opposite the visitor center across CA 180 to the west side of the road and a trail sign. A very short path leads downhill from there to a marked junction, ▶2 where you turn left to follow a trail that parallels the highway toward Sunset Campground. Soon cross the campground access road and proceed to a T-junction between the Azalea and Sunset Trails. ▶3

Turn right and follow the Sunset Trail over a low hill, and then make a short descent on indistinct tread to the bottom of a swale. After a very brief climb away from the swale, break out into a small clearing, where the trail is lined with manzanita. From the clearing, the route of the trail becomes more obvious again, as you begin a steady descent that lasts until the park boundary near Sequoia Lake. Weave down the hillside over slabs and around boulders through a light, mixed forest to a bridge over a tributary of Sequoia Creek, and then continue to a signed, four-way junction with an old road from the Swale Work Center. ▶4

Turn left (south) at the junction and follow the old road on a mild descent through moderate forest for 0.2 mile to where the road bends east. A small

> While Viola Falls may seem a bit tame, Ella presents the sights and sounds one expects from a significant waterfall.

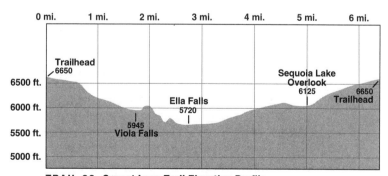

TRAIL 32 Sunset Loop Trail Elevation Profile

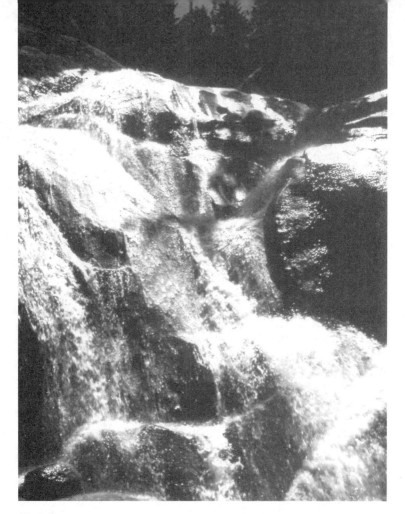

Ella Falls

sign marked VIOLA FALLS directs foot traffic straight ahead onto singletrack trail that soon leads alongside Sequoia Creek. The narrow and somewhat faint path ends at the base of a hill, from where you can work your way to an overlook directly above Viola Falls.

Waterfall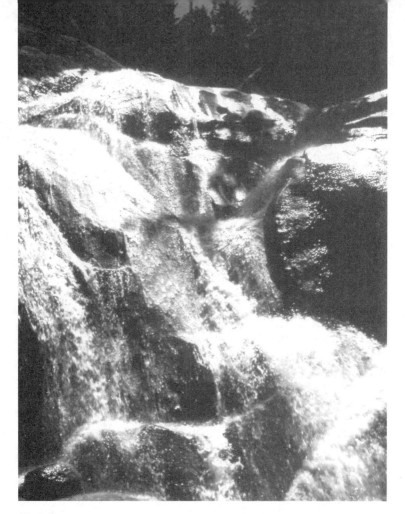

▶5 Don't expect the scenic drama of a Yosemite-type waterfall; Viola Falls is more like a series of cataracts pouring swiftly down a narrow channel into the swirling pools of basins that have been scoured out of solid rock. Early-season wildflowers add a lovely touch of color to the stream banks.

 Wildflowers

Retrace your steps back to the four-way junction ▶6 and turn left toward Ella Falls. A steady descent through light to moderate forest leads to a series of switchbacks that take you across a seasonal stream, over a seep, and down to Ella Falls. ▶7 While Viola Falls may seem a bit tame, Ella presents the sights and sounds one expects from a significant waterfall. In spring and early summer, Sequoia Creek plunges raucously down a sheer face into a whirling pool before resuming a cacophonous journey toward Sequoia Lake.

 Waterfall

Proceed a quarter mile beyond Ella Falls to a junction ▶8 between the boundary of Kings Canyon National Park and the private property of the YMCA camps around Sequoia Lake. The YMCA has granted permission to pass over their land to hikers who wish to continue ahead a short distance to an overview of the lake. Those who choose to do so should remain on the trail and out of the camps.

Following a sign marked GRANT TREE, angle away from the trail to Sequoia Lake and follow the continuation of the Sunset Trail on a moderately steep climb to an old road ▶9 that used to be the main access into the park via Sequoia Lake. Once at the road, turn right and proceed on broken asphalt on a steady, winding ascent that leads through the partial shade of a mixed forest. Pass by a couple of

HISTORY

Sequoia Lake

Although at first glance the body of water before you appears natural, Sequoia Lake was created in the late 1800s as a millpond to provide water for a flume that carried lumber to a mill in Sanger in the San Joaquin Valley below. Today the lake is home to a number of summer camps.

roads on the left coming from the vicinity of the lake and continue the climb to the top of a hill and a junction with the Dead Giant Loop Trail on the left, ►10 4.75 miles from the trailhead.

Turn left at the junction and follow the upper part of the Dead Giant Loop across a lightly forested hillside above verdant Lion Meadow. Continue a short distance past the far edge of the meadow to the Dead Giant, a very large sequoia that met an untimely demise at the hands of axe-wielding loggers. Careful inspection of the trunk reveals axe marks encircling the trunk that basically sheared off the cambium layer, permanently interrupting the flow of nutrients up the tree. Without such life-giving sustenance, the tree eventually succumbed, providing a visual memorial to modern-day visitors of an age-old truth: Nature's greatest enemy is man himself. Leaving the Dead Giant behind, climb a hillside to the crest of an open ridge, and then follow this spine southwest to an unmarked junction. ►11 Continue straight ahead a short distance to where the ridge begins to fall away, soon arriving at Sequoia Lake Overlook.

After fully enjoying the view, backtrack the short distance to the junction ►11 and, following a sign marked simply TRAIL, proceed eastbound on the return leg of the loop back to the junction with the Sunset Trail. ►12

From the Dead Giant Loop junction, resume the climb along the old roadbed, passing around the edge of Lion Meadow. After 0.25 mile you pass the first junction ►13 of the North Grove Trail and then the second junction ►14 0.25 mile farther. A short distance from the second junction, you reach the edge of a large parking lot for the popular General Grant Tree area. Stroll across the lot to the far side and the resumption of trail near a restroom building and a grove of sequoias known as the Happy Family, passing the General Grant Trailhead along the way.

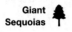
Giant Sequoias

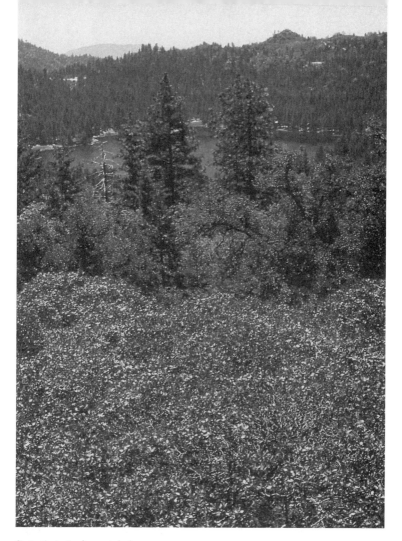

Sequoia Lake *from overlook*

Walk along a split-rail fence just to the left of Big Tree Creek, a delightful rivulet lined with verdant plants. Cross the tiny stream on a wood-plank bridge and pass by the Michigan Tree, a huge, toppled-over giant sequoia that lies in broken sections beside the trail. The fence ends just beyond the tree, but you continue up the trail to a crossing of the Grant Tree road. A short climb through light forest away from the road leads past Columbine Picnic Area and into Azalea Campground. Pass through the campground, negotiating a number of access-road crossings, walk across a plank bridge, and then ascend the hillside to the junction across from the visitor center at the close of your loop. ►15 From there, retrace your steps the short distance to the parking lot. ►16

🚶 MILESTONES

►1	0.0	Start at Grant Grove Visitor Center
►2	0.01	Left at junction
►3	0.3	Right at Azalea-Sunset junction
►4	1.5	Left at junction
►5	1.75	Viola Falls
►6	2.0	Left at junction
►7	2.75	Ella Falls
►8	3.0	Right at junction
►9	3.03	Right at old road
►10	4.75	Left at Dead Giant junction
►11	5.0	Straight ahead at Sequoia Lake Overlook junction
►11	5.05	Veer right at junction
►12	5.4	Left at Sunset Trail junction
►13	5.65	Straight at first North Grove Trail junction
►14	5.9	Straight at second North Grove Trail junction
►15	6.39	Left at junction
►16	6.4	End at Grant Grove Visitor Center

General Grant Tree

With a height of 268 feet and a base diameter of more than 40 feet (as measured in 2002), the General Grant Tree has the distinction of being the second-largest living tree in the world. Additional prestige is attached to the Grant Grove area as being the oldest parcel of land in Kings Canyon National Park, set aside as General Grant National Park in 1890 by the same congressional bill that established Yosemite National Park and greatly enlarged Sequoia National Park. Such notoriety has resulted in making Grant Grove one of the area's most popular tourist attractions and the easy half-mile loop around the namesake tree one of the area's most popular trails. Be sure to pick up a leaflet at the visitor center or the trailhead.

Best Time

While the trail is generally free of snow from mid-May to mid-October, weekends between the Fourth of July and Labor Day see big crowds. Even weekdays can be very busy during that period, with hordes of tourists craning their necks to see the namesake tree. During peak season an early-morning or early-evening visit may alleviate the congestion somewhat.

Finding the Trail

Public transportation to Grant Grove Market is available from stops in Fresno, Sanger, and Squaw Valley/Clingan's Junction on the Fresno/Sanger Shuttle. The round-trip cost is $15, and reservations

TRAIL USE
Day Hike, Child Friendly, Handicapped Access
LENGTH
0.5 mile, ½ hour
VERTICAL FEET
+100/-100/±200
DIFFICULTY
– **1** 2 3 4 5 +
TRAIL TYPE
Loop

FEATURES
Giant Sequoias

FACILITIES
Lodging
Store
Café
Visitor Center
Post Office
Restrooms
Water
Picnic Area
Campgrounds
Stables
Shuttle Bus Stop

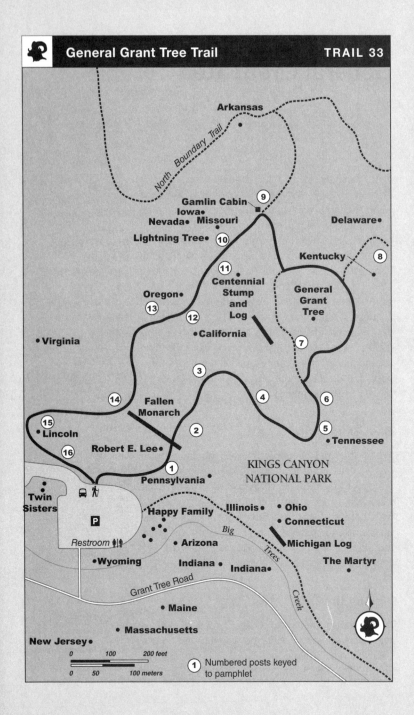

Arkansas

North Boundary Trail

⑨ Gamlin Cabin
Iowa•
Nevada• •Missouri
Lightning Tree• ⑩

Delaware•

Kentucky ⑧

⑪
Centennial
Stump
and
Log

General
Grant
Tree

Oregon•
⑬
⑫
•California

⑦

• Virginia

③
④ ⑥

⑤
•Tennessee

⑭
Fallen
Monarch

② ⑮
•Lincoln
Robert E. Lee•
⑯
① Pennsylvania•

KINGS CANYON
NATIONAL PARK

Twin
Sisters•

P

Restroom

Happy Family
•

Illinois• •Ohio
•Connecticut

Big

•Arizona

Trees

•Michigan Log

•Wyoming
Indiana •
Indiana•

The Martyr

Grant Tree Road

Creek

•Maine

•Massachusetts

New Jersey•

| 0 | 100 | 200 feet |
| 0 | 50 | 100 meters |

① Numbered posts keyed
to pamphlet

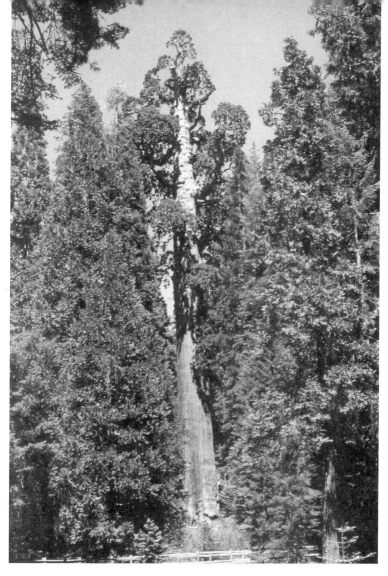

General Grant Tree

are required. Call 800-325-RIDE (7433). From the vicinity of the Grant Grove Market, catch the free Big Tree Shuttle and ride to the Grant Tree trailhead.

Private vehicles should follow CA 180 east from Fresno and, just north of the Grant Grove Visitor

Center, turn west at the well-signed junction with the road to the General Grant Tree. Follow the access road 0.7 mile to the large parking lot. Grant Grove has three campgrounds—Azalea, Crystal Springs, and Sunset (fee, flush toilets, and bear boxes). John Muir Lodge and Grant Grove Cabins offer accommodations, and the village has a restaurant, general store, gift shop, and showers.

Trail Description

▶1 Head in a counterclockwise direction on the paved loop trail, weaving your way up to the area's centerpiece attraction, the General Grant Tree. ▶2 A short climb from this immense monarch takes you past the Gamlin Cabin, followed by a mild descent beside more giant sequoias back to the trailhead. ▶3 Trail extensions north of the grove are far less traveled, providing options for further wanderings.

🚶	**MILESTONES**	
▶1	0.0	Begin at trailhead
▶2	0.2	Walk around General Grant Tree
▶3	0.5	End at trailhead

North Grove Loop

A fairly short trail leads away from the usual hubbub around General Grant Tree and heads down into a more secluded grove of the Big Trees. The route starts by following a paved section of the road that once served as the main entrance into the park from Sequoia Lake. These days, the cars are gone and so are most of the tourists, allowing hikers to visit these sequoias with a higher dose of solitude. Adding the nearby Dead Giant Loop, which is described in Trail 32, easily creates a longer trip than the one described here.

Best Time

Trails in this area are usually free of snow from late May until the first major snowfall in autumn, usually by November. Wildflowers reach the peak of bloom in late spring and early summer; watch for the crescendo of autumn color in mid- to late October.

Finding the Trail

Public transportation to Grant Grove Market is available from stops in Fresno, Sanger, and Squaw Valley/Clingan's Junction on the Fresno/Sanger Shuttle. The round-trip cost is $15, and reservations are required. Call 800-325-RIDE (7433). From the vicinity of the Grant Grove Market, catch the free Big Tree Shuttle and ride to the Grant Tree trailhead.

Private vehicles should follow CA 180 east from Fresno and, just north of the Grant Grove Visitor Center, turn west at the well-signed junction with the road to the General Grant Tree. Follow the

TRAIL USE
Day Hike, Run
LENGTH
1.5 miles, 1 hour
VERTICAL FEET
+350/-350/±700
DIFFICULTY
– 1 **2** 3 4 5 +
TRAIL TYPE
Loop

FEATURES
Giant Sequoias
Secluded

FACILITIES
Lodging
Store
Café
Visitor Center
Post Office
Restrooms
Water
Picnic Area
Campground
Stables
Shuttle Bus Stop

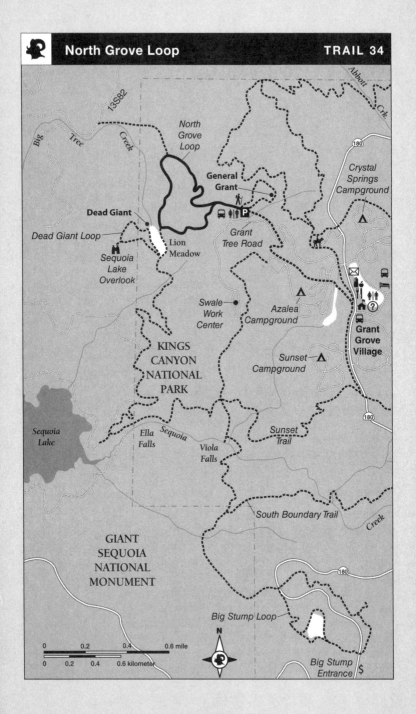

North Grove Loop

13S82

Big Tree Creek

North Grove Loop

General Grant

Dead Giant

Dead Giant Loop

Lion Meadow

Sequoia Lake Overlook

Grant Tree Road

Crystal Springs Campground

180

Swale Work Center

Azalea Campground

KINGS CANYON NATIONAL PARK

Sunset Campground

Grant Grove Village

180

Sequoia Lake

Ella Falls

Sequoia

Viola Falls

Sunset Trail

South Boundary Trail

Creek

GIANT SEQUOIA NATIONAL MONUMENT

180

Big Stump Loop

Big Stump Entrance $

| 0 | 0.2 | 0.4 | 0.6 mile |

| 0 | 0.2 | 0.4 | 0.6 kilometer |

N

access road 0.7 mile to the large parking lot. Grant Grove has three campgrounds—Azalea, Crystal Springs, and Sunset (fee, flush toilets, and bear boxes). John Muir Lodge and Grant Grove Cabins offer accommodations, and the village has a restaurant, general store, gift shop, and showers.

Trail Description

▶1 Head west from the parking lot, through the RV and bus parking area, and then to the closed road at the far end. Follow this road 0.1 mile to a signed junction ▶2 with the North Grove Trail. Leaving the road, turn right (west) and begin a moderate, winding descent through mixed forest. Eventually the trail draws near a trickling stream on the left, which provides enough moisture to sustain a number of large sequoias, as well as an assortment of shrubs and seasonal wildflowers. Where the descent bottoms out, the trail veers west and merges with an overgrown old wagon road.

Giant
Sequoias

The immediate task is to regain all the lost elevation on the way back toward the old entrance road. Eventually, you leave the mighty sequoias behind and continue through lesser conifers. The grade eases just past the 1-mile mark, as the trail intersects the old road. ▶3 From here, the optional Dead Giant

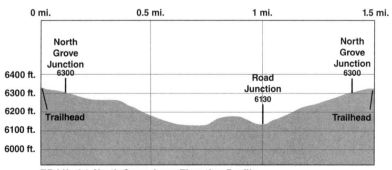

TRAIL 34 North Grove Loop Elevation Profile

Loop is only 0.25 mile down the Sunset Trail on the right (see Trail 32). To return to the General Grant parking lot, turn left and follow the road to the first intersection, ►4 and then retrace your steps to the parking lot. ►5

🚶	**MILESTONES**	
►1	0.0	Start at General Grant Tree parking lot
►2	0.1	Right at North Grove Trail junction
►3	1.0	Left at old road junction
►4	1.4	Left at Sunset Trail junction
►5	1.5	General Grant Tree parking lot

Panoramic Point and Park Ridge Lookout

This fine trip begins with a short walk to the view-packed tourist destination of Panoramic Point, where visitors are treated to outstanding views of the Great Western Divide, Sierra Crest, and Monarch Divide. From there, the pleasant loop combines a hiking trail and a fire road to access one of the few remaining operational fire lookouts in the Sierra, where hikers will have far fewer elbows to rub while admiring vistas of the Great Western Divide and San Joaquin Valley. Alternating between mixed forest and shrub-covered clearings, the route along Park Ridge is fairly gently graded.

Best Time

The view from Panoramic Point is extraordinary at any time of the year, although you may need cross-country skis or snowshoes in winter. Hikers will find snow-free trails to the lookout from late May through October.

Finding the Trail

From Fresno, follow CA 180 east into Kings Canyon National Park and, just north of Grant Grove Visitor Center, turn east at the well-signed junction with Panoramic Point Road. Proceed on paved road for 2.3 miles to the trailhead. Restrooms and a picnic area are nearby. Grant Grove has three campgrounds—Azalea, Crystal Springs, and Sunset (fee, flush toilets, and bear boxes). John Muir Lodge and Grant Grove Cabins offer accommodations, and the village has a restaurant, general store, gift shop, and showers.

TRAIL USE
Day Hike, Run

LENGTH
5.6 miles, 2½–3 hours

VERTICAL FEET
+1430/-1430/±2860

DIFFICULTY
– 1 2 **3** 4 5 +

TRAIL TYPE
Loop

FEATURES
Great Views

FACILITIES
Lodging
Store
Café
Visitor Center
Post Office
Restrooms
Water
Picnic Area
Campgrounds
Stables

237

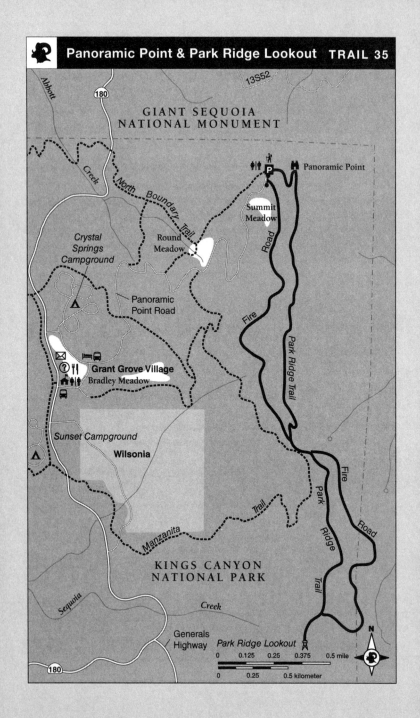

Panoramic Point & Park Ridge Lookout TRAIL 35

13S52

GIANT SEQUOIA NATIONAL MONUMENT

Abbott

180

Creek

North

Boundary

Trail

Panoramic Point

Summit Meadow

Crystal Springs Campground

Round Meadow

Road

Panoramic Point Road

Fire

Park Ridge Trail

Grant Grove Village

Bradley Meadow

Sunset Campground

Wilsonia

Manzanita

Trail

Park

Ridge

Fire

Road

KINGS CANYON NATIONAL PARK

Sequoia

Creek

Park Ridge Trail

Generals Highway

Park Ridge Lookout

| 0 | 0.125 | 0.25 | 0.375 | 0.5 mile |

| 0 | 0.25 | 0.5 kilometer |

N

180

Trail Description

▶1 Follow paved trail bordered by a split rail fence for about 300 yards to Panoramic Point, ▶2 where a magnificent view unfolds. Metal signs help identify some of the numerous peaks of the Monarch Divide, Great Western Divide, and Sierra Crest seen from this spectacular vista point.

 Great Views

Leaving the vast majority of sightseers behind, continue up the trail away from Panoramic Point, following a winding climb that weaves in and out of scattered to light forest, with an understory of manzanita and azalea. Scarred trunks on many of the conifers provide evidence of a recent fire. Where the forest parts, views northeast of the Monarch Divide alternate with views southeast of the Great Western Divide and views west toward San Joaquin Valley. Reach the crest of a knoll past the 1-mile mark, and then begin a moderate descent to a junction where the trail merges with a fire road at 1.6 miles. ▶3

The view from the lookout—from the San Joaquin Valley to the Great Western Divide and points in between—is quite rewarding.

Walk along the fire road for about 50 yards to a signed junction with the resumption of singletrack trail. ▶4 The trail follows a mildly undulating course for another mile before merging with the fire road again. ▶5 Follow the road for approximately 250 yards to the vicinity of the fire lookout tower, ▶6 where transformers, power

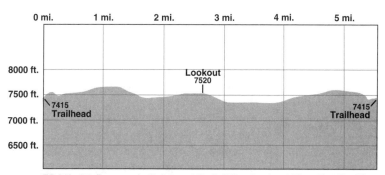

TRAIL 35 Panoramic Point and Park Ridge Lookout Elevation Profile

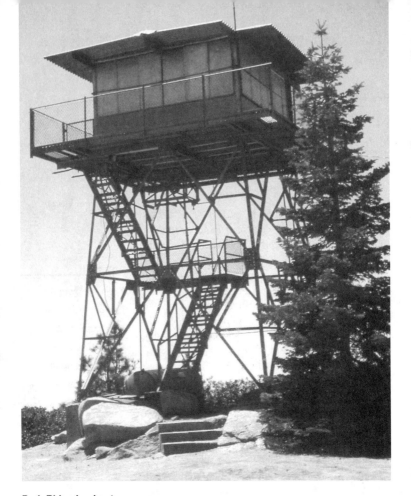

Park Ridge Lookout

poles, communication towers, weather-monitoring equipment, and a concrete-block building litter the edge of the ridge. Despite the human-made features, the view from the lookout—from the San Joaquin Valley to the Great Western Divide and points in between—is quite rewarding.

 Great Views

After fully enjoying the view, retrace your steps 250 yards to the trail junction ▶7 and veer right to continue along the fire road. Proceed on the gently graded road through a light, mixed forest, wrapping around a hillside above Log Corral Meadow to the junction with the singletrack trail that heads south toward the lookout. ►8 Continue on the road another 50 yards to the next junction ►9 of singletrack trail and, remaining on the road, you make a general ascent for about 0.8 mile across open slopes dotted with fire-scarred trees and covered with shrubs. A final half-mile descent leads past a small meadow to a closed gate. From there, follow a short stretch of paved road back to the parking lot. ►10

		MILESTONES
►1	0.0	Start at trailhead
►2	0.1	Panoramic Point
►3	1.6	Straight at fire road
►4	1.63	Straight at junction
►5	2.7	Straight at fire road
►6	2.75	Lookout
►7	2.8	Veer right at junction
►8	4.05	Straight at junction
►9	4.1	Straight at junction
►10	5.6	Return to trailhead

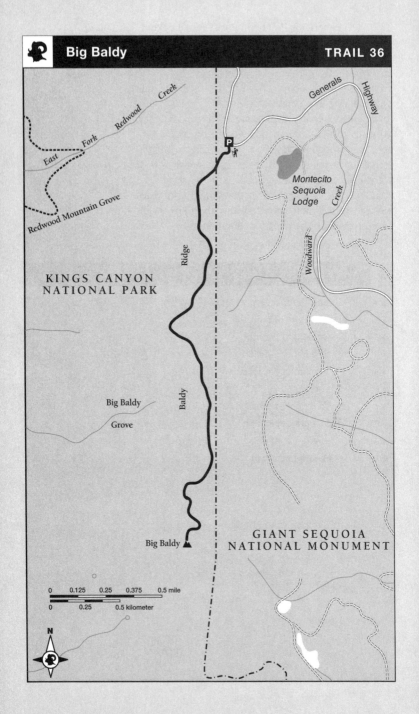

Generals Highway

P

Montecito
Sequoia
Lodge

Woodward Creek

East Fork Redwood Creek

Redwood Mountain Grove

Ridge

KINGS CANYON
NATIONAL PARK

Big Baldy
Grove

Baldy

Big Baldy ▲

GIANT SEQUOIA
NATIONAL MONUMENT

| 0 | 0.125 | 0.25 | 0.375 | 0.5 mile |

| 0 | 0.25 | 0.5 kilometer |

N

Big Baldy

Several granite domes rise above the forested terrain on the west side of Kings Canyon and Sequoia National Parks, offering inspirational views to those who can gain their summits. At 8,209 feet, Big Baldy is one such dome, offering hikers a 360-degree view east toward the Sierra and west across the San Joaquin Valley as the reward for a mere 2.2-mile trip to the summit. Bring along plenty of water because none is available at the trailhead or along the trail.

Best Time

Snow melts from the Big Baldy Trail by the beginning of June in years of average snowfall. As with most vista points on the west side of the parks, the view across the San Joaquin Valley is best following a rare cleansing rainstorm.

TRAIL USE
Day Hike, Run

LENGTH
4.4 miles, 2 hours

VERTICAL FEET
+975/-450, ±2850

DIFFICULTY
– 1 2 **3** 4 5 +

TRAIL TYPE
Out-and-back

FEATURES
Summit
Great Views

FACILITIES
None

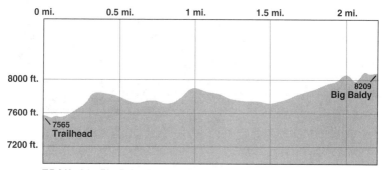

TRAIL 36 Big Baldy Elevation Profile

243

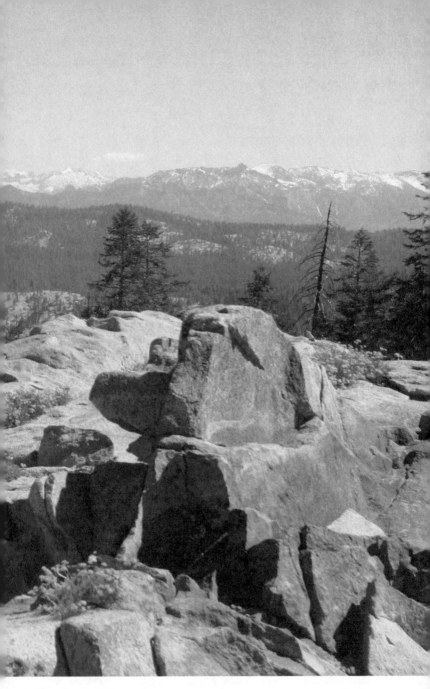

View *from Big Baldy*

Finding the Trail

From Fresno, drive CA 180 to the Y-junction with Generals Highway, turn right, and follow Generals Highway 6.3 miles to the start of the Big Baldy Trail (16.9 miles northwest of Lodgepole). Park your vehicle along the shoulder of the highway as space allows. Giant Sequoia National Monument has a number of campgrounds not far from the trailhead: Stony Creek (fee, flush toilets, running water, and bear boxes) is accessed from Generals Highway, while Horse Camp (vault toilets and no fee), Buck Rock (vault toilets and no fee), and Big Meadow (vault toilets, phone, and no fee) are accessed from Big Meadow Road. Privately run Montecito Sequoia Lodge is a year-round lodge about 1 mile from the trailhead just off Generals Highway. Stony Creek Village (guest rooms, market, restaurant, showers, and gasoline) is about 4 miles farther southbound on Generals Highway.

On a rare clear day, the view extends all the way west to the coastal hills.

Trail Description

▶1 From the vicinity of a wood trail sign on the west side of the highway, follow singletrack trail through a sparse fir forest, soon crossing the boundary into Kings Canyon National Park and following near the crest of an undulating, south-trending ridge. From the top of a granite outcrop, about a half mile from the trailhead, the trees part enough to allow a fine view down into neighboring Redwood Canyon.

Continue along the ridge for the next 1.5 miles, passing in and out of light mixed forest, with the sporadic openings offering a tantalizing foretaste of the view waiting ahead at the top of Big Baldy. Nearing the summit, you pass below a television tower and a concrete-block building before a final, winding ascent over rocks leads to the top of the exposed granite dome. ▶2

 Summit

The view from the apex of Big Baldy is grand indeed, with the serrated summits of peaks belonging to the Kings-Kaweah and Great Western Divides beyond Little Baldy to the east. Westward, across Redwood Canyon and Redwood Mountain, lie the foothills and the usually smoggy air above the San Joaquin Valley. On a rare clear day, the view extends all the way west to the coastal hills.

Great Views

🚶 MILESTONES

▶1   0.0   Start at trailhead
▶2   2.2   Big Baldy

Buena Vista Peak

The short 1-mile distance, combined with easy access immediately off Generals Highway, makes this trip to the top of Buena Vista Peak relatively popular. The view from the summit is quite rewarding, especially when the atmospheric conditions are favorable.

Best Time

Snow clears the area relatively soon in the lower elevations on the west side of Kings Canyon, opening up the trail to Buena Vista Peak usually by early June. Cold weather and snowstorms generally return to the area by early November.

Finding the Trail

From the Y-junction of Generals Highway and Kings Canyon Highway (CA 180), the trailhead is 5.8 miles east on Generals Highway, across from Kings Canyon Overlook. Park your vehicle on the highway shoulder as space allows.

TRAIL USE
Day Hike, Run

LENGTH
2.0 miles, 1 hour

VERTICAL FEET
+1000/-450/±2900

DIFFICULTY
– 1 **2** 3 4 5 +

TRAIL TYPE
Out-and-back

FEATURES
Summit
Great Views

FACILITIES
None

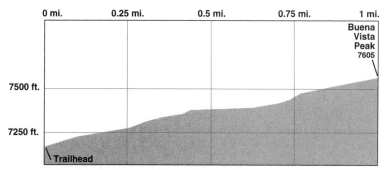

TRAIL 38 **Buena Vista Peak Elevation Profile**

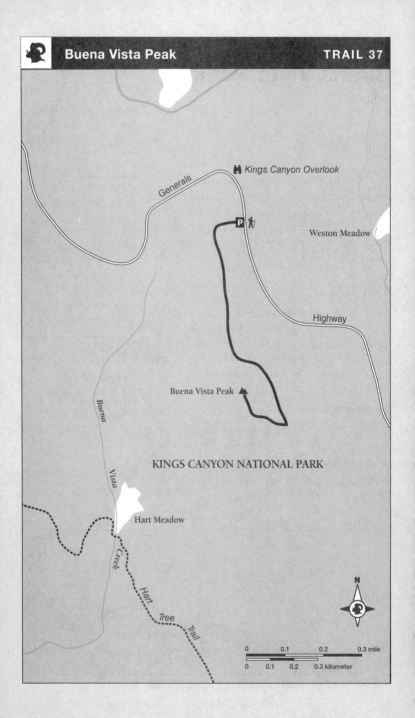

Kings Canyon Overlook

Weston Meadow

Generals

Highway

Buena Vista Peak

Buena

Vista

KINGS CANYON NATIONAL PARK

Hart Meadow

Creek

Hart

Tree

Trail

N

| 0 | 0.1 | 0.2 | 0.3 mile |
| 0 | 0.1 | 0.2 | 0.3 kilometer |

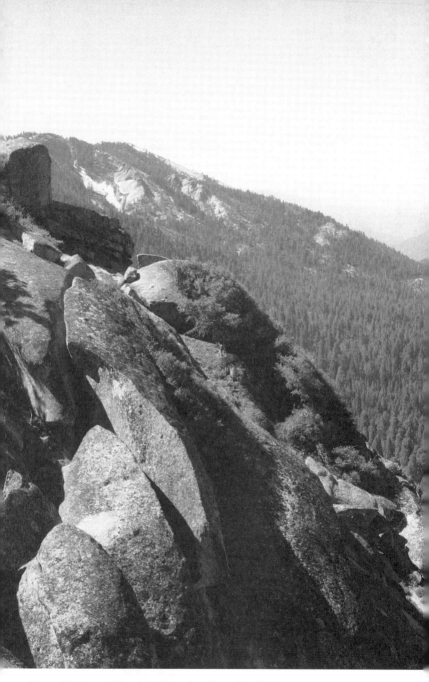

View of Redwood Mountain Grove *from Buena Vista Peak*

Trail Description

▶1 From the edge of the highway, follow a dirt path that climbs moderately through mostly open terrain of large boulders, manzanita, and an occasional incense cedar or fir. Coming close to the domelike summit, scamper over granite slabs and follow an ascending traverse across the east side of a ridge through light fir forest to a series of switchbacks leading up the southeast ridge to the top of Buena Vista Peak. ▶2

On a rare, smogless day, the westward view can be quite exhilarating, extending all the way across the San Joaquin Valley to the coastal hills. During times of less idyllic atmospheric conditions, successful peak baggers have a splendid view of nearby landmarks, including Redwood Mountain, Mount Baldy, Buck Rock, and the deep cleft of Kings Canyon to the northeast.

🚶	MILESTONES		
▶1	0.0	Start at Buena Vista Peak Trailhead	
▶2	1.0	Summit of Buena Vista Peak	

Hart Tree Loop

The Redwood Mountain Grove represents the largest intact grove of giant sequoias in the world, and this 7-plus-mile loop leads visitors past many distinguished monarchs, as well as to lush riparian habitats along Redwood Creek and its tributaries, and to the pastoral surroundings of beautiful Hart Meadow. Trails in the grove are relatively lightly used, thanks in part to access via a dirt road and a lack of signs pointing the way. Visitors should appreciate the opportunity to stand among the giant sequoias in quiet reverence, an experience contrary to more popular groves in the park.

TRAIL USE
Day Hike, Backpack, Run

LENGTH
7.25 miles, 4 hours

VERTICAL FEET
+2050/-2050/±4100

DIFFICULTY
– 1 2 **3** 4 5 +

TRAIL TYPE
Loop

FEATURES
Fall Colors
Wildflowers
Giant Sequoias
Great Views
Camping
Secluded

FACILITIES
Restrooms

Best Time

Generally by the end of April or the beginning of May, the trails of Redwood Mountain Grove start to shed their covering of winter snow. Somewhat off the beaten path, the trails are host to the highest number of visitors between Fourth of July and Labor Day weekend. Springtime offers the added bonus of blooming dogwoods, while fall offers leaves ablaze with autumn color.

Finding the Trail

From Fresno, follow CA 180 to the Y-junction with Generals Highway, turn right, and follow Generals Highway 3.4 miles to Quail Flat. Directly opposite Tenmile Road, turn south and follow a narrow dirt road with turnouts for 1.7 miles to a junction. Bear left at the junction, signed for Redwood Mountain Grove, and drive 0.1 mile to the entrance into the

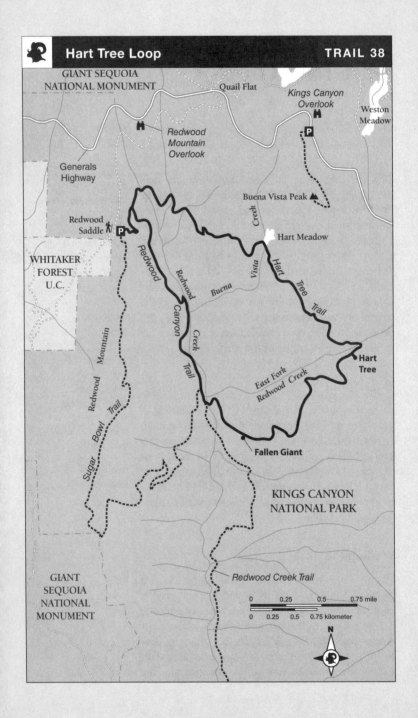

Hart Tree Loop

TRAIL 38

GIANT SEQUOIA
NATIONAL MONUMENT

Quail Flat

*Kings Canyon
Overlook*

Weston
Meadow

*Redwood
Mountain
Overlook*

Generals
Highway

Buena Vista Peak

Hart Meadow

Redwood
Saddle

WHITAKER
FOREST
U.C.

Redwood

Redwood

Buena

Hart

Vista

Creek

Tree

Redwood Mountain

Canyon

Trail

Creek

Trail

Hart
Tree

Sugar Bowl Trail

East Fork
Redwood Creek

Fallen Giant

KINGS CANYON
NATIONAL PARK

GIANT
SEQUOIA
NATIONAL
MONUMENT

Redwood Creek Trail

| 0 | 0.25 | 0.5 | 0.75 mile |

| 0 | 0.25 | 0.5 | 0.75 kilometer |

N

large parking area at Redwood Saddle. Tenmile and Landslide (fee and vault toilets) are U.S. Forest Service campgrounds located nearby on Tenmile Road.

Logistics

Backpackers must obtain a wilderness permit for all overnight visits. See page 210 for more details about how to obtain one.

Trail Description

▶1 From the trailhead, take the left-hand trail, signed HART TREE, REDWOOD CANYON TRAIL, and head north. Descend into a mixed forest of firs, pines, and giant sequoias while following the course of an old roadbed to a junction in a small ravine. ▶2 Bear left and proceed under cool and shady forest on soft dirt tread past lush ground cover, winding down to an easy boulder-hop of a wildflower- and fern-lined tributary of Redwood Creek. From the creek, a mild climb leads to the next delightful, flower-lined branch, where you can see Redwood Cabin above the far bank.

Giant Sequoias

Wildflowers

The climb continues away from the cabin for another 0.2 mile to yet another stream crossing. Leave the stream and most of the redwoods behind

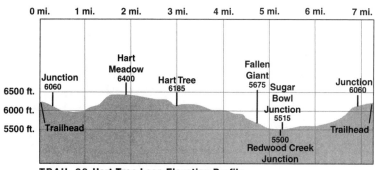
TRAIL 38 Hart Tree Loop Elevation Profile

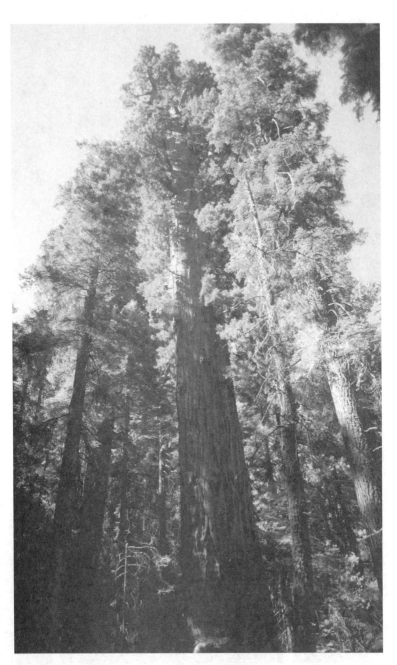

Hart Tree, *Redwood Canyon*

as the trail climbs more moderately. Through infrequent gaps in the forest, you catch fleeting glimpses of Redwood Mountain to the west before reaching a granite outcrop with an unobstructed view of the mountain and Big Baldy to the southeast. A mild climb from the outcrop leads to the fringe of Hart Meadow, ▶3 a sloping, verdant glade picturesquely backdropped by the west face of Buena Vista Peak. After stepping across twin channels of Buena Vista Creek, you bid farewell to this pastoral scene.

 Great Views

A general descent leads away from the meadow and back into the mighty presence of the Big Trees, reaching the Fallen Tunnel Tree, where the trail passes directly through the hollowed core of this downed giant sequoia. The mostly gentle descent continues through the cool forest, eventually drawing alongside a trickling seasonal stream followed by lushly lined East Fork Redwood Creek, spilling serenely over moss-covered rocks and swirling gently through diminutive pools—a quite pleasant forest scene. A brief climb from the East Fork brings you to a junction with a short spur to the Hart Tree, ▶4 the 24th-largest giant sequoia in the world. Black scars 20 to 30 feet up the trunk show evidence that this immense redwood has withstood some significant fires in the past.

 Giant Sequoias

Gently descending tread leads away from the Hart Tree spur past a thin ribbon of water from a seasonal stream cascading down a rock cleft into a pool lined with lush foliage and wildflowers. Proceed through a mixed forest of incense cedars, white firs, and a smattering of sequoias, interrupted briefly by a sunny clearing filled with drier vegetation, on the way to a junction with a spur to a huge downed sequoia known as the Fallen Giant. ▶5

 Wildflowers

Another half mile leads to a crossing of the main branch of Redwood Creek, a crossing that may prove a little difficult in early season. Just over the creek, you reach a junction with Redwood Canyon

Fire Ecology

Over the last few decades, biologists have learned a great deal about the relationship between fire and the giant sequoia through experimental burns performed in research areas within Redwood Mountain Grove. For instance, the thick bark of sequoias protects them from the ravages of a forest fire while other coniferous species are burned, thereby creating space on the forest floor for new sequoia saplings. The tiny sequoia cone also releases its seeds when heated by fire.

Camping

Giant Sequoias

Trail, ▶6 where backpackers should head downstream to campsites farther down the canyon.

Turn right and head upstream along Redwood Canyon Trail on a mild climb through a mixed forest, including towering sequoias, soon passing a junction with the Sugar Bowl Trail on your left. ▶7 Continue ahead, following Redwood Creek upstream past more magnificent sequoias for another 0.75 mile until the trail forsakes the creek in favor of an ascent of the hillside above. Reach the close of the loop at a junction between the Redwood Canyon and Hart Tree Trails at 6.9 miles. ▶8

From the junction, retrace your steps 0.3 mile to the trailhead at Redwood Saddle. ▶9

MILESTONES

▶1	0.0	Head left at Redwood Saddle Trailhead
▶2	0.3	Bear left at junction
▶3	1.9	Hart Meadow
▶4	3.0	Hart Tree
▶5	4.75	Fallen Giant
▶6	5.25	Right at Redwood Canyon Trail junction
▶7	5.3	Straight at Sugar Bowl Trail junction
▶8	6.9	Left at junction
▶9	7.25	Redwood Saddle Trailhead

Sugar Bowl Loop

Redwood Mountain Grove represents the largest intact grove of giant sequoias in the world. Although lacking the number of notable sequoia landmarks found on the Hart Tree Loop, the Sugar Bowl Loop exposes hikers to plenty of stately trees and also passes through an interesting work in progress—a hillside covered with young sequoias planted on the site of an old burn. Biologists have learned a great deal about the relationship between sequoias and fire through experimental burns in research areas within the Redwood Mountain Grove. In addition, the loop follows a stretch of Redwood Creek, where the pleasant stream tumbles down a canyon carpeted with lush foliage and towering sequoias. Backpackers have the opportunity to camp farther down Redwood Creek. Trails in the grove are relatively lightly used, thanks in part to access via a dirt road and a lack of signs pointing the way. Visitors should appreciate the opportunity to stand among the giant sequoias in quiet reverence, an experience contrary to more popular groves in the park.

TRAIL USE
Day Hike, Backpack, Run

LENGTH
6.6 miles, 3½ hours

VERTICAL FEET
+2150/-2150/±4300

DIFFICULTY
– 1 2 **3** 4 5 +

TRAIL TYPE
Loop

FEATURES
Fall Colors
Wildflowers
Giant Sequoias
Great Views
Camping
Secluded

FACILITIES
Restrooms

Best Time

Generally by the end of April or the beginning of May, the trails of Redwood Mountain Grove start to shed their covering of winter snow. Somewhat off the beaten path, the trails are host to the highest number of visitors between Fourth of July and Labor Day weekend. Springtime offers the added bonus of blooming dogwoods, while fall offers leaves ablaze with autumn color.

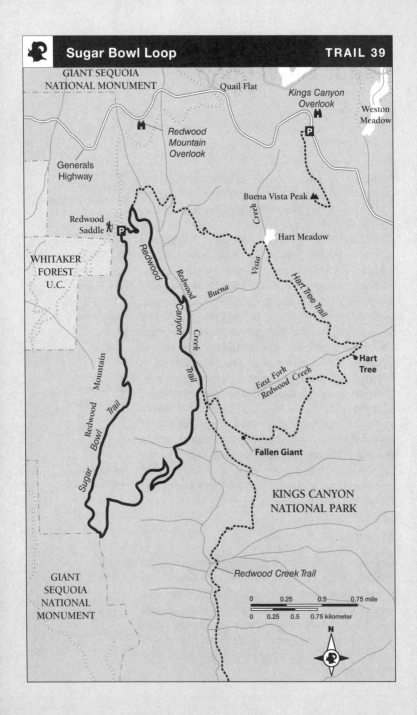

Sugar Bowl Loop   TRAIL 39

GIANT SEQUOIA
NATIONAL MONUMENT   Quail Flat

Kings Canyon
Overlook

Weston
Meadow

Redwood
Mountain
Overlook

Generals
Highway

Buena Vista Peak ▲

Vista Creek

Hart Meadow

Redwood
Saddle

Redwood Saddle

WHITAKER
FOREST
U.C.

Redwood Canyon Trail

Redwood Creek

Buena

Hart Tree Trail

Redwood Mountain Trail

East Fork Redwood Creek

Hart
Tree

Sugar Bowl Trail

Fallen Giant

KINGS CANYON
NATIONAL PARK

GIANT
SEQUOIA
NATIONAL
MONUMENT

Redwood Creek Trail

| 0 | 0.25 | 0.5 | 0.75 mile |

| 0 | 0.25 | 0.5 | 0.75 kilometer |

N

Finding the Trail

From Fresno, follow CA 180 to the Y-junction with Generals Highway, turn right, and follow Generals Highway 3.4 miles to Quail Flat. Directly opposite Tenmile Road, turn south and follow a narrow dirt road with turnouts for 1.7 miles to a junction. Bear left at the junction, signed for Redwood Mountain Grove, and drive 0.1 mile to the entrance into the large parking area at Redwood Saddle. Tenmile and Landslide (fee and vault toilets) are U.S. Forest Service campgrounds located nearby on Tenmile Road.

Logistics

Backpackers must obtain a wilderness permit for all overnight visits. See page 210 for more details about how to obtain one.

Trail Description

►1 From the trailhead, take the left-hand trail, signed HART TREE, REDWOOD CANYON TRAIL, and head north. Descend into a mixed forest of firs, pines, and giant sequoias while following the course of an old roadbed to a junction in a small ravine. ►2 Bear right at the junction and follow the Redwood

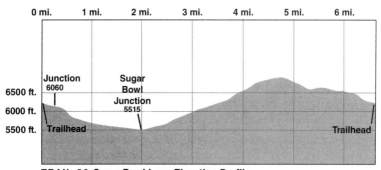

TRAIL 39 Sugar Bowl Loop Elevation Profile

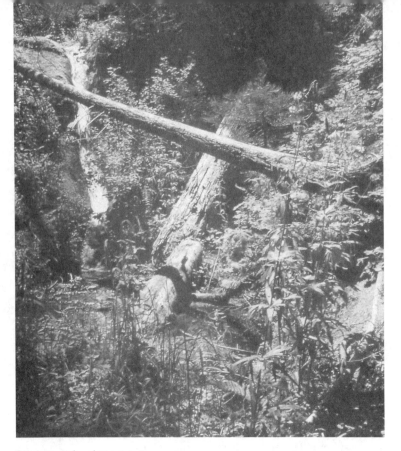

Rivulet *in Redwood Mountain Grove*

Canyon Trail initially on a gentle descent that soon becomes moderate. A mile or so from the junction, you reach the west bank of enchanting Redwood Creek and proceed downstream through lush vegetation past a number of stately sequoias. The path stays reasonably close to the stream for a while, veers away briefly, and then follows the creek to a junction with the Sugar Bowl Trail. ▶3

Turn right and head southwest from the junction on a moderate climb up the hillside. Beyond a pair of short-legged switchbacks, you continue the climb across a slope covered with myriad young sequoias and dotted with a few widely scattered old

Giant Sequoias

giants. Over the tops of the young trees, the granite dome of Big Baldy puts in an appearance. Cross a seasonal stream, where the increase in moisture has given rise to more mature trees that provide a pocket of welcome shade. Beyond the stream the moderate ascent continues across open slopes via a set of switchbacks climbing across a hillside covered with drought-tolerant shrubs, such as manzanita and huckleberry oak. As you climb, views continue to improve of Big Baldy, Buena Vista Peak, and the surrounding terrain. The moderate climb abates where the trail gains the crest of Redwood Mountain's lengthy ridge.

 Great Views

Now the trail turns north and follows the ridge into the cover of a mixed forest, where giant sequoias once again tower over their lower counterparts. As you proceed amid these majestic monarchs on soft tread, you may eventually notice the end of the Big Trees near the east end of the ridge, further evidence that sequoias require specialized conditions for their growth and survival. Most likely the soil on this side of the ridge doesn't receive a suitable amount of moisture for the sequoias to flourish. Climb mildly to the high point of the journey, weaving in and out of forest cover along the way, where good views from the clearings span across Redwood Canyon to the granite domes of Buena Vista Peak and Big Baldy. A gradual descent leads away from the high point through mixed forest to close the loop at the parking area. From there, retrace your steps to the trailhead at Redwood Saddle. ▶4

 Giant Sequoias

MILESTONES

▶1	0.0	Head left at Redwood Saddle Trailhead
▶2	0.3	Right at Redwood Canyon Trail junction
▶3	2.0	Right at Sugar Bowl Trail junction
▶4	6.6	Redwood Saddle Trailhead

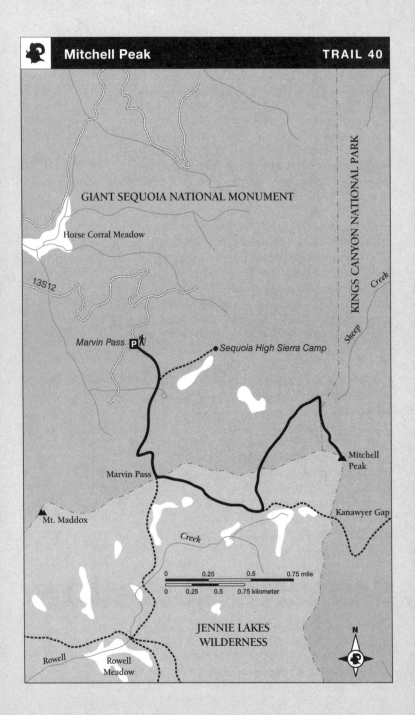

Mitchell Peak

Straddling the border between Kings Canyon National Park and Jennie Lakes Wilderness, 10,356-foot Mitchell Peak affords peak baggers a supreme vista of the deep cleft of Kings Canyon, as well as numerous Sierra summits along the crest, Great Western and Monarch Divides, and the Kaweahs. A high expectation of solitude enhances the marvelous view.

Best Time

Following winters of average snowfall, the trail to Mitchell Peak is usually open by sometime in July and remains so until the first snowstorm in fall. Wildflowers reach their peak during the month of July.

Finding the Trail

Leave Generals Highway, 6.4 miles southeast of the Y-intersection with CA 180, and head northeast on Big Meadows Road. After 9.7 miles, turn onto a single-lane dirt road (FS 13S12), signed MARVIN PASS TRAILHEAD, and travel 2.5 miles to the trailhead, remaining on the most well-traveled road at all junctions.

Trail Description

▶1 From the trailhead, proceed uphill on singletrack tread through a mixed forest of white firs, lodgepole pines, and western white pines. A healthy understory of shrubs includes chinquapin, manzanita, and currant. A moderately steep climb gains the top

TRAIL USE
Day Hike, Run
LENGTH
6.6 miles, 3–4 hours
VERTICAL FEET
+2100/-350/±4900
DIFFICULTY
– 1 2 3 **4** 5 +
TRAIL TYPE
Out-and-back

FEATURES
Mountain
Summit
Wildflowers
Great Views
Secluded

FACILITIES
None

263

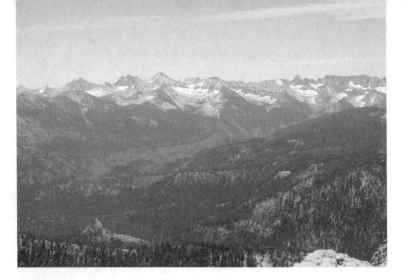

View *from Mitchell Peak*

of a ridge, where the grade eases on the way to a junction ►2 with a lateral from Sequoia High Sierra Camp, a walk-in resort 0.3 mile east.

Continue straight ahead from the junction, immediately crossing a small fern- and flower-lined rivulet. Pass above a pocket of lush foliage dotted with an array of colorful wildflowers, including shooting stars, corn lilies, buttercups, and monkeyflowers. **Wildflowers** Away from the verdant surroundings, the steady climb continues via some switchbacks on the way to the signed Jennie Lakes Wilderness boundary and a junction ►3 at Marvin Pass, 1 mile from the trailhead.

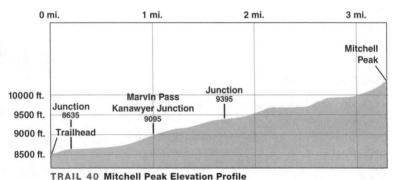

TRAIL 40 Mitchell Peak Elevation Profile

From the junction, turn left and head southeast along the Kanawyer Gap Trail across the south side of a ridge through scattered to light forest above shrubs and boulders. Lupine and paintbrush add splashes of color in early season. A gently graded traverse leads to a junction ►4 in a swath of chinquapin, 0.7 mile from Marvin Pass.

Turn left (north) and ascend a mostly open slope back to and across the ridge crest. Follow the trail as it veers northeast on an ascending traverse across the northwest flank of Mitchell Peak through a light forest of red firs, western white pines, and Jeffrey pines. Eventually, the grade increases on a winding climb toward the blocky summit. Leaving the last of the conifers behind, weave southeast among a sea of boulders to the summit of Mitchell Peak. ►5

Perhaps the most impressive view from the top is the foreground terrain to the northeast plummeting steeply into the yawning chasm of Kings Canyon, backdropped by the rising profile of the Monarch Divide. A vast array of summits fills the horizon, including the Palisades and Mount Goddard to the northeast, the Great Western Divide, and the multi-hued Kaweah Peaks to the southeast. Remnants of an old fire lookout lie scattered about, a silent reminder of the days when rangers once had the privilege of this amazing view on a daily basis. When the time comes, retrace your steps to the trailhead.

👤 MILESTONES

►1	0.0	Start at Marvin Pass Trailhead
►2	0.2	Straight at Sequoia High Sierra Camp junction
►3	1.0	Left at Marvin Pass/Kanawyer Gap Trail junction
►4	1.7	Left at junction
►5	3.3	Mitchell Peak

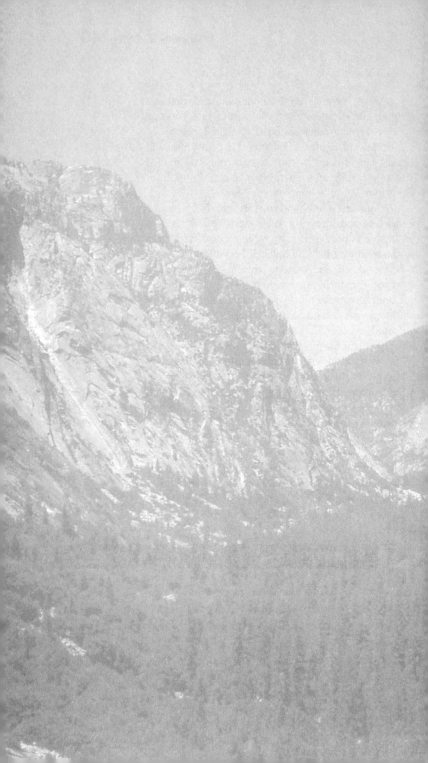

CHAPTER 5

Kings Canyon

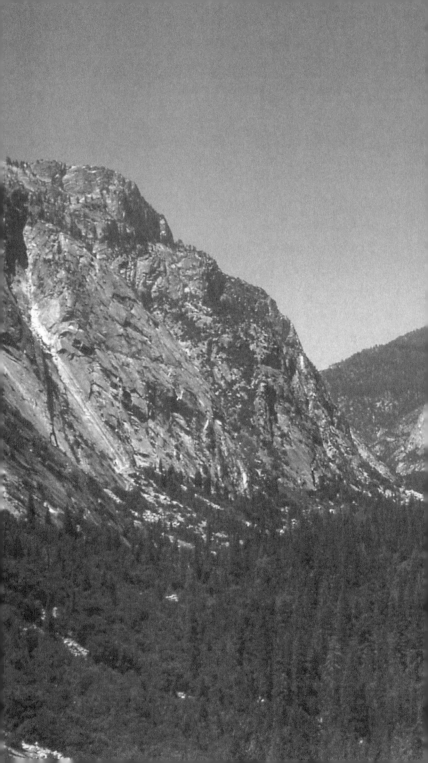

Kings Canyon

One of America's deepest gorges, Kings Canyon rivals the more popular Yosemite Valley for mountain grandeur. When measured from the top of Spanish Mountain, Kings Canyon is more than 8,000 feet deep, second only to Hells Canyon, where the Snake River forms part of the boundary between Oregon and Idaho. Born in the uppermost region of the High Sierra, South Fork Kings River flows through the sheer granite walls of the canyon on the way toward the San Joaquin Valley below. Towering granite features such as Grand Sentinel stand guard over the river valley in dramatic fashion. From Cedar Grove and Roads End, a network of recreational trails climb out of the valley destined for the high country beyond, luring hikers, backpackers, and equestrians from around the world.

While three of the trails featured in this chapter are short and without much elevation gain (42–44), the topography forces most of the trails to climb stiffly out of the deep cleft of Kings Canyon in order to go anywhere. Fortunately, the destinations are well worth the effort, including supreme views of the canyon from Lookout Peak (Trail 41) and Cedar Grove Overlook (Trail 47), beautiful Mist Falls (Trail 45), and the classic High Sierra landscapes on the extended Rae Lakes Loop (Trail 46).

CA 180 provides the only access into Kings Canyon; the road is usually open from late April to mid-November. Motorists should plan on a one-hour drive from the Big Stump Entrance because portions of the highway are steep and winding. Cedar Grove offers a visitor center, general store, gift shop, snack bar, laundromat, showers, stables, motel-style lodging, and four campgrounds.

Visitors will see extensive damage from the 2015 Rough Fire on the drive down to the floor of the canyon and on the north wall above Cedar Grove.

Overleaf and opposite: *Kings Canyon View, Bubbs Creek Trail*

Permits

Permits are not required for day hikes. Backpackers must obtain a wilderness permit for all overnight trips. Between late May and late September, a quota system is in place, with a $15 fee per group. Outside the quota period, permits are free, self-issue, and available 24 hours a day. Advance reservations are available for approximately 75% of the quota, with the remainder set aside for walk-in permits. All permits must be picked up from the Roads End Permit Station between 7 a.m. and 3:45 p.m. Applications for advance reservations are accepted only by fax or mail, no earlier than midnight March 1 and no later than two weeks prior to the start of the trip. Visit the park website to download a permit application and to check on quota availability.

Maps

For the Kings Canyon area, the U.S. Geological Survey 7.5-minute (1:24,000 scale) topographic maps are listed below, corresponding to the trails described in this section. Sequoia Natural History Association (SNHA) publishes *Cedar Grove*, a handy foldout map for the trails in the Kings Canyon area. The SNHA also publishes an interpretive guide to the Zumwalt Meadow Nature Trail with map. Trail users also may want to consider using Tom Harrison's map, *Sequoia & Kings Canyon National Parks* (1:125,000), or *Kings Canyon High Country* (1:63,360).

Trails 41–42 and 47–48: *Cedar Grove*

Trails 43–45: *The Sphinx*

Trail 46: *The Sphinx, Mt. Clarence King*

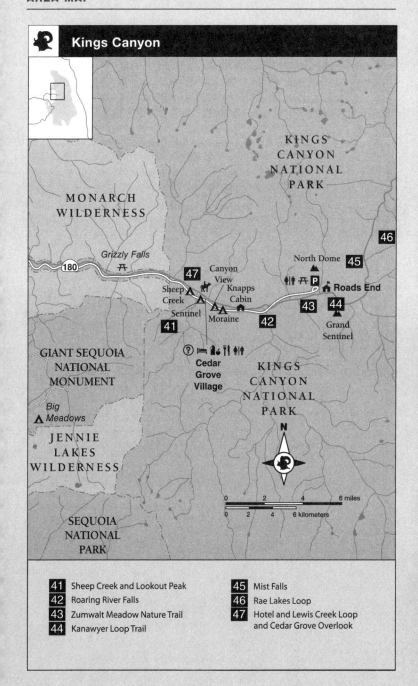

Kings Canyon

MONARCH
WILDERNESS

KINGS
CANYON
NATIONAL
PARK

Grizzly Falls

180

46

North Dome 45

47 Canyon
View
Knapps
Sheep Cabin
Creek
Sentinel
43
Moraine 42
44
Grand
Sentinel

41

GIANT SEQUOIA
NATIONAL
MONUMENT

Cedar
Grove
Village

KINGS
CANYON
NATIONAL
PARK

Big
Meadows

N

JENNIE
LAKES
WILDERNESS

0   2   4   6 miles
0   2   4   6 kilometers

Roads End

SEQUOIA
NATIONAL
PARK

41 Sheep Creek and Lookout Peak
42 Roaring River Falls
43 Zumwalt Meadow Nature Trail
44 Kanawyer Loop Trail

45 Mist Falls
46 Rae Lakes Loop
47 Hotel and Lewis Creek Loop
and Cedar Grove Overlook

TRAIL FEATURES TABLE

Kings Canyon

TRAIL	DIFFICULTY	LENGTH	TYPE	USES & ACCESS	TERRAIN	FLORA & FAUNA	OTHER
41	3 and 4	1.8, 10.0	⟋	🚶🏃	🏔△◪	✳	⋔🏊
42	1	0.5	⟋	🚶👫	◫		
43	1	1.5	⟳	🚶👫	◪		⋔
44	2	4.7	⟳	🚶🏃🐎👫	◪		⋔🎣
45	3	7.8	⟋	🚶🏃🐎	◩◪◫		🎣
46	4 and 5	41.6	⟳	🏃🐎🐕	◩🏔≋◪◫	✳	⋔△⇌⚓🎣
47	4	4.8, 6.4	⟲⟳	🚶🏃🐎	◩◪	✳	⋔

USES & ACCESS	TYPE	TERRAIN	FLORA & FAUNA	OTHER
🚶 Day Hiking	⟳ Loop	◩ Canyon	🍂 Fall Colors	⋔ Great Views
🎒 Backpacking	⟋ Out-and-back	🏔 Mountain	✳ Wildflowers	△ Camping
🏃 Running	⟍ Point-to-point	△ Summit	🌲 Giant Sequoias	⇌ Swimming
🐎 Horses	DIFFICULTY	≋ Lake		⬱ Secluded
🐕 Dogs Allowed	- 1 2 3 4 5 +	◪ Stream		⚲ Steep
👫 Child Friendly	less more	◫ Waterfall		🎣 Fishing
♿ Wheelchair-Access				🏛 Historical Interest

Kings Canyon

Sheep Creek and Lookout Peak ... 275

Follow the Don Cecil Trail on a climb from Cedar Grove to a verdant grotto along Sheep Creek for a short out-and-back hike, or continue the ascent all the way to one of the park's best views of Kings Canyon from the summit of Lookout Peak. The 4,000-foot elevation gain may be taxing, but the amazing vista is a more than adequate reward for all the hard work.

TRAIL 41

Day Hike, Run
1.8 miles, Out-and-back to Sheep Creek
10.0 miles, Out-and-back to Lookout Peak
Difficulty: 1 2 **3-4** 5

Roaring River Falls 280

Before Roaring River empties into South Fork Kings River near Cedar Grove, the waters spill down the south wall of Kings Canyon in a pair of scenic falls. A very short stroll leads to a viewpoint of the lower falls, a magnificent sight, especially in late spring when the river is swollen with snowmelt from the high mountains above.

TRAIL 42

Day Hike, Child Friendly
0.5 mile, Out-and-back
Difficulty: **1** 2 3 4 5

Zumwalt Meadow Nature Trail 284

A great place to acquaint yourself with the ecology of Kings Canyon, Zumwalt Meadow Nature Trail circles a grass- and flower-covered meadow near the banks of the mighty South Fork Kings River. The self-guiding trail has numbered posts corresponding to information in a pamphlet describing the natural and human history of the area. Fine views of the canyon walls are an added bonus.

TRAIL 43

Day Hike, Child Friendly
1.5 miles, Loop
Difficulty: **1** 2 3 4 5

TRAIL 44

Day Hike, Run, Horse,
Child Friendly
4.7 miles, Loop
Difficulty: 1 **2** 3 4 5

Kanawyer Loop Trail 288

This pleasantly graded trail across the upper floor of Kings Canyon forms a loop through mixed forest and clearings along the South Fork Kings River, which is a fine introduction to the area for trail users of all skill levels.

TRAIL 45

Day Hike, Run, Horse
7.8 miles, Out-and-back
Difficulty: 1 2 **3** 4 5

Mist Falls 292

A great hike along the South Fork Kings River leads to aptly named Mist Falls, where summertime visitors can feel cool and refreshed from the mist created by the river's water cascading over a cliff and crashing into granite boulders.

TRAIL 46

Backpack, Horse
41.6 miles, Loop
Difficulty: 1 2 3 **4-5**

Rae Lakes Loop 296

Considered by many to be Kings Canyon's quintessential backpack, this extended trip circles through some of the park's most sublime backcountry. Highly popular, the route travels along the upper reaches of South Fork Kings River through Paradise Valley and the Woods Creek drainage on the way to the subalpine wonderland of Rae Lakes Basin. After climbing to 11,960-foot Glen Pass, the trail drops to Bubbs Creek and heads downstream back to Kings Canyon.

TRAIL 47

Day Hike, Run, Horse
4.8 miles, Out-and-back to Cedar Grove Overlook
6.4 miles, Loop
Difficulty: 1 2 3 **4** 5

Hotel and Lewis Creeks Loop and Cedar Grove Overlook 309

Any trail leaving the floor of Kings Canyon must climb steeply to get out of the valley, and this trip is no exception. This steep ascent leads to a commanding view of Kings Canyon from Cedar Grove Overlook, which makes a fine out-and-back hike. For those up to the task, the full 6.4-mile Hotel and Lewis Creeks Loop offers stunning views of the canyon below and the Monarch Divide above. The route passes through an area burned in the 2015 Rough Fire, offering an opportunity to witness the regeneration process firsthand.

Sheep Creek and Lookout Peak

This trip follows the Don Cecil Trail to the top of Lookout Peak, from which hikers have a bird's-eye view of the deep cleft of Kings Canyon and an impressive vista of the peaks and ridges in the back-country of Kings Canyon National Park. While a few tourists may hike the first part of the trail to the cool grotto of Sheep Creek, the remaining 4 miles of trail sees little use—a definite bonus for solitude seekers. The steady, 4,000-foot climb seems more than enough to deter the average park visitor. Although stiff, the ascent can be done in a few hours by hikers in reasonable condition. Be sure to shoot for an early start, however, as temperatures at these relatively low elevations can become hot during the heat of the day.

Best Time

The route to the 8,485-foot summit is usually free of snow from June to mid-October. Wildflowers along Sheep Creek are usually at their peak sometime in early summer.

Finding the Trail

From Fresno, follow CA 180 east into Kings Canyon National Park and continue past Grant Grove into Kings Canyon. Park your vehicle along the shoulder of the highway near the trailhead, 0.15 mile east of the turnoff into Cedar Grove. The National Park Service has four campgrounds in the Cedar Grove area: Sentinel, Sheep Creek, Canyon View, and Moraine (all of which have fees, flush toilets, running water,

TRAIL USE
Day Hike, Run

LENGTH
1.8 miles, 1 hour to
Sheep Creek
10.0 miles, 5 hours to
Lookout Peak

VERTICAL FEET
+600/-600/±1200
+4000/-225/±8450

DIFFICULTY
– 1 2 **3 4** 5 +

TRAIL TYPE
Out-and-back

FEATURES
Mountain
Summit
Stream
Wildflowers
Great Views
Steep

FACILITIES
Lodging
Store
Visitor Center
Snack Bar
Restrooms
Showers
Laundromat
Water
Picnic Area
Campground
Stables

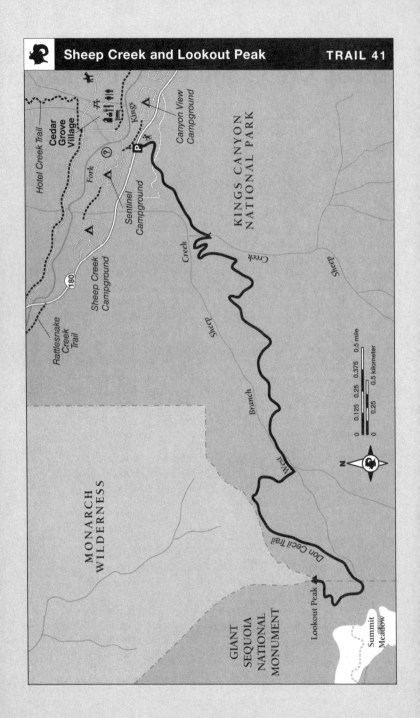

Cedar Grove Village

Hotel Creek Trail

Kings

Canyon View Campground

KINGS CANYON NATIONAL PARK

Sentinel Campground

P

Fork

Creek

Creek

Sheep

Sheep Creek Campground

180

Rattlesnake Creek Trail

Sheep

Branch

West

0   0.125 0.25 0.375 0.5 mile

0   0.25   0.5 kilometer

N

Don Cecil Trail

MONARCH WILDERNESS

Lookout Peak

GIANT SEQUOIA NATIONAL MONUMENT

Summit Meadow

and bear boxes). Cedar Grove has a motel, showers, general store, restaurant, and laundry facilities.

Trail Description

▶1 The trail begins by climbing the south wall of the canyon on a moderately steep grade through a light, mixed forest of black oaks, incense cedars, ponderosa pines, and white firs. Careful perusal of the trunks reveals black scars, indicating that this area has seen its share of forest fires. Soon the trail bends west to cross an access road for the Cedar Grove heliport and then resumes the stiff ascent before shortly dropping to Sheep Creek at 0.9 mile, ▶2 where the cool and refreshing waters cascade picturesquely down a series of rock slabs. As Sheep Creek is the domestic water source for Cedar Grove, do not contaminate the water in any way. Fortunately for solitude seekers, most sightseers go no farther than the bridge over the creek.

Beyond the creek, a series of switchbacks leads through scattered forest, with periodic breaks that allow fine views of Kings Canyon below, the Monarch Divide to the north, and the Sierra Crest to the east—precursors of the much more excellent view waiting at the top of Lookout Peak. The forest thickens a tad on the approach to the west branch

> Nearly 4,000 feet straight below is the South Fork Kings River, tumbling through the rugged and deep gorge of Kings Canyon.

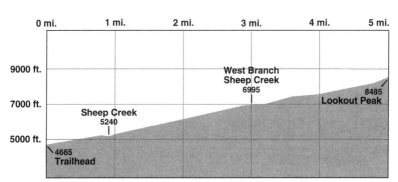

TRAIL 41   Sheep Creek and Lookout Peak Elevation Profile

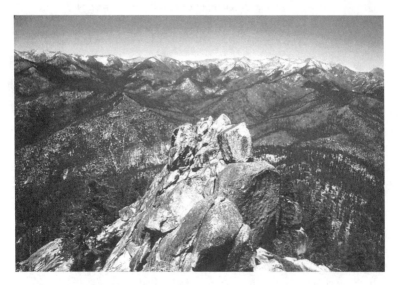

The Monarch Divide *from Lookout Peak*

Wildflowers

of Sheep Creek, which is lined with a verdant assortment of wildflowers, ferns, and small plants. After a short stroll alongside this pleasant stream, you cross the creek on a flat-topped log. ▶3

Steep

After following the north bank for a while, the trail veers away from the creek and then climbs across the east slope of Lookout Peak through more drought-tolerant vegetation. A protracted climb leads to a saddle at the signed boundary of Kings Canyon National Park and Sequoia National Forest. ▶4

Beyond the boundary, the condition of the trail deteriorates to a faint path that leads up to the crest of the peak's west ridge and then follows the ridge to the summit. In the absence of well-defined tread, small ducks may help guide you up the ridge, but the route is quite obvious. The path becomes more distinct again as the trail dips shortly, winds across a shrub-covered slope, and then zigzags toward the summit. Nearing the top, pick your way around large slabs and over boulders to emerge triumphantly on top of Lookout Peak. ▶5

Summit

Although a large microwave telephone reflector anchored to the top of the peak may detract from the sense of wildness, the view is nonetheless dramatic. Nearly 4,000 feet straight below is the South Fork Kings River, tumbling through the rugged and deep gorge of Kings Canyon. Across the canyon to the north, the Monarch Divide cuts a jagged profile across the azure Sierra sky. Looking east, the peaks of the Sierra Crest span the horizon. If you're fortunate enough to be here on a rare clear day following a cleansing summer rain, even the view across the San Joaquin Valley can be impressive.

 Great Views

🚶	**MILESTONES**	
▶1	0.0	Start at trailhead
▶2	0.9	Sheep Creek
▶3	3.0	West Branch Sheep Creek
▶4	4.3	Saddle at park boundary
▶5	5.0	Lookout Peak

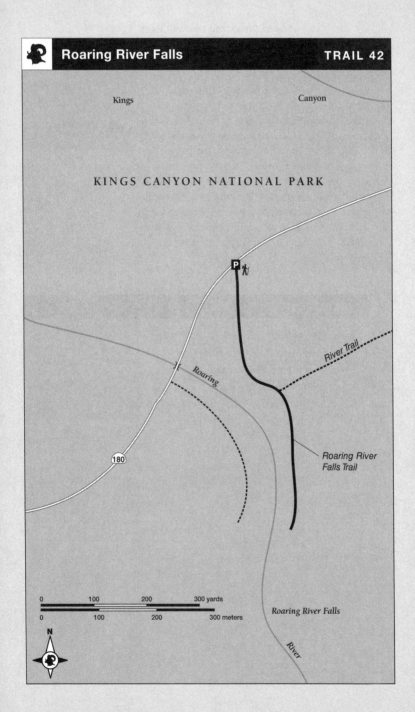

Kings

Canyon

KINGS CANYON NATIONAL PARK

River Trail

Roaring

180

Roaring River
Falls Trail

0   100   200   300 yards

0   100   200   300 meters

N

Roaring River Falls

River

Roaring River Falls

While the short trip to a view of Roaring River Falls is not much of a hike by most standards, the falls are impressive and should be seen at least once by anyone visiting Kings Canyon.

Best Times

While the highway into Cedar Grove is open from late April to mid-November, Roaring River Falls is best appreciated in late spring and early summer, when snowmelt in the higher elevations swells Roaring River into a wild torrent and the falls into a turbulent, raging, two-tiered cascade. However, the falls are still reasonably scenic later in the season because Roaring River always seems to have a dependable supply of water.

Finding the Trail

From Fresno, follow CA 180 east into Kings Canyon National Park and continue past Grant Grove into Kings Canyon. Drive 2.8 miles past the Cedar Grove turnoff to the signed parking area on the right. The National Park Service has four campgrounds in the Cedar Grove area: Sentinel, Sheep Creek, Canyon View, and Moraine (all of which have fees, flush toilets, running water, and bear boxes). Cedar Grove has a motel, showers, general store, restaurant, and laundry facilities.

TRAIL USE
Day Hike, Child Friendly

LENGTH
0.5 mile, ¼ hour

VERTICAL FEET
+100/-100/±200

DIFFICULTY
– **1** 2 3 4 5 +

TRAIL TYPE
Out-and-back

FEATURES
Waterfall

FACILITIES
Lodging
Store
Visitor Center
Post Office
Restrooms
Water
Picnic Area
Campgrounds
Stables

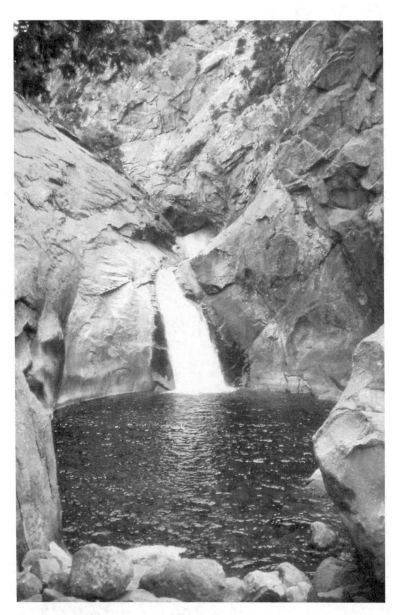

Roaring River Falls

Trail Description

▶1 Follow a paved path away from the parking area on the east side of Roaring River through mixed forest and foliage typical of Kings Canyon. A short, mild climb leads to a junction with the River Trail on the left, where you continue straight ahead a short distance to a viewpoint of the falls. ▶2

An alternate route heads west from the parking area and across the highway bridge to the start of dirt tread on the west side of Roaring River. The path heads above the west bank to a series of rock steps that lead down to a fenced viewpoint.

 Waterfall

🚶	**MILESTONES**	
▶1	0.0	Start at trailhead
▶2	0.25	Roaring River Falls viewpoint

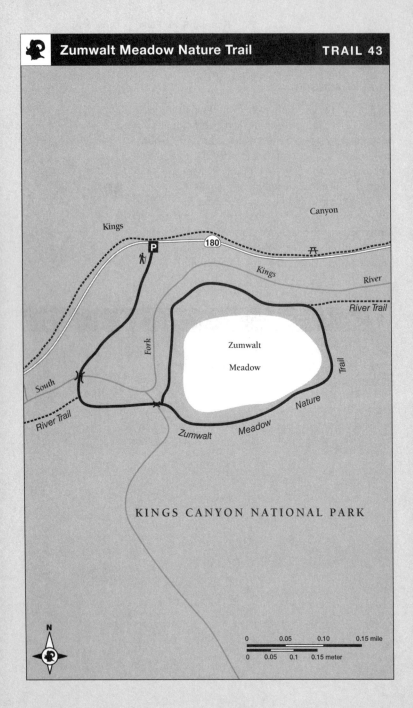

Canyon

Kings

P

180

Kings

River

Kings   River Trail

Fork

Zumwalt
Meadow

Trail

South

River Trail

Nature

Zumwalt   Meadow

KINGS CANYON NATIONAL PARK

N

| 0 | 0.05 | 0.10 | 0.15 mile |

| 0 | 0.05 | 0.1 | 0.15 meter |

Zumwalt Meadow Nature Trail

The easy 1.5-mile loop around Zumwalt Meadow provides a leisurely way to get acquainted with the ecology of Kings Canyon. An inexpensive pamphlet filled with interesting tidbits about the natural history of the immediate area is a fine complement to the journey around the meadow. Along with surveys of the verdant, grass- and flower-filled meadow, the short path offers plenty of additional scenery, from glimpses of the scenic South Fork Kings River to impressive views of the glistening granite spires and cliffs on the canyon walls, including Grand Sentinel and North Dome.

TRAIL USE
Day Hike, Child Friendly
LENGTH
1.5 miles, 1 hour
VERTICAL FEET
+100/-100/±200
DIFFICULTY
– **1** 2 3 4 5 +
TRAIL TYPE
Loop

FEATURES
Stream
Great Views

FACILITIES
Lodging
Store
Visitor Center
Post Office
Restrooms
Water
Picnic Area
Campgrounds
Stables

Best Time

The road into Kings Canyon is usually open from late May to mid-November, with the majority of tourists visiting the area between Memorial Day and Labor Day weekends. South Fork Kings River is a raging torrent in late spring, when the meadow grass is green and wildflowers add splashes of color. Summer temperatures can be hot; an afternoon dip in the reduced river flow offers a refreshing alternative for beating the heat. Autumn, when many of the tourists are gone and the weather is pleasant, can be a fine time for a visit as well.

Finding the Trail

From Fresno, follow CA 180 east into Kings Canyon National Park and continue past Grant Grove into Kings Canyon. Continue up-canyon to the Zumwalt Meadow parking lot, 4.25 miles east of the turnoff

Daniel K. Zumwalt

Daniel K. Zumwalt was a land agent and attorney for the Southern Pacific Railroad who, along with his employee Jesse Agnew acquired 120 acres of land near Cedar Grove. Zumwalt was a strong advocate for preserving the natural heritage of the area, influencing the decision to set aside land for General Grant (subsequently incorporated into the much larger Kings Canyon National Park) and Sequoia National Parks in 1890.

to Cedar Grove. The National Park Service has four campgrounds in the Cedar Grove area: Sentinel, Sheep Creek, Canyon View, and Moraine (all of which have fees, flush toilets, running water, and bear boxes). Cedar Grove has a motel, showers, general store, restaurant, and laundry facilities.

Trail Description

▶1 Your first stop along the Zumwalt Meadow Nature Trail should be at the trailhead signboard, where, for a nominal fee, you can purchase a pamphlet with a map and detailed information corresponding to the 18 numbered posts placed along the self-guiding trail. Once you're armed with a pamphlet, follow a wide path to a suspension bridge spanning South Fork Kings River. Along the way and on the bridge, you have fine views of verdant Zumwalt Meadow, the river, and Grand Sentinel rising sharply above the canyon floor. Immediately beyond the bridge is a junction with the River Trail. ▶2

> Along the way and on the bridge, you have fine views of verdant Zumwalt Meadow, the river, and Grand Sentinel.

Turn left (east) and proceed upstream on the River Trail through cool forest, soon arriving at the westernmost junction with the Zumwalt Meadow Nature Trail. ▶3 Proceed straight ahead at the junction, leaving the forest canopy behind to follow a brief climb across an exposed talus field above the meadow. From this slightly higher vantage, you have fine views across the meadow and the river

Great Views

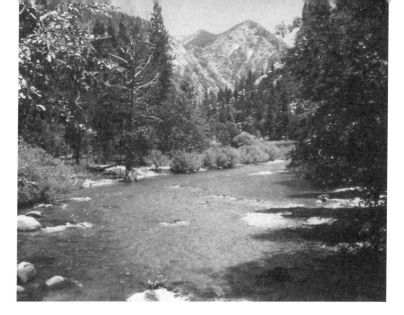

South Fork Kings River

to the far canyon wall. Soon, reach the easternmost junction of the nature trail. ▶4

Turn left at the junction, leaving the River Trail to skirt the fringe of the grassy meadow on the way toward the riverbank. Then follow the meandering river downstream, aided by a section of boardwalk, to the close of the loop at the westernmost junction of the nature trail. ▶5 From there, retrace your steps to the junction near the bridge. ▶6 Turn right at the junction, cross the bridge, and then retrace your steps back to the parking lot. ▶7

🚶	**MILESTONES**	
▶1	0.0	Start at trailhead
▶2	0.25	Left at junction
▶3	0.35	Straight at junction
▶4	0.65	Left at junction
▶5	1.1	Right at junction
▶6	1.25	Right at junction
▶7	1.5	End at trailhead

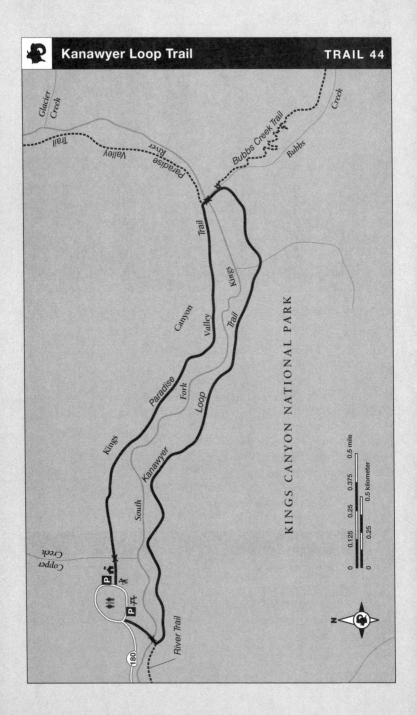

Kanawyer Loop Trail

Roads End is a very popular trailhead for the army of recreationists bound for trips into the heart of the southern Sierra. Chances are you will share the first half of this loop trip with plenty of backpackers, day hikers, and equestrians headed for popular destinations accessed by the Paradise Valley and Bubbs Creek Trails. However, on the second half of the journey the troops drop off considerably, allowing the notion of quiet solitude in the upper end of Kings Canyon to be a real possibility. The loop is an easy stroll across the nearly level valley floor, making this a trip well suited for hikers at any level of skill and fitness. Be prepared for hot afternoon temperatures in summer, but relief via a refreshing dip in the chilly waters of South Fork Kings River is never too far away.

Best Time

The road into Kings Canyon is usually open from late May to mid-November, with the majority of tourists visiting the area between Memorial Day and Labor Day weekends. South Fork Kings River is a raging torrent in late spring, when the meadow grass is green and wildflowers add splashes of color. Summer temperatures can be hot; an afternoon dip in the reduced river flow offers a refreshing alternative for beating the heat. Autumn, when many of the tourists are gone and the weather is pleasant, can be a fine time for a visit as well.

TRAIL USE
Day Hike, Run, Horse, Child Friendly

LENGTH
4.7 miles, 2½ hours

VERTICAL FEET
+275/-275/±550

DIFFICULTY
– 1 **2** 3 4 5 +

TRAIL TYPE
Loop

FEATURES
Stream
Great Views
Fishing

FACILITIES
Lodging
Store
Visitor Center
Post Office
Restrooms
Water
Picnic Area
Campgrounds
Stables

Finding the Trail

From Fresno, follow CA 180 east into Kings Canyon National Park and continue past Grant Grove into Kings Canyon. Continue up-canyon to the day-use parking area at Roads End, 5 miles east of the turnoff to Cedar Grove. The National Park Service has four campgrounds in the Cedar Grove area: Sentinel, Sheep Creek, Canyon View, and Moraine (all of which have fees, flush toilets, running water, and bear boxes). Cedar Grove has a motel, showers, general store, restaurant, and laundry facilities.

Trail Description

From the parking area, walk to the well-signed trailhead ▶1 at the east end of the paved turnaround at Roads End, near the rustic cabin that serves as the wilderness permit office. Follow a wide, sandy, gently ascending path that parallels the river through a mixed forest of incense cedars, ponderosa pines, black oaks, sugar pines, and white firs to a bridge across Copper Creek. Continue up-canyon into thinning forest cover, with occasional views of the impressive granite walls of Kings Canyon, which are often compared favorably to the more

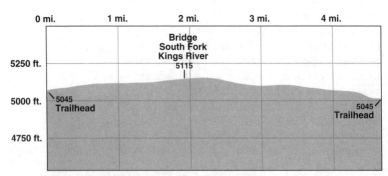

TRAIL 44 Kanawyer Loop Elevation Profile

famous walls of Yosemite Valley. Soon you enter a shady forest of ponderosa pines, sugar pines, white firs, and alders on the way to a Y-junction with the Paradise Valley Trail. ▶2

Turn right (south) at the junction and immediately cross a bridge over the river, just downstream from its confluence with Bubbs Creek. Soon, you reach another junction, ▶3 this one between the Bubbs Creek Trail headed southeast and the Kanawyer Trail headed southwest.

Turn right and follow the Kanawyer Trail, where you may notice evidence of a recent fire. Cross Avalanche Creek on a pair of logs and follow gently graded trail through dense forest. Past a small meadow, the trail draws closer to the south bank of the river, where anglers can easily drop a line. As you continue downstream, the forest parts just enough on occasion to allow grand views of the canyon walls. A very brief climb through a boulder field leads to a junction ▶4 with the River Trail near a bridge across the river.

Turn right, cross the bridge, and follow gently ascending trail through dense forest and lush ground cover to the day-use parking lot. ▶5

> The loop is an easy stroll across the nearly level valley floor, making this a trip well suited for hikers at any level of skill and fitness.

 Fishing

🔭 Great Views

	MILESTONES	
▶1	0.0	Start at trailhead
▶2	1.9	Right at Paradise Valley Trail junction
▶3	2.0	Right at Kanawyer Trail junction
▶4	4.5	Right at River Trail junction
▶5	4.7	End at parking area

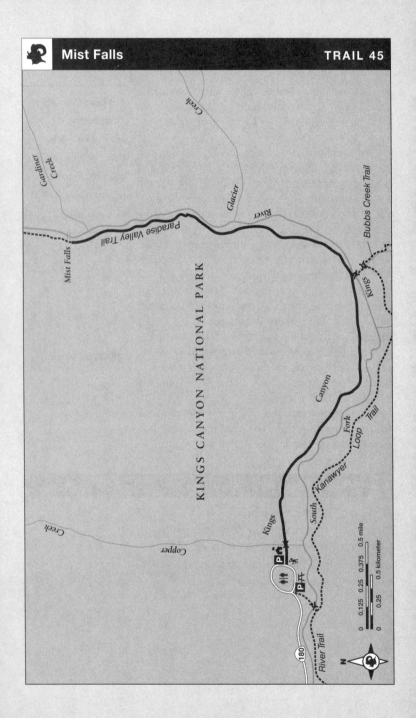

Mist Falls **TRAIL 45**

Gardiner Creek

Creek

Glacier

River

Mist Falls

Paradise Valley Trail

Bubbs Creek Trail

Kings

KINGS CANYON NATIONAL PARK

Canyon

Fork Loop Trail

Kanawyer

South

Kings

Copper Creek

0 0.125 0.25 0.375 0.5 mile

0 0.25 0.5 kilometer

180

River Trail

N

Mist Falls

The nearly 4-mile trek to Mist Falls is a must-do hike for anyone visiting Kings Canyon, especially early in the season when the falls are at peak glory. The first half of the trail follows the relatively flat floor of Kings Canyon, with the second half climbing moderately up the South Fork Kings River gorge toward Paradise Valley. The trail is a popular one, not only with day hikers, but also with backpackers on the Rae Lakes Loop. Consequently, you shouldn't expect a high dose of solitude.

TRAIL USE
Day Hike, Run, Horse
LENGTH
7.8 miles, 4 hours
VERTICAL FEET
+775/-775/±1550
DIFFICULTY
– 1 2 **3** 4 5 +
TRAIL TYPE
Out-and-back

FEATURES
Canyon
Stream
Waterfall
Fishing

FACILITIES
Lodging
Store
Visitor Center
Post Office
Restrooms
Water
Picnic Area
Campgrounds
Stables

Best Time

The falls are best appreciated in late spring and early summer, when South Fork Kings River is swollen with snowmelt. By midsummer the falls become fairly tame.

Finding the Trail

From Fresno, follow CA 180 east into Kings Canyon National Park and continue past Grant Grove into Kings Canyon. Continue up-canyon to the day-use parking area at Roads End, 5 miles east of the turnoff to Cedar Grove. The National Park Service has four campgrounds in the Cedar Grove area: Sentinel, Sheep Creek, Canyon View, and Moraine (all of which have fees, flush toilets, running water, and bear boxes). Cedar Grove has a motel, showers, general store, restaurant, and laundry facilities.

Trail Description

The aptly named falls tumbles over a precipitous cliff and smashes into boulders and rocks near the base.

From the parking area, walk to the well-signed trailhead ▶1 at the east end of the paved turnaround at Roads End, near the rustic cabin that serves as the wilderness permit office. Follow a wide, sandy, gently ascending path that parallels the river through a mixed forest of incense cedars, ponderosa pines, black oaks, sugar pines, and white firs to a bridge across Copper Creek. Continue up-canyon into thinning forest cover, which allows occasional views of the impressive granite walls of Kings Canyon, which are often compared favorably to the more famous walls of Yosemite Valley. Soon you enter a shady forest on the way to a Y-junction with the Bubbs Creek Trail. ▶2

Veer left at the junction and follow ascending trail through a mixed forest of alders, black oaks, canyon live oaks, incense cedars, ponderosa pines, and white firs. Occasional clearings in the forest are carpeted with manzanita and mountain mahogany, while ferns and thimbleberries thrive in damper soils. The trail follows the course of the river past delightful pools and tumbling cascades, arcing around the base of Beck Peak. Anglers can work their way down to the bank and ply the waters for rainbow and brown trout. Buck, Sphinx, and

Fishing 🎣

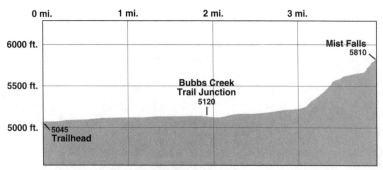

TRAIL 45 Mist Falls Elevation Profile

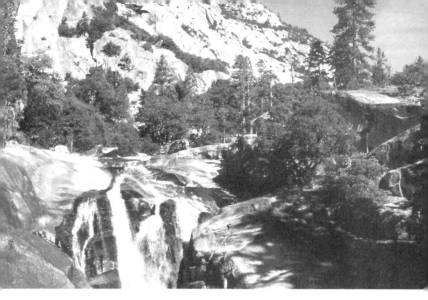

Mist Falls

Avalanche Peaks play hide and seek through gaps in the forest cover. Ascending over rock steps and slabs, continue up the narrow chasm of the canyon with occasional views of the dramatic canyon topography. Following a long, forested stretch of trail, the thundering roar from Mist Falls becomes progressively louder the farther up the trail you travel. Soon a use trail splits away from the Paradise Valley Trail to the right and leads over large boulders to a viewpoint near the base of Mist Falls. ►3

The aptly named falls tumbles over a precipitous cliff and smashes into boulders and rocks near the base, creating a spray of mist that catapults down-canyon and coats everything in its path. Even on hot summer days, you can feel cool and moist below the falls, an attribute that must certainly add to this destination's popularity.

 Waterfall

🚶	**MILESTONES**	
►1	0.0	Start at trailhead
►2	1.9	Left at junction
►3	3.9	Mist Falls

Rae Lakes Loop

Many consider the Rae Lakes Loop the quintessential High Sierra backpacking trip, and the stiff competition for wilderness permits would certainly indicate such. The Rae Lakes Basin is blessed with beautiful subalpine scenery as fine as any in the High Sierra, with crystalline lakes reflecting a bevy of glacier-sculpted domes and serrated peaks. Getting to the basin has its own rewards, including visits to Mist Falls, Paradise Valley, Castle Domes Meadow, and Woods Crossing. An easy cross-country jaunt through picturesque Sixty Lake Basin is a must-do extension from Rae Lakes. Beyond Rae Lakes the trail climbs to a high point at Glen Pass and then descends to lovely Vidette Meadows before a long descent along Bubbs Creek leads back to Kings Canyon.

TRAIL USE
Backpack, Horse

LENGTH
41.6 miles, 3–6 days

VERTICAL FEET
+7500/-7500/±15000

DIFFICULTY
– 1 2 3 **4-5** +

TRAIL TYPE
Loop

FEATURES
Canyon
Mountain
Lakes
Streams
Waterfall
Wildflowers
Great Views
Camping
Swimming
Steep
Fishing

FACILITIES
Lodging

Best Time

Snow leaves the higher elevations by mid-July following an average winter, and the typically sunny and mild Sierra weather continues through summer. Early autumn can be a pleasant time for this loop, when the crowds diminish and the weather, although cooler, is oftentimes mild and sunny during the day. The first significant snowfall at these elevations usually comes sometime by late October or early November.

Finding the Trail

From Fresno, follow CA 180 east into Kings Canyon National Park and continue past Grant Grove into Kings Canyon. Continue up-canyon to the overnight parking lot at Roads End, 5 miles from the turnoff to Cedar Grove. The National Park Service has four campgrounds in the Cedar Grove area: Sentinel, Sheep Creek, Canyon View, and Moraine (all of which have fees, flush toilets, running water, and bear boxes). Cedar Grove has a motel, showers, general store, restaurant, and laundry facilities.

Logistics

Wilderness permits are at a premium for this extremely popular route. Make advance reservations as soon as possible. Walk-in permits are easier to procure for trips not starting on weekends. Two-night camping limits are in place for Paradise Valley, Rae Lakes Basin (including Dollar and Arrowhead Lakes), and Charlotte Lake. Bear canisters are required. Campfires are not allowed above 10,000 feet.

Trail Description

►1 The well-signed trail begins at the east edge of the paved turnaround, near the wilderness permit station. Follow wide, sandy, gently ascending tread, roughly paralleling South Fork Kings River, through a mixed forest of incense cedars, ponderosa pines,

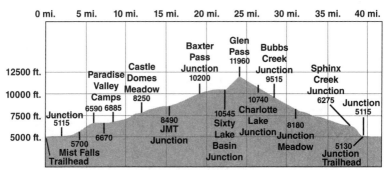

TRAIL 46 Rae Lakes Loop Elevation Profile

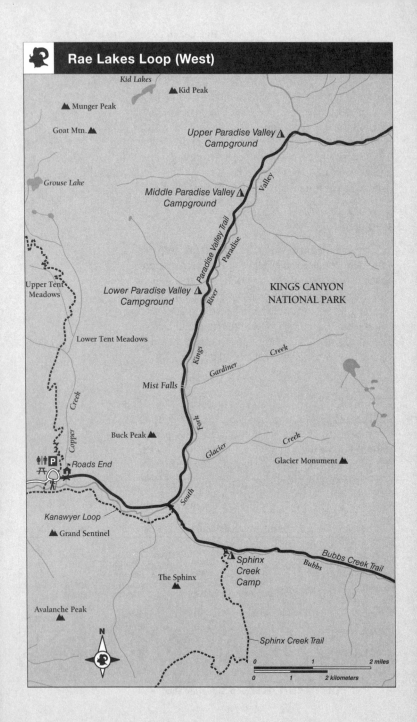

Rae Lakes Loop (West)

Kid Lakes

▲ Kid Peak

▲ Munger Peak

Goat Mtn. ▲

Upper Paradise Valley ▲
Campground

Valley

Grouse Lake

Middle Paradise Valley ▲
Campground

Paradise

Paradise Valley Trail

Upper Tent
Meadows

Lower Paradise Valley ▲
Campground

KINGS CANYON
NATIONAL PARK

River

Kings

Lower Tent Meadows

Gardiner   Creek

Creek

Mist Falls

Fork

Copper

Buck Peak ▲

Glacier   Creek

Glacier Monument ▲

⚥ P
⛺ Roads End

South

Kanawyer Loop

▲ Grand Sentinel

Sphinx
Creek
Camp

Bubbs

Bubbs Creek Trail

The Sphinx ▲

Avalanche Peak
▲

N

Sphinx Creek Trail

| 0 | | 1 | | 2 miles |
| 0 | 1 | | 2 kilometers | |

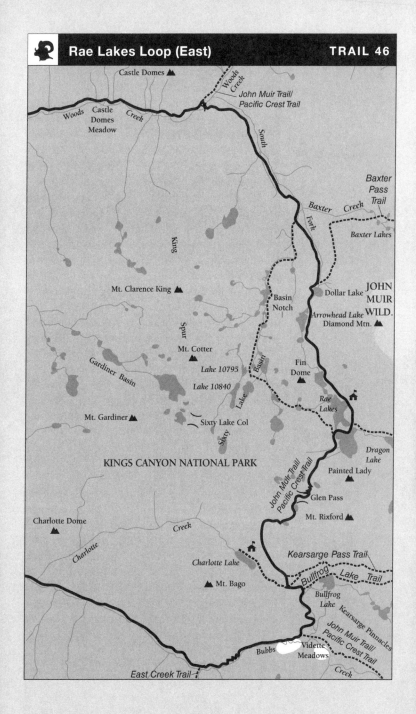

Castle Domes ▲

Woods Creek

John Muir Trail/
Pacific Crest Trail

Woods Creek

Castle
Domes
Meadow

South

Baxter
Pass
Trail

Baxter Creek

Fork

Baxter Lakes

King

Dollar Lake

JOHN
MUIR
WILD.

Mt. Clarence King ▲

Basin
Notch

Arrowhead Lake
Diamond Mtn. ▲

Spur

Mt. Cotter ▲

Lake 10795

Lake 10840

Basin

Fin
Dome

Rae
Lakes

Gardiner Basin

Lake

Mt. Gardiner ▲

Sixty Lake Col

Sixty

Dragon
Lake

KINGS CANYON NATIONAL PARK

Painted Lady ▲

John Muir Trail/
Pacific Crest Trail

Glen Pass

Mt. Rixford ▲

Charlotte Dome
▲

Creek

Kearsarge Pass Trail

Charlotte

Charlotte Lake

Bullfrog Lake Trail

▲ Mt. Bago

Bullfrog
Lake

Kearsarge Pinnacles

John Muir Trail/
Pacific Crest Trail

Bubbs Vidette
Meadows

East Creek Trail

Creek

black oaks, sugar pines, and white firs. Soon cross a wood bridge over Copper Creek and proceed up the canyon into thinning forest cover, which allows views of the impressive granite walls forming the canyon. Enter cool forest on the way to a signed Y-junction ▶2 with the Bubbs Creek Trail, 2 miles from the trailhead.

Great Views 🔭

Veer left at the junction and ascend through a mixed forest of alders, black oaks, canyon live oaks, incense cedars, white firs, and ponderosa pines. Sunny slopes are covered with manzanita and mountain mahogany, while ferns and thimbleberries thrive in the damper, shady soils. Follow the course of South Fork Kings River past delightful pools and tumbling cascades, while arcing around the base of Buck Peak, which, along with The Sphinx and Avalanche Peak on the opposite side of the canyon, plays hide and seek through gaps in the forest cover. Ascending rock slabs and steps, continue up the narrow chasm with periodic views of the dramatic canyon topography. After a long, forested stretch, you begin to hear the thunderous roar emanating from Mist Falls. ▶3 Soon, you reach a use trail branching to the right, which leads toward the river and a scramble over large boulders to a view of the falls near the base.

Waterfall 🏞

Aptly named Mist Falls tumbles over a precipitous cliff and smashes into the boulders and rocks at the bottom. A spray of mist catapults down the canyon, coating everything in its path. Even later in summer, when days are characteristically hot, the area around the falls is cool and moist. As with most Sierra waterfalls, Mist Falls is best appreciated in early summer, when the river is swollen with snowmelt and the falls are pouring hard and fast. By mid- to late summer, the falls become fairly tame.

From Mist Falls, continue upstream on a moderate climb following the course of the river up the canyon. One section of the river is quite picturesque, where the water dances over granite slabs before tumbling into a sculpted pool. Follow the well-used trail past large boulders and up rock-stepped switchbacks, with occasional views of the canyon and the towering peaks above. Just before the lip of Paradise Valley, the grade eases on the way into a mixed forest of red firs, lodgepole and Jeffrey pines, stands of aspen, and an occasional western juniper. A tangle of driftwood chokes the slow-moving river, heralding your arrival at the lower end of the valley. A short distance ahead is Lower Paradise Valley Camp, ▶4 5.8 miles from Roads End. The camp has designated sites, a pit toilet, and bear boxes.

 Camping

Continue through Paradise Valley on a gentle stroll alongside the river through a mixed forest to Middle Paradise Valley Camp, ▶5 7.25 miles from the trailhead, where more designated campsites (bear boxes) provide overnight possibilities.

Proceed upstream on gently graded trail through stands of conifers alternating with clearings with grand views of the steep-walled South Fork canyon. After a while, a more moderate ascent ensues, followed by a stretch of nearly level tread across a flower-filled meadow. At 8.4 miles, reach the final camping area in the valley at Upper Paradise Valley Camp, ▶6 with more designated campsites and bear boxes.

 Great Views

 Wildflowers

 Camping

Immediately beyond the camp, a system of logs allows for a straightforward crossing to the east bank of South Fork Kings River, just upstream from the confluence of Woods Creek. This crossing may be difficult in early season. The first half mile beyond the crossing is a gentle climb away from Woods Creek, but then the trail draws nearer to the creek and begins a moderate climb up the steep-walled valley for the next couple of miles. Along the way, periodic avalanches have swept the slope, allowing good views of the granite canyon walls and domes above. After the crossings of two side streams,

 Great Views

emerge into Castle Domes Meadow, ▶7 where campsites (bear box) can be found near the east edge, 12 miles from the trailhead.

Camping Λ

Beyond the meadow, gently ascending tread heads east toward a junction with the John Muir Trail (JMT) through primarily lodgepole pine forest. Reach the well-signed JMT junction, ▶8 15.4 miles from the trailhead. Just up a hillside, about 150 yards to the north, is an open-air pit toilet.

Turn right (south) at the junction and soon arrive at roaring Woods Creek. Fortunately, a suspension bridge, built in 1988, provides a welcome alternative to an otherwise difficult ford. Previously built bridges across the creek were subject to periodic washouts. Cross the lively bridge, one person at a time, and reach the overused campsites above the south bank

Camping Λ

(bear boxes). Although the area has numerous fire rings, finding enough wood for a fire will be an increasing challenge as the season progresses at this extremely popular overnight destination.

Away from Woods Creek Crossing, curve around the north end of King Spur and begin a moderate climb up the lightly forested canyon of South Fork Woods Creek, passing through stands of red fir, lodgepole pine, and aspen alternating with sagebrush-covered slopes and pockets of verdant foliage. The steady ascent continues well above the creek, leading across a stream draining a pair of unnamed tarns below King Spur and across exposed, rocky terrain to a boggy meadow. Beyond the meadow, pass through a gap in a drift fence, ascend over a rocky ridge, and come to a pair of campsites near the crossing of the willow- and wildflower-lined stream draining Sixty Lake Basin. A mile-long ascent through diminishing forest cover leads to a junction ▶9 with the Baxter Pass Trail, just north of Dollar Lake, 19.1 miles from the trailhead, where an old post marks the junction. Solitude seekers, perhaps weary of the heavy traffic on the

JMT, should find the 2-plus-mile climb to decent campsites on the shore of the largest Baxter Lake a worthy diversion.

Although Dollar Lake has a few passable camp-sites, better sites can be found a short distance ahead at Arrowhead Lake. Leaving Dollar Lake, continue the ascent on the JMT with improving scenery, including views of King Spur and Fine Dome, on the way past a small waterfall and to a crossing of the creek. Just beyond the crossing, a use trail veers around the north end of Arrowhead Lake to campsites (bear box).

Waterfall

Away from Arrowhead Lake, a short climb through widely scattered lodgepole pines and past a small, unnamed lake, leads over the lip of Rae Lakes Basin and the first of the three Rae Lakes. Campsites (bear boxes) are along the shore of the first lake and also at the middle lake, where a ranger cabin is tucked into the pines above the northeast shore. Gently ascending tread leads across the basin around the east side of the first two lakes to upper Rae Lake, where a trail heads east to more-secluded campsites near Dragon Lake. The trail then bends around the north shore of the upper lake and fords a short stretch of creek between the two uppermost lakes.

Lake

Camping

Lake

Camping

The Rae Lakes Basin is one of the most scenic areas of the Sierra Nevada, with great views of monolithic Fin Dome, rugged King Spur, multihued Painted Lady, and rugged peaks along the Sierra Crest a fine complement to the sparkling, island-dotted lakes, bordered by glistening granite slabs and pockets of verdant, flower-carpeted meadows. Fishing for brook and rainbow trout is reported to be fair, despite the obvious pressure the area receives. Swimmers will find the waters chilly but refreshing. Although the stunning scenery is more than worthy of a multiday visit, park regulations limit camping to two nights only. Just past the ford

Great Views

Wildflowers

Fishing

Swimming

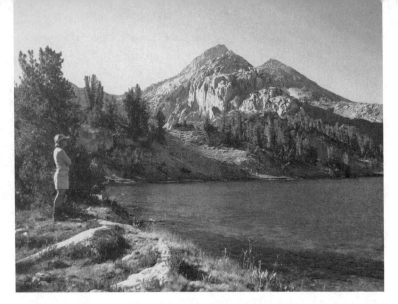

Sixty Lake Basin

between the two uppermost lakes, reach a junction ▶10 with the Sixty Lake Basin Trail, 22.2 miles from the trailhead.

SIDE TRIP TO SIXTY LAKE BASIN: Any trip to Rae Lakes without a visit to Sixty Lake Basin would be incomplete. Although the trail is unmaintained, the route through the basin has been so well used over the years that defined tread is easy to follow. Once hikers reach the mostly open basin, cross-country travel between the lakes is fairly straightforward, with plenty of nooks and crannies awaiting exploration.

From the junction at the northwest shore of upper Rae Lake, head south along the southwest shore of the middle lake, traverse a marshy clearing, and climb northwest to the lip of a small basin overlooking a tarn below. The view of Rae Lakes during this ascent is superb. Drop around the north side of the tarn and climb shortly up to a saddle in the ridge dividing Rae Lakes and Sixty Lake Basins, where Mount Clarence King and Mount Cotter dominate the impressive view to the northwest. A winding, rocky descent leads to the shore of an irregular-shaped lake (10,925'±), with campsites near the outlet.

Continuing northwest, round a ridge and enter the heart of Sixty Lake Basin, approaching a sizable, island-dotted lake (10.795'±), 1.9 miles from the junction. The trail continues north from here, eventually deteriorating to a cross-country route following the basin's outlet stream to a junction with the JMT, just south of Baxter Creek. You also have the option of returning to the JMT over Basin Notch, via a straightforward route through a gap in a ridge about 1 mile north of Fin Dome. From the notch, descend to the west shore of Arrowhead Lake and work around the lake to the JMT above the east shore. **END SIDE TRIP**

From the Sixty Lake Basin junction, pass above the west shore of upper Rae Lake and then begin a 2-mile climb to Glen Pass, switchbacking through diminishing vegetation on the way to a tarn-dotted, rock-filled bench. From there, a winding ascent leads to the crest of a ridge, which is followed for a short distance to 11,978-foot Glen Pass, ►11 24.1 miles from the trailhead. The view is rather scanty compared to other High Sierra passes, hemmed in by the topography, but you do have a fine farewell vista of Rae Lakes.

 Great Views

From Glen Pass, the trail makes a rocky, switchbacking descent; passes a pair of greenish-colored, rockbound tarns; and then crosses a seasonal stream with a pair of poor campsites nearby. The descent continues beside more rocks and boulders until reaching more-hospitable terrain farther down the slope, where the trail veers southeast. The grade eases on a descending traverse across a lodgepole pine–covered hillside above Charlotte Lake, where brief gaps in the forest allow views of the lake and Charlotte Dome farther down Charlotte Creek canyon. At 2 miles from the pass, reach a junction ►12 with a connector to the Kearsarge Pass Trail.

Continue south on the JMT, breaking out of the trees to a good view of Mount Bago, and then stroll across a sandy flat to a four-way junction, ▶13 0.3 mile from the previous junction. Here, the Kearsarge Pass Trail heads northeast and the Charlotte Lake Trail heads northwest 0.8 mile to excellent campsites (bear boxes) around the lake (two-night camping limit).

Camping

Remaining on the JMT, head away from the junction and climb east over a low rise. From there, short-legged switchbacks lead downhill through dense forest to a junction ▶14 with the Bullfrog Lake Trail, which climbs northeast to the picturesque lake (no camping) and continues east to Kearsarge Lakes (two-night camping limit).

From the junction, the descent continues, crossing Bullfrog Lake's outlet twice on the way to Lower Vidette Meadow and a junction ▶15 with the Bubbs Creek Trail, 4.1 miles from Glen Pass.

Turn away from the JMT and head west on Bubbs Creek Trail on a short descent to the north edge of expansive Lower Vidette Meadow. Overnighters will find excellent, but heavily used, campsites (bear box) nestled beneath lodgepole pines along the meadow's fringe.

Camping

Leaving the gently graded trail along the meadow behind, follow a more-pronounced descent as the now tumbling creek plunges down the gorge. Momentarily break out into the open, where a large hump of granite provides an excellent vantage from which to survey the surrounding terrain. Head back into forest cover and continue down the canyon, stepping over a number of lushly lined freshets along the way. The forest breaks enough on occasion to allow views of the dramatic topography above East Creek canyon, including Mount Brewer, North Guard, and Mount Farquhar. Farther down Bubbs Creek, picturesque waterfalls and cascades provide additional visual treats. The stiff descent

Great Views

eventually eases near the edge of grassy, fern-filled, and wildflower-covered Junction Meadow. Stroll across the meadow to a signed, three-way junction ►16 of the East Creek Trail, 2.9 miles from the JMT junction. Campsites can be found shortly down this trail on either side of a ford of Bubbs Creek, and farther west on the Bubbs Creek Trail, past the horse camp.

 Wildflowers

Head away from Junction Meadow, as the moderate descent down the canyon resumes alongside turbulent Bubbs Creek through the moderate cover of a white-fir forest. After nearly 2 miles of steady descent, the creek mellows and the grade eases through an aspen grove with a floor of ferns on the way to a log crossing over Charlotte Creek. Nearby, a short lateral leads to campsites near Bubbs Creek, where fishing for rainbow, brook, and brown trout is reportedly good.

 Camping

 Camping

Gently graded trail continues for a while beyond Charlotte Creek, as you hop across a trio of side streams and stroll through shoulder-high ferns, before Bubbs Creek returns to its tumultuous course down the gorge. A steady, moderate descent follows the course of the creek for the next several miles. Farther down the canyon, moderate forest gives way to a light covering of trees, composed mainly of Jeffrey pines, with lesser amounts of firs, incense cedars, and black oaks. Reach Sphinx Creek Camp and a junction of the Sphinx Creek Trail, 9.7 miles from the JMT. ►17

 Fishing

 Camping

Away from Sphinx Creek, the trail descends moderately through coniferous forest and then mixed forest on the way to a series of switchbacks that zigzag down the east wall of Kings Canyon. Reach the floor of the canyon, cross a series of short wood bridges across multiple channels of Bubbs Creek, and reach a junction ►18 with the Kanawyer Loop Trail on the left. Continue ahead from the junction, cross South Fork Kings River on a bridge, and immediately reach a junction ▶19 with the Paradise Valley Trail, closing the loop. From there, retrace your steps 2 miles to the Roads End trailhead. ▶20

| 🚶 | **MILESTONES** |

▶1	0.0	Start at Roads End trailhead
▶2	2.0	Left at Bubbs Creek/Paradise Valley junction
▶3	3.9	Mist Falls
▶4	5.8	Lower Paradise Valley Camp
▶5	7.25	Middle Paradise Valley Camp
▶6	8.4	Upper Paradise Valley Camp
▶7	12.0	Castle Domes Meadow
▶8	15.4	Right at John Muir Trail junction
▶9	19.1	Baxter Pass Trail
▶10	22.2	Sixty Lake Basin junction
▶11	24.1	Glen Pass
▶12	26.1	Straight at connector junction
▶13	26.4	Straight at Charlotte Lake/Kearsarge Pass junction
▶14	26.9	Straight at Bullfrog Lake junction
▶15	28.2	Right at Bubbs Creek Trail junction
▶16	31.1	Straight at Junction Meadow junction
▶17	37.8	Straight at Sphinx Creek Camp junction
▶18	39.5	Straight at Kanawyer Loop junction
▶19	39.6	Left at Bubbs Creek/Paradise Valley junction
▶20	41.6	Roads End trailhead

Hotel and Lewis Creeks Loop and Cedar Grove Overlook

Consumed by the 2015 Rough Fire, the slopes on the north side of Kings Canyon once boasted a very diverse flora, from the riparian woodland community along the banks of South Fork Kings River to the mixed coniferous forest and chaparral communities of the canyon rim. Hikers now have the opportunity to watch the regeneration of these communities during the plant succession following such a major fire. Whether opting for the out-and-back hike to Cedar Grove Overlook or the full loop, trail users will experience extraordinary views of Kings Canyon and the surrounding terrain, including the Monarch Divide. Check with the National Park Service about current conditions.

Best Time

Snow usually leaves the trail by sometime in early May and generally doesn't return until November. Since the trail is located on a south-facing slope, an early start to beat the heat will be appreciated on the stiff climb out of Kings Canyon.

Finding the Trail

From Fresno, follow CA 180 east into Kings Canyon National Park and continue past Grant Grove into Kings Canyon. Continue up-canyon to the signed turnoff to Cedar Grove, turn left, and follow signs for the pack station. At 0.5 mile from the highway, turn right and immediately come to the Hotel Creek Trailhead on the left. If you have the luxury of two vehicles, or can arrange for someone to pick you

TRAIL USE
Day Hike, Run, Horse
LENGTH
4.8 miles, 3 hours to
Cedar Grove Overlook
6.4 miles, 3–4 hours
for loop
VERTICAL FEET
+1525/-125/±3300
+2100/-2100/±4200
DIFFICULTY
– 1 2 3 **4** 5 +
TRAIL TYPE
Out-and-back, Loop

FEATURES
Canyon
Streams
Wildflowers
Great Views

FACILITIES
Lodging
Store
Visitor Center
Post Office
Restrooms
Water
Picnic Area
Campgrounds
Stables

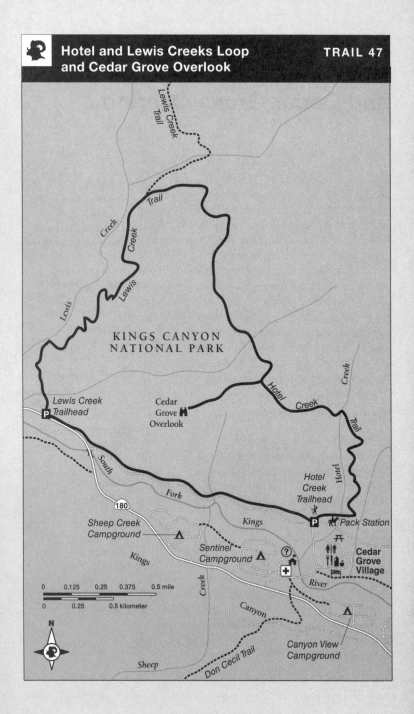

KINGS CANYON NATIONAL PARK

Lewis Creek Trail

Creek

Lewis Creek

Lewis

Lewis Creek Trailhead

Cedar Grove Overlook

Hotel Creek

Creek

Trail

Hotel

South Fork

Kings

Hotel Creek Trailhead

Pack Station

180

Sheep Creek Campground

Kings

Sentinel Campground

Cedar Grove Village

Creek

River

Canyon

Canyon View Campground

Sheep

Don Cecil Trail

0   0.125   0.25   0.375   0.5 mile
0   0.25   0.5 kilometer

N

up, 1.4 miles of uninteresting hiking can be saved by ending the trip at the Lewis Creek Trailhead, which is on the north shoulder of CA 180 (0.4 mile east of the park boundary and 1.3 miles west of the Cedar Grove junction). The National Park Service has four campgrounds in the Cedar Grove area: Sentinel, Sheep Creek, Canyon View, and Moraine (all of which have fees, flush toilets, running water, and bear boxes). Cedar Grove has a motel, showers, general store, restaurant, and laundry facilities.

Trail Description

▶1 Follow the Hotel Creek Trail up a hillside to a junction with a lateral from the pack station. Continue the ascent on the main trail, soon hearing the roar of the creek ahead. Reach the west bank of Hotel Creek, where a short use trail heads down to the water's edge, a convenient spot from which to filter water for the stiff and exposed climb above. The trail veers away from the creek and attacks the hillside on a series of switchbacks up the north wall of Kings Canyon. The switchbacks eventually end, where the trail veers west away from the creek and the steep ascent is mercifully replaced by a mild to moderate

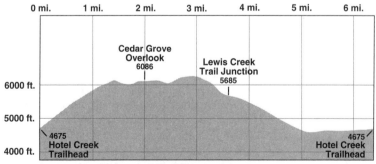

TRAIL 47 Hotel and Lewis Creeks Loop and Cedar Grove Overlook Elevation Profile

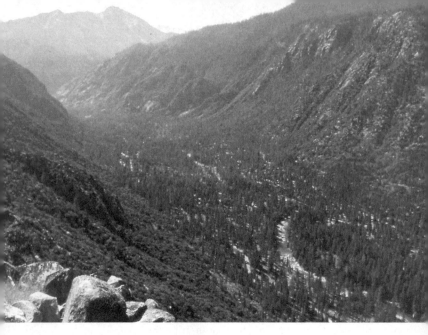

Kings Canyon *from Cedar Grove Overlook*

climb that leads to a junction ▶2 with a trail on the left to Cedar Grove Overlook.

A half-mile detour from the loop route allows you to enjoy a supreme view of Kings Canyon and the Monarch Divide. Turn left (west) at the junction and gently descend through scattered pines with views to the north of Monarch Divide. After a quarter mile, you reach a low spot on a ridge and then begin a mild, short climb toward the overlook, ▶3 a knob of granite near the end of a ridge. From this aerie, you gaze spellbound straight down 1,500 feet to Cedar Grove at the bottom of Kings Canyon. The bird's-eye view of South Fork Kings River is expansive, spanning from the western foothills to the confluence of Bubbs Creek. To the north, peaks of the Monarch Divide are quite impressive as well. After fully appreciating the view, retrace your steps to the junction. If you're just doing the out-and-back hike, retrace your steps from the junction and return to the Hotel Creek Trailhead.

For anyone taking the full loop, turn left at the overlook junction and proceed generally north on a mild descent. After crossing a couple of seasonal drainages, a moderate climb leads to the high point of the trip on the top of a ridge. Along the way are good views of the Monarch Divide. From the ridgetop, the long descent back to Kings Canyon begins, proceeding through burned forest and paralleling an unnamed tributary of Lewis Creek on the way to a junction ▶4 with the Lewis Creek Trail.

 Great Views

Turn left (southwest) at the junction and head downhill. High above Lewis Creek, you follow numerous switchbacks down-canyon. The protracted descent ends at the Lewis Creek Trailhead. ▶5

Without the benefit of a second vehicle or someone to pick you up, you must walk southeast from the trailhead on a section of seldom-used trail that parallels the road toward Cedar Grove Village. The 1.4-mile trail seems to needlessly undulate across the hillside above the nearly level road, but the trail does provide a straightforward return route to the Hotel Creek Trailhead. ▶6

🚶	**MILESTONES**	
▶1	0.0	Start at Hotel Creek Trailhead
▶2	1.9	Left at Cedar Grove Overlook junction
▶3	2.4	Cedar Grove Overlook
▶4	4.2	Left at Lewis Creek Trail junction
▶5	5.0	Left at Lewis Creek Trailhead
▶6	6.4	Hotel Creek Trailhead

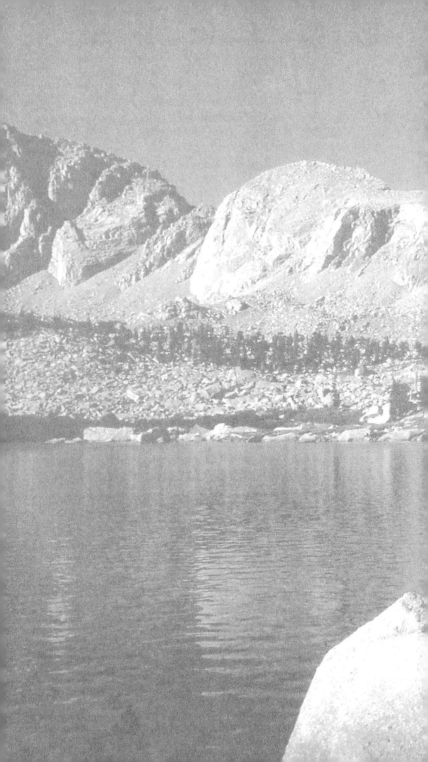

Eastern Sierra: Mount Whitney Ranger District

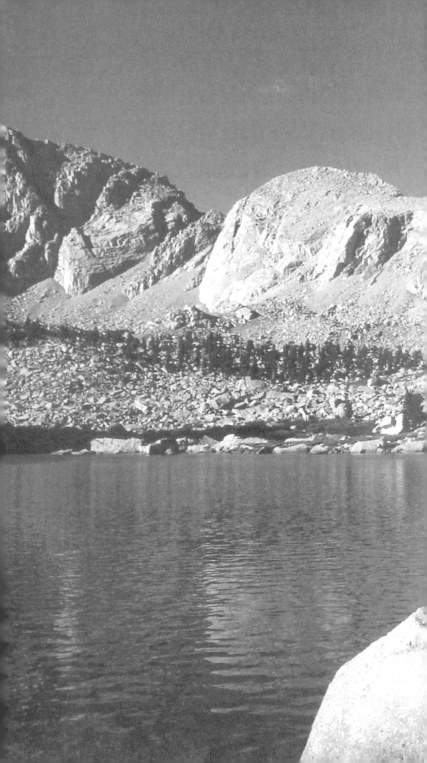

Eastern Sierra: Mount Whitney Ranger District

I n sharp contrast to the gently rising western side of the Sierra, the east side soars up from the floor of Owens Valley in rapid fashion to form the apex of the High Sierra, a seemingly impenetrable wall of serrated peaks thousands of feet above the valley, a barrier seemingly able to bar all westward penetration. Trails on this side generally adopt one of two forms: Many paths make no attempt at conquering the crest, instead following raucous streams that terminate in steep, dead-end canyons. A few other paths actually ascend over the towering east face of the Sierra on stiff, protracted climbs topping out at passes more than 11,000 or 12,000 feet high. Along this section of the High Sierra's spine is the highly coveted 14,494-foot summit of Mount Whitney—the highest point in the contiguous United States. A handful of other peaks in the area exceed 14,000 feet, with several more than 13,000 feet high. With such high altitudes and steep topography, recreationists should not only be well acclimatized but also in excellent physical condition.

The high and rugged terrain in the Mount Whitney Ranger District limits the number of trail crossings of the Sierra crest to five (from south to north): Cottonwood Pass, New Army Pass, Trail Crest, Shepherd Pass, and Kearsarge Pass. Consequently, available wilderness permits for overnight backpackers are oftentimes hard to obtain. Even more so, demand for the 100 day permits and 60 overnight permits for the Mount Whitney Trail is so competitive that applications must be made through a lottery system. With the exception of the Mount Whitney Trail, day trips into the Golden Trout Wilderness and John Muir Wilderness are far more easily arranged than backpacks.

Trails 48–50 all begin from the Horseshoe Meadow/Cottonwood Lakes Trailheads, with the first trip traveling through Golden Trout Wilderness and over Cottonwood Pass to scenic Chicken Spring Lake in the southeastern part of Sequoia National Park. Trail 49 is a relatively short journey to

Overleaf and opposite: *Cottonwood Lakes Basin*

several beautiful lakes lying in the eastern shadow of the Sierra crest. The six Cottonwood Lakes, accessed by a relatively short trail described in Trail 50, offer excellent opportunities for anglers, as well as hikers, backpackers, and equestrians. Most trail users heading to Whitney Portal are ultimately bound for the summit of Mount Whitney (Trail 52), but the previous journey to Meysan Lake sees much less traffic and is well worth the time and effort.

Trails 53–55 begin from trailheads at the end of Onion Valley Road, where short climbs lead to Robinson and Golden Trout Lakes, and a longer journey over Kearsarge Pass provides access to the highly scenic Kearsarge Lakes nestled below Kearsarge Pinnacles.

Permits

Wilderness permits are required for all overnight stays in the backcountry of Golden Trout Wilderness, John Muir Wilderness, Sequoia National Park, and Kings Canyon National Park. Trailhead quotas are in effect from the last Friday in June to September 15 into Golden Trout Wilderness and from May 1 to November 1 for eastside entry into John Muir Wilderness. Sixty percent of the daily quota is available by advance reservation with a $6 reservation fee and a $5 per-person fee. To make an advance reservation for trails described in this chapter, go to **recreation.gov** and enter "Inyo National Forest wilderness permit" in the search window. The remaining 40% of the daily quota is available as walk-in permits. These free permits can be picked up the day before the start of a trip at U.S. Forest Service offices during normal business hours. All permits can be picked up at either the Eastern Sierra Interagency Visitor Center (Lone Pine), White Mountain Ranger Station (Bishop), Mammoth Ranger Station (Mammoth Lakes), or Mono Basin Scenic Area Visitor Center (Lee Vining). For more information, call the wilderness permit information line at 760-873-2483 between 8 a.m. and 4:30 p.m.

Mount Whitney Zone: Both day hikers and overnight backpackers entering the Mount Whitney Zone from any trailhead within Inyo National Forest must pay a $6 permit fee and a $15 per-person fee (all fees are nonrefundable). Applications for reservations are accepted from February 1 to March 15 through **recreation.gov** and are awarded through a lottery system. Although 100% of the quota can be reserved, fewer than 50% of applicants are successful. Permits can be picked up only at the Eastern Sierra Interagency Visitor Center near Lone Pine. As the permit process is somewhat complicated and special rules apply to both hikers and backpackers in the Mount Whitney Zone, consult the Inyo National Forest website for more information at **fs.usda.gov/inyo,** or call the wilderness permit information line at 760-873-2483 between 8 a.m. and 4:30 p.m.

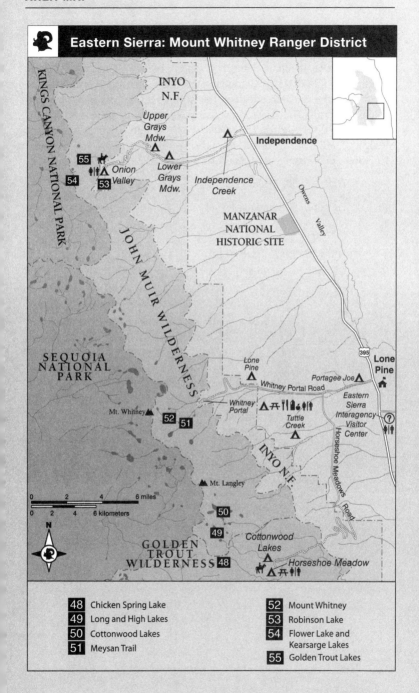

Eastern Sierra: Mount Whitney Ranger District

KINGS CANYON NATIONAL PARK

INYO N.F.

Upper Grays Mdw.

Independence

Lower Grays Mdw.

Onion Valley

55

54

53

Independence Creek

MANZANAR NATIONAL HISTORIC SITE

Owens Valley

JOHN MUIR WILDERNESS

SEQUOIA NATIONAL PARK

Lone Pine

395

Lone Pine

Whitney Portal Road

Portagee Joe

Eastern Sierra Interagency Visitor Center

Mt. Whitney

52 51

Whitney Portal

Tuttle Creek

Horseshoe Meadows Road

INYO N.F.

Mt. Langley

0   2   4   6 miles

0   2   4   6 kilometers

N

50

49

48

GOLDEN TROUT WILDERNESS

Cottonwood Lakes

Horseshoe Meadow

48	Chicken Spring Lake	
49	Long and High Lakes	
50	Cottonwood Lakes	
51	Meysan Trail	

52	Mount Whitney
53	Robinson Lake
54	Flower Lake and Kearsarge Lakes
55	Golden Trout Lakes

Maps

For the Mount Whitney Ranger District, the U.S. Geological Survey 7.5-minute (1:24,000 scale) topographic maps are listed below, corresponding to the trails described in this section. Trail users also may want to consider using Tom Harrison's maps, *Sequoia & Kings Canyon National Parks* (1:125,000), *Golden Trout Wilderness* (1:63,360), *Mt. Whitney Zone* (1:31,680), *Mt. Whitney High Country* (1:63,360), *Kings Canyon High Country* (1:63,360), or *Kearsarge Pass-Rae Lakes Loop* (1:42,240).

Trails 48–50: *Cirque Peak*

Trails 50–51: *Mt. Langley*

Trail 52: *Mt. Whitney*

Trails 53–55: *Kearsarge Peak*

TRAIL FEATURES TABLE

Eastern Sierra: Mt. Whitney Ranger District

TRAIL	DIFFICULTY	LENGTH	TYPE	USES & ACCESS	TERRAIN	FLORA & FAUNA	OTHER
48	3	8.2	↗	🚶👣🏃🏇	⛰🌊		🔭 ⛺ ⊃•
49	3	13.0	↗	🚶👣🏃🏇🐕	⛰🌊		⛺ ⊃•
50	3	11.8	↗	🚶👣🏃🏇🐕	⛰🌊		⛺ ⊃• 🎣
51	4	9.0	↗	🚶👣🏃	🏞⛰🌊	✳	⛺ ⊃• 👣
52	5	22.0	↗	🚶👣🏃	🏞⛰🔺🌊	✳	🔭 ⛺ 👣
53	3	3.0	↗	👣👣🏃 🐕	⛰🌊 ⧘		⛺ ⊃• 👣 🎣
54	3 and 4	5.0, 12.2	↗	🚶👣🏃🏇🐕	⛰🌊	✳	🔭 ⛺ ⊃• 👣 🎣
55	3	4.4	↗	🚶👣🏃🏇🐕	⛰🌊	✳	⛺ ⊃• 🎣

USES & ACCESS	TYPE	TERRAIN	FLORA & FAUNA	OTHER
🚶 Day Hiking	↻ Loop	🏞 Canyon	✳ Fall Colors	🔭 Great Views
👣 Backpacking	↗ Out-and-back	⛰ Mountain	✳ Wildflowers	⛺ Camping
🏃 Running	↘ Point-to-point	🔺 Summit	🌲 Giant Sequoias	⊃• Swimming
🏇 Horses		🌊 Lake		👣 Secluded
🐕 Dogs Allowed	DIFFICULTY	⧘ Stream		👣 Steep
👣👣 Child Friendly	- 1 2 3 4 5 +	⧘ Waterfall		🎣 Fishing
♿ Wheelchair-Access	less more			🏛 Historical Interest

Eastern Sierra:
Mount Whitney Ranger District

TRAIL 48

Day Hike, Backpack,
Run, Horse
8.2 miles, Out-and-back
Difficulty: 1 2 **3** 4 5

Chicken Spring Lake............ 324
Good views and an attractive lake make this
4-mile hike through Golden Trout Wilderness over
Cottonwood Pass to Chicken Spring Lake a worthy
goal for both day-trippers and overnighters.

TRAIL 49

Day Hike, Backpack,
Run, Horse,
Dogs Allowed
13.0 miles,
Out-and-back
Difficulty: 1 2 **3** 4 5

Long and High Lakes 328
Two fine lakes provide handsome destinations for
this trip into the southern extremity of John Muir
Wilderness, where open, rock-strewn basins and
grassy meadows provide excellent views of the
Sierra crest.

TRAIL 50

Day Hike, Backpack,
Run, Horse, Dogs
Allowed
11.8 miles,
Out-and-back
Difficulty: 1 2 **3** 4 5

Cottonwood Lakes 334
While most eastside High Sierra trails are generally
quite steep, the trail to Cottonwood Lakes is, for the
most part, a pleasantly graded exception, with only
about one-third of the route ascending at a moderate
grade. The relative ease of the trail combined with
outstanding scenery and a notable golden-trout fishery
make the area a popular destination for a wide range of
recreationists. Despite such popularity, the high number of lakes in Cottonwood Lakes Basin allows visitors
the opportunity to spread out quite easily.

TRAIL 51

Day Hike, Backpack, Run
9.0 miles, Out-and-back
Difficulty: 1 2 3 **4** 5

Meysan Trail 340
While hundreds toil along the nearby Mount
Whitney Trail, a relative few hike this neighboring
path up the canyon of Meysan Creek to a string of
attractive lakes east of the Sierra crest.

Mount Whitney 344

Despite the hassle of entering the lottery and angling for a permit with far too many would-be Whitney pilgrims, hiking the 11-mile one-way trail to the top of the Lower 48's loftiest summit remains one of the High Sierra's most notable achievements. The view from the summit is sublime, but the scenery along the way is equally rewarding.

Day Hike, Backpack, Run
22.0 miles,
Out-and-back
Difficulty: 1 2 3 4 **5**

Robinson Lake 354

A steep but short hike leads to a beautiful lake beneath towering peaks in the Inyo National Forest. Despite the short distance, the lake is not heavily visited because most trail users starting out from Onion Valley are destined for more-far-flung locations accessed from the Kearsarge Pass Trail.

Day Hike, Backpack, Run, Dogs Allowed
3.0 miles, Out-and-back
Difficulty: 1 2 **3** 4 5

Flower Lake and Kearsarge Lakes . 358

The Kearsarge Pass Trail offers one of the least-difficult crossings of the Sierra crest from an eastside trailhead, which partially accounts for the trail's popularity and the corresponding competition for wilderness permits. A quintet of scenic lakes graces the trail on the east side of the pass, offering opportunities for short day hikes and overnight backpacks. The stunning scenery from the pass and beyond around Kearsarge Lakes will tempt those seeking a longer adventure.

Day Hike, Backpack, Run, Horse, Dogs Allowed (east of Kearsarge Pass only)
5.0 miles, Out-and-back to Flower Lake
12.2 miles, Out-and-back to Kearsarge Lakes
Difficulty: 1 2 **3-4** 5

Golden Trout Lakes.............. 366

A short trail away from the usual hubbub found on the popular Kearsarge Pass Trail nearby leads to a trio of high lakes in the shadow of the eastern Sierra crest. Along with the stunning terrain, the area offers anglers the chance to fish for the namesake trout.

Day Hike, Backpack, Run, Horse, Dogs Allowed
4.4 miles, Out-and-back
Difficulty: 1 2 **3** 4 5

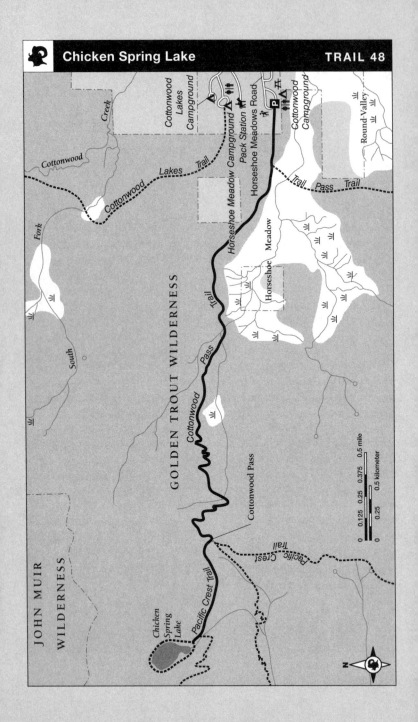

Chicken Spring Lake

Aside from a 0.75-mile switchbacking climb to an 11,000-foot pass, the grade of the trail is gentle, offering recreationists a relatively easy 4-plus-mile trip to scenic Chicken Spring Lake. Views along the way from Cottonwood Pass of the Great Western Divide to the west and the Panamint and Inyo Mountains to the east are quite scenic. Although the trail is straightforward and the distance is short, the lake sees far fewer visitors than expected, helping to make this a fine destination for hikers, backpackers, anglers, and swimmers.

TRAIL USE
Day Hike, Backpack, Run, Horse
LENGTH
8.2 miles, 4 hours
VERTICAL FEET
+1400/-100/±3000
DIFFICULTY
– 1 2 **3** 4 5 +
TRAIL TYPE
Out-and-back

FEATURES
Mountain
Lake
Great Views
Camping
Swimming

FACILITIES
Campground
Picnic Area
Stables

Best Time

With a location in the High Sierra, trails are usually snow-free by mid-July and remain so through mid-October.

Finding the Trail

In the town of Lone Pine, turn west from US 395 and follow Whitney Portal Road 3 miles to a left-hand turn onto Horseshoe Meadows Road. Head south 18.5 miles, passing the turnoff to Cottonwood Lakes, to the Horseshoe Meadows parking lot at the end of the road. The trailhead has vault toilets, running water, and a walk-in campground nearby (one-night limit, fee, vault toilets, running water, bear boxes, and phone).

Logistics

Backpackers must obtain a wilderness permit for all
overnight visits. See page 318 for more details about
how to obtain one.

Trail Description

▶1 The well-signed trail begins by an interpretive
signboard near the restrooms and follows gently
graded, wide, and sandy tread through scattered
lodgepole and foxtail pines. The sandy soil is nearly
barren of ground cover. Shortly cross the Golden
Trout Wilderness boundary and reach a junction
▶2 with trails heading south to Trail Pass and
north to the pack station. Continue ahead (west)
from the junction along the fringe of expansive
Horseshoe Meadow on nearly level and sandy tread
that may remind you of trudging through beach
sand. Where the forest thickens, come alongside
and then across a stream. On the far bank, a use
trail leads to the remains of a dilapidated cabin
(no camping). The trail shortly crosses back over
the stream, leaves Horseshoe Meadow behind,
and then begins a moderate ascent. Farther along,
a series of switchbacks leads up a rock-strewn
hillside along a willow-lined drainage, eventually

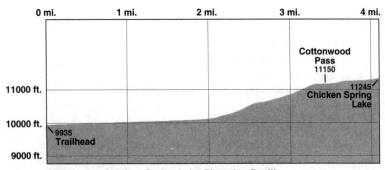

TRAIL 48 Chicken Spring Lake Elevation Profile

zigzagging up to 11,200-foot Cottonwood Pass. The fine view includes Horseshoe Meadow back-dropped picturesquely by the Panamint and Inyo Mountains to the east and the southern tip of the Great Western Divide to the west. A very short distance beyond the pass is a junction ►3 with the Pacific Crest Trail (PCT) and a path heading south-west toward Big Whitney Meadow.

 Great Views

Following a sign toward Rock Creek, turn right on the PCT to proceed northwest on an easy half-mile traverse to Chicken Spring Lake's seasonal outlet and a use-trail junction. ►4 Leave the PCT here and follow the use trail upstream to the south shore of the lake. ►5

Tucked into a cirque bowl, Chicken Spring Lake is nearly surrounded by rugged granite cliffs. The shoreline is peppered with foxtail pines, with several weather-beaten snags adding a little character to the picture-postcard scene. Several good campsites (no fires) occupy sandy patches around a small bay on the south side near the outlet and in scattered pines above the west shore. A use trail nearly encircles the shoreline, providing access to the cool waters for both anglers and swimmers.

 Lake

 Camping

🚶	**MILESTONES**	
►1	0.0	Start at trailhead
►2	0.35	Straight at junction
►3	3.4	Right on Pacific Crest Trail
►4	4.0	Right at use trail
►5	4.1	Chicken Spring Lake

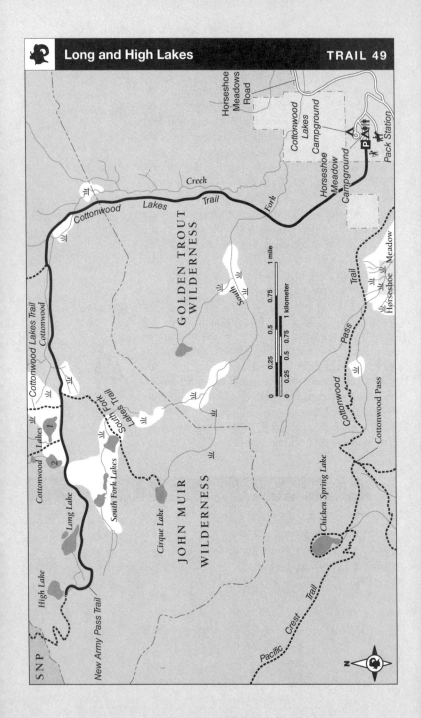

Long and High Lakes

The gently graded trails into this area provide a reasonably easy trip to a handful of scenic lakes along the Cottonwood Lakes and New Army Pass Trails, where a plethora of open, rock-strewn basins and grassy meadows permit fine views of the rugged eastern Sierra Crest. Although this picturesque area is quite popular during the height of summer, many of the more-far-flung lakes are lightly visited.

Best Time

Snow leaves the area by mid-July following an average winter, and the typically sunny and mild Sierra weather continues through summer. Autumn can be a pleasant time for a hike because the crowds diminish and the weather is cooler but generally sunny. The first significant snowfall at these elevations usually comes sometime by late October or early November.

Finding the Trail

In the town of Lone Pine, turn west from US 395 and follow Whitney Portal Road for 3 miles to a left-hand turn onto Horseshoe Meadows Road. Head south 18.5 miles and turn right toward Cottonwood Lakes. Pass the Cottonwood Lakes walk-in campground (one-night limit, fee, vault toilets, running water, bear boxes, and phone) and continue to the trailhead parking area, 0.5 mile from Horseshoe Meadows Road. The trailhead has vault toilets and running water.

TRAIL USE
Day Hike, Backpack, Run, Horse, Dogs Allowed

LENGTH
13.0 miles, 7 hours

VERTICAL FEET
+1650/-235/±3770

DIFFICULTY
– 1 2 **3** 4 5 +

TRAIL TYPE
Out-and-back

FEATURES
Mountain
Lake
Camping
Swimming

FACILITIES
Campground
Picnic Area
Stables

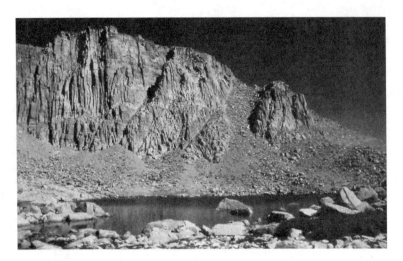

High Lake

Logistics

Backpackers must obtain a wilderness permit for all overnight visits. See page 318 for more details about how to obtain one.

Trail Description

▶1 The Cottonwood Lakes Trail begins somewhat auspiciously as a short, brick-lined path near a restroom building and a trailhead signboard. Sandy tread leads away from the trailhead on a gentle ascent through widely scattered foxtail and

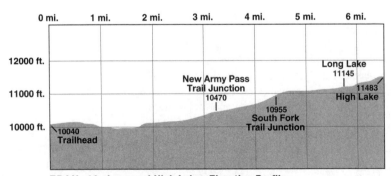

TRAIL 49 Long and High Lakes Elevation Profile

Cottonwood Lakes

Backpackers blessed with an extra day or two can easily journey to the neighboring Cottonwood Lakes, as described in Trail 50 (see page 335).
The relatively easy travel combined with outstanding scenery and a noteworthy golden-trout fishery make the area quite popular with a wide range of outdoor enthusiasts. However, solitude seekers should not despair because the bounty of lakes tends to disperse visitors around the basin. The extensive network of trails and easy cross-country jaunts makes travel from one lake to another fairly easy. Anglers should stay abreast of fishing regulations, which limit Lakes 1–4 to catch-and-release only. All lakes in the basin are restricted to artificial lures or flies with barbless hooks, with a limit of five fish.

lodgepole pines, where virtually no ground cover is able to take root in the sandy soil. Soon cross into Golden Trout Wilderness and pass a spur trail on the left headed toward the pack station. ▶2 From there, an equally gentle ascent leads down to a crossing of South Fork Cottonwood Creek, 1 mile from the trailhead, where a few campsites are found on the far bank. The lush vegetation along the banks of the creek seems especially vibrant after the dearth of plant life in the first mile.

Camping

From the creek, the trail climbs gently through more scattered pines to the main branch of Cottonwood Creek and then follows this stream up a broad valley for the next 1.5 miles. Along the way, you cross the boundary separating the Golden Trout and John Muir wilderness areas, in the shadow of steep rock cliffs on the left and within view of the wood structures of Golden Trout Camp across a meadow on the right. Beyond the boundary, the trail veers west on a more moderate ascent up the narrowing canyon. At 2.5 miles, cross the creek on a beveled

South Fork and Cirque Lakes

A side trip to these lakes is a fine diversion for those with the extra time and energy. From the junction, head south along the fringe of a sloping meadow lined with willows and then veer southwest on a gentle climb through foxtail pines. A short descent leads to a crossing of South Fork Cottonwood Creek, and then the trail slices across a large meadow to the east side of the easternmost South Fork Lake. The roughly oval-shaped lake, splendidly backdropped by rocky ridges and craggy peaks, offers backpackers a few choice campsites on a hill above the southwest shore. A straightforward cross-country jaunt leads to the upper South Fork Lakes.

To visit Cirque Lake, follow the continuation of the trail on a moderate climb through scattered foxtail pines to the apex of a ridge, and then descend shortly to the northeast shore. The lake has a decidedly alpine ambience, nestled at the base of steep cliffs below the rugged profile of Cirque Peak. A few campsites are scattered around the sparsely forested shoreline, but the number seems more than adequate for the few adventurous souls who travel this far off the Cottonwood Lakes and New Army Pass Trails.

Camping log and pass more campsites near the meadow-lined stream. Just after the crossing of a side stream is a junction of the Cottonwood Lakes and New Army Pass Trails. ▶3

Leaving the Cottonwood Lakes Trail, veer left at the junction, soon cross to the south side of Cottonwood Creek, and then climb moderately for a little more than a mile to a junction with South Fork Lakes Trail beside a large meadow. ▶4

To continue toward Cottonwood Lakes, proceed ahead (west) at the South Fork Lakes Trail junction and make a short climb up a hillside to a Y-junction with a connector to the Cottonwood Lakes Trail. ▶5 Keep heading west on the New Army Pass Trail, skirting the edge of a large meadow surrounding Cottonwood Lake 1 and continuing past Lake 2. Leaving the meadowland behind, make a short climb to a desolate area filled with scads of large granite boulders, where only a few scattered pockets of pines seem able to gain a foothold in this sea of rock. Eventually the boulders are left behind as gently graded trail arcs around a lightly forested hillside. Below, a meadow-lined, refreshing-looking stream rushes toward the westernmost South Fork Lake. A faint use trail leads across the stream to forested campsites between this lake and Long Lake above. A more moderate climb then leads up through thinning forest to the south shore of Long Lake, ▶6 where the best campsites are found beneath a stand of pines near the southwest shore, with a few less-protected sites above the north shore.

 Camping

From the east shore of Long Lake, the New Army Pass Trail climbs steeper toward High Lake and the pass beyond. Through grasses, low-growing alpine plants, and widely scattered dwarf pines, you climb to timberline and then wind up rocky switchbacks to High Lake. ▶7 The lake is set in a rocky, open bowl rimmed by steep cliffs, the rocky terrain severely limiting the opportunity for decent campsites. For those interested in additional pursuits, the moderately graded mile climb to New Army Pass at the boundary of Sequoia National Park offers wide-ranging views.

🚶	**MILESTONES**	
▶1	0.0	Start at trailhead
▶2	0.1	Ahead at pack station spur
▶3	3.25	Left at New Army Pass Trail junction
▶4	4.4	Ahead at South Fork Lakes Trail junction
▶5	4.5	Ahead at connector junction
▶6	5.75	Long Lake
▶7	6.5	High Lake

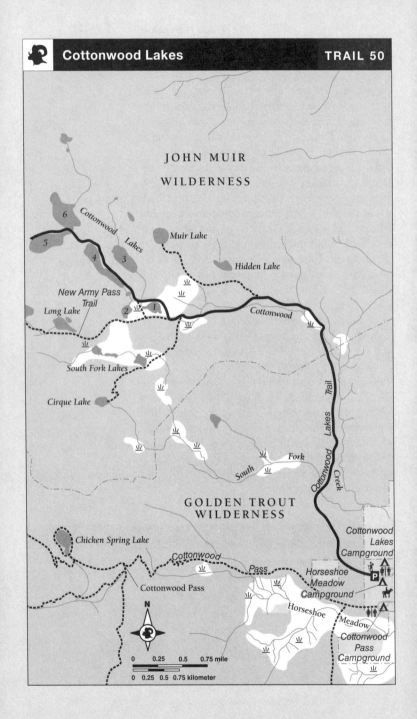

JOHN MUIR

WILDERNESS

Cottonwood Lakes

6

5

4

3

Muir Lake

Hidden Lake

New Army Pass
Trail

Long Lake

2

1

Cottonwood

South Fork Lakes

Cirque Lake

South

Fork

Cottonwood Lakes Trail

Cottonwood Creek

GOLDEN TROUT
WILDERNESS

Chicken Spring Lake

Cottonwood

Pass

Cottonwood Pass

Horseshoe

Meadow

Cottonwood
Lakes
Campground

Horseshoe
Meadow
Campground

Cottonwood
Pass
Campground

N

0   0.25   0.5   0.75 mile

0   0.25   0.5   0.75 kilometer

Cottonwood Lakes

Aside from a 1.75-mile stretch of moderate climbing, the journey to Cottonwood Lakes is on gently graded trail. The relatively easy trail, outstanding scenery, and noted golden trout fishery combine to make this area a popular destination for a wide range of recreationists. Travel between the lakes via a fine network of trails and easy cross-country routes makes getting around fairly straightforward. Solitude seekers should be able to find some secluded spots away from the main thoroughfare.

Best Time

Snow leaves the area by mid-July following an average winter, and the typically sunny and mild Sierra weather continues through summer. Autumn can be a pleasant time for a hike because the crowds diminish and the weather is cooler but generally sunny. The first significant snowfall at these elevations usually comes sometime by late October or early November.

Finding the Trail

In the town of Lone Pine, turn west from US 395 and follow Whitney Portal Road 3 miles to a left-hand turn onto Horseshoe Meadows Road. Head south 18.5 miles and turn right toward Cottonwood Lakes. Pass the Cottonwood Lakes walk-in campground (one-night limit, fee, vault toilets, running water, bear boxes, and phone) and continue to the trailhead parking area, 0.5 mile from Horseshoe Meadows Road. The trailhead has vault toilets and running water.

TRAIL USE
Day Hike, Backpack, Run, Horse, Dogs Allowed

LENGTH
11.8 miles, 6 hours

VERTICAL FEET
+1450/-300/±3500

DIFFICULTY
– 1 2 **3** 4 5 +

TRAIL TYPE
Out-and-back

FEATURES
Mountain
Lake
Camping
Swimming
Fishing

FACILITIES
Campground
Picnic Area
Stables

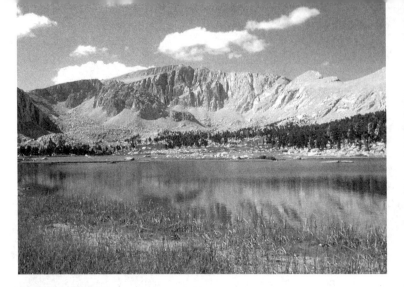

Cottonwood Lake 3

Logistics

Backpackers must obtain a wilderness permit for all overnight visits. See page 318 for more details about how to obtain one.

Trail Description

▶1 The Cottonwood Lakes Trail begins somewhat auspiciously as a short, brick-lined path near a restroom building and a trailhead signboard. Sandy tread leads away from the trailhead on a

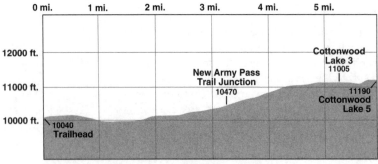

TRAIL 50 Cottonwood Lakes Elevation Profile

gentle ascent through widely scattered foxtail and lodgepole pines, where virtually no ground cover is able to take root in the sandy soil. Soon cross into Golden Trout Wilderness and pass a spur trail on the left headed toward the pack station. ▶2 From there, an equally gentle grade leads down to a crossing of South Fork Cottonwood Creek, 1 mile from the trailhead, where a few campsites are found on the far bank. The lush vegetation along the banks of the creek seems especially vibrant after the dearth of plant life in the first mile.

 Camping

From the creek, the trail climbs gently through more scattered pines to the main branch of Cottonwood Creek and then follows this stream up a broad valley for the next 1.5 miles. Along the way, you cross the boundary separating the Golden Trout and John Muir wilderness areas, in the shadow of steep rock cliffs on the left and within view of the wood structures of Golden Trout Camp across a meadow on the right. Beyond the boundary, the trail veers west on a more moderate ascent up the narrowing canyon. At 2.5 miles, cross the creek on a beveled log and pass more campsites near the meadow-lined stream. Just after the crossing of a side stream is a junction of the Cottonwood Lakes and New Army Pass Trails. ▶3

The relatively easy trail, outstanding scenery, and noted golden trout fishery combine to make this area a popular destination for a wide range of recreationists.

Veer right at the junction and continue up the Cottonwood Lakes Trail on a moderate climb through lodgepole- and foxtail-pine forest on an ascent that leads well above the creek to a series of switchbacks. Through the trees you have occasional views up the canyon to Cirque Peak and the east Sierra Crest. At the eastern edge of an expansive meadow, near the lip of the Cottonwood Lakes Basin, you reach a signed junction with a lateral to Muir Lake. ▶4

Continue ahead (west) from the Muir Lake junction on gently graded trail well to the right of Cottonwood Lake 1. The trail soon bends northwest up a low, forested rise (campsites), crosses a stream, and then heads across a grassy meadow dotted with

OPTIONS

Muir Lake

Muir Lake makes a fine diversion for those with extra time and energy. The beginning of the trail is somewhat difficult to discern, but the designated route follows a faint path that skirts the northeast side of the meadow and then bends north toward the lake (in spite of some indication that the trail heads northeast up a low hill on the right, which is the beginning of a cross-country route to Hidden Lake). Follow the path around the meadow and then ascend north through pines and scattered boulders to a flower-lined rivulet. From there, continue on a sometimes indistinct path toward the lake, which is hard to miss, despite the periodically disappearing nature of the trail due to the lake being tucked into a horseshoe-shaped cirque at the base of an unnamed peak (3913).

Muir Lake is quite scenic, with rugged cliffs partially encircling the basin and the upper slopes of Mount Langley towering over the terrain to the northwest. Judging by the condition of the trail, the lake appears to see few visitors, in spite of the pleasant scenery and a selection of fine campsites shaded by scattered pines.

boulders, clumps of willow, and widely scattered pines. From the meadow, the massive east wall of the Sierra Crest looms over the surroundings. Pass by a corrugated metal shed on the left and a small tarn on the right before arriving at willow-rimmed Cottonwood Lake 3. ▶5 Fine campsites on a forested rise between Lakes 3 and 4 will lure overnighters.

Camping

Lake

From the northwest end of Lake 3, the trail briefly skirts a meadow and then follows a gentle course through mostly open terrain to the north tip of Lake 4. Here, indistinct tread marked by a sign simply reading TRAIL, marks a faint path that follows the east shore of Lake 4 southeast for a mile to a junction with the New Army Pass Trail near Lake 1. To visit Lake 5, ▶6 head northwest up a steep hillside to a short stretch of creek connecting two large bodies of water, rimmed by steep cliffs and talus piles, and meadows with scattered clumps of willows. A lack of trees leaves the handful of campsites sprinkled around the shoreline exposed to the elements—much better sites can be found on the rise between Lakes 3 and 4. A straightforward, mile-long cross-country jaunt leads to the seldom-visited and diminutive upper lake. While golden trout can be found in all the Cottonwood Lakes, the upper lakes are the only ones that are not catch-and-release. All lakes in Cottonwood Lakes Basin are restricted to artificial lures or flies with barbless hooks, and the limit is 5.

 Camping

 Fishing

🚶	MILESTONES	
►1	0.0	Start at trailhead
►2	0.1	Ahead at pack station spur
►3	3.25	Right at New Army Pass Trail junction
►4	4.5	Straight at lateral to Muir Lake
►5	5.25	Cottonwood Lake 3
►6	5.9	Cottonwood Lake 5

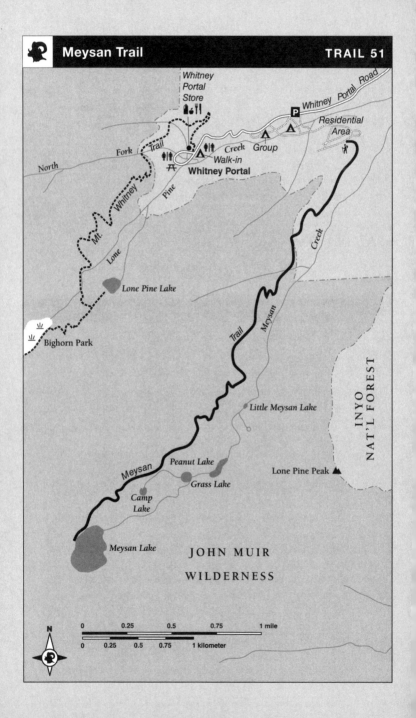

Meysan Trail

TRAIL 51

Whitney
Portal
Store

Whitney Portal Road

P

Residential
Area

North

Fork

Whitney Trail

Creek

Group

Walk-in
Whitney Portal

Lone

Mt.

Pine

Lone Pine Lake

Meysan Creek

Bighorn Park

Trail

Meysan

Little Meysan Lake

INYO NAT'L FOREST

Meysan

Peanut Lake

Grass Lake

Camp
Lake

Lone Pine Peak ▲

Meysan Lake

JOHN MUIR

WILDERNESS

N

| 0 | 0.25 | 0.5 | 0.75 | 1 mile |

| 0 | 0.25 | 0.5 | 0.75 | 1 kilometer |

Meysan Trail

While hundreds toil along the nearby Mount Whitney Trail, a relative few hike this neighboring path up the canyon of Meysan Creek to a string of attractive lakes east of the Sierra Crest. Once the typical hubbub of Whitney Portal is left behind, visitors experience quiet serenity on the ascent up Meysan Creek canyon to the end of the trail at Meysan Lake, a fine destination for lunch or for an overnight camp.

Best Time

The Meysan Trail, in the rain shadow of lofty Mount Whitney, is usually snow-free by early July.

Finding the Trail

From Lone Pine, head west from US 395 on the Whitney Portal Road, and drive 13 miles to Whitney Portal, parking your vehicle either in the day-use or overnight parking lots. Campgrounds, a picnic area, restrooms, a store, and a café are all nearby. To begin the hike you must descend the old service road from the parking area to the Whitney Portal Campground (fee, flush toilets, running water, bear boxes, and phone). Following a series of signs, walk along the campground loop road across Lone Pine Creek to an intersection. Turn left, pass some summer homes, and make a steep climb to the official trailhead on your right.

TRAIL USE
Day Hike, Backpack, Run

LENGTH
9.0 miles, 5 hours

VERTICAL FEET
+3850/-300/±8300

DIFFICULTY
– 1 2 3 **4** 5 +

TRAIL TYPE
Out-and-back

FEATURES
Canyon
Mountain
Lake
Wildflowers
Camping
Swimming
Steep

FACILITIES
Campground
Picnic Area
Store
Café
Showers

Logistics

At the first of many switchbacks to come, you have good views to the northeast of Alabama Hills and Owens Valley.

Backpackers must obtain a wilderness permit for all overnight visits. See page 318 for more details about how to obtain one.

Trail Description

▶1 From the official trailhead, follow singletrack trail on a steep climb up the hillside. Fortunately, the steep grade is short-lived, as the trail soon merges with another section of road that leads past more summer homes to the resumption of trail.

Having left the last vestiges of civilization behind, you embark on a more moderate climb that leads across a dry hillside dotted with firs, pinyon pines, Jeffrey pines, and mountain mahogany. Soon the trail bends into the canyon of Meysan Creek and curves southwest, slicing across a steep hillside well above the creek. At the first of many switchbacks to come, you have good views to the northeast of Alabama Hills and Owens Valley. Cross into the signed John Muir Wilderness at 1.5 miles.

Continue the switchbacking climb up the canyon, drawing slightly closer to the level of the creek as you go. Along the way is a fine view of a pretty cascade gliding down a rock slab into a delightful

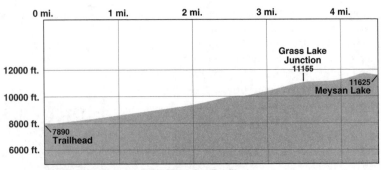

TRAIL 51 Meysan Trail Elevation Profile

pool. More switchbacks lead to even better views farther up the canyon, including another cascade dropping down the headwall of the lake-filled basin above. Scattered foxtail pines start to appear just before a grassy meadow. Nearby, a trail sign directs traffic ahead to Grass Lake and to Meysan Lake to the right. ▶2

The tread is a little indistinct beyond the junction, but ducks periodically mark the faint trail on the final climb to Meysan Lake. Bend around a large meadow bordering Camp Lake and then ascend a grassy couloir. Where the slope ahead becomes steeper, veer southwest and climb over rock slabs to a gap above the lake. A short descent from there leads to the northwest shore of Meysan Lake, ▶3 where small pockets of flower-filled meadows dot the otherwise rocky shore, and the dramatic headwall formed by Mounts Irvine and Mallory form a picturesque backdrop. The marginal campsites may be unattractive to backpackers—better sites can be found below, near Camp Lake.

 Camping

 Lake

 Wildflowers

🚶	**MILESTONES**	
▶1	0.0	Start at trailhead
▶2	3.5	Right at Grass Lake junction
▶3	4.5	Meysan Lake

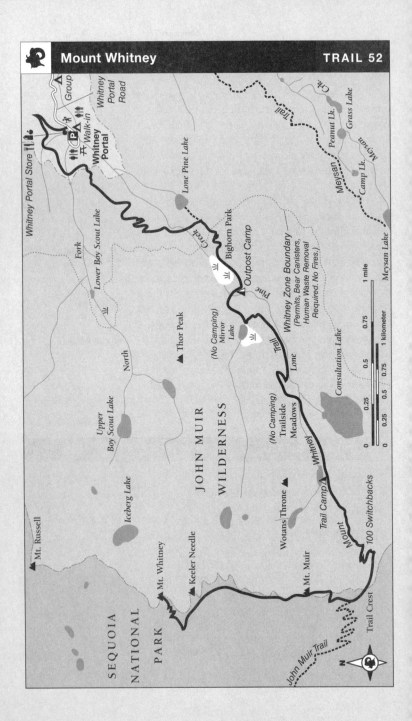

Mount Whitney

With a dramatic, towering, and vertical east face that cuts a familiar alpine profile as seen from the town of Lone Pine, more than 10,750 feet below, Mount Whitney is one of North America's most impressive mountains. Not only is the view of the mountain quite exceptional, but the vista from the summit is equally impressive, a reward commensurate with the diligence required to reach the climax of the Sierra. To stand on top of the 14,494-foot summit is an extraordinary accomplishment.

While defined trail leads all the way to the summit, a Whitney climb is not necessarily a walk in the park. You must be in good physical condition to reach the summit and enjoy the journey along the way. Altitude is certainly a consideration, especially for those who reside at or near sea level. Spending a night in the campground at Whitney Portal prior to the start of a trip is a good way to begin the acclimatization process. Once on the trail, drink plenty of fluids, consume lots of high-energy foods, and continuously monitor your condition, as well as that of any companions. Slow your rate of ascent upon noticing any signs of mild altitude sickness. If symptoms persist, or worsen, make an immediate descent to lower altitudes. The proper equipment (including sunglasses, sunblock, and plenty of food and water) and the appropriate clothing for the wide range of temperatures and weather conditions you might experience on this mountain are essential. Weather conditions run the gamut from intense sunlight and heat to sudden thunderstorms with torrential rains or hail. Snow can fall on Mount Whitney during any month of the year!

TRAIL USE
Day Hike, Backpack, Run

LENGTH
22.0 miles, 11–15 hours

VERTICAL FEET
+7830/-1870/±19,400

DIFFICULTY
– 1 2 3 4 **5** +

TRAIL TYPE
Out-and-back

FEATURES
Canyon
Mountain
Summit
Lake
Wildflowers
Great Views
Camping
Steep

FACILITIES
Campground
Picnic Area
Store
Café
Showers

To stand on top of the 14,494-foot summit is an extraordinary accomplishment.

Saying that Mount Whitney is a coveted ascent is a huge understatement. So many wish to climb the highest summit in the Lower 48 that the U.S. Forest Service long ago implemented a strict quota system to try to stem the tide of hordes of devotees attempting to reach the summit. Even with 100 day hiker and 60 backpacker permits available per day ($15 per person), competition is so fierce that permits are granted by lottery (see page 318 for more information). In addition to the quota permit system, the U.S. Forest Service also has instituted a mandatory pack-out system within the Whitney Zone for removal of all human waste.

The first question you need to answer before embarking on a Whitney climb is whether to do the ascent as a one-day hike or an overnight (or longer) backpack. The benefit of the one-day option is not having to carry a heavy backpack up the steep trail to base camp. However, the 22-mile round trip demands that you be in top condition and get an early start for the long day ahead. Backpacking obviously requires you to carry more gear, but it allows you more time to acclimatize and to get up and down the mountain.

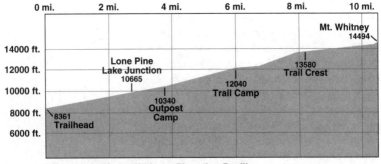

TRAIL 52 Mount Whitney Elevation Profile

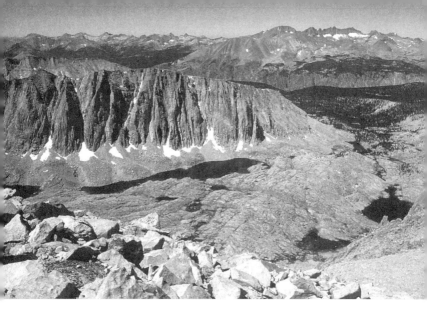

Western view *from summit of Mount Whitney*

Best Time

Sunny and mild days between mid-July and mid-September are the ideal times for a climb of Mount Whitney. Afternoon thunderstorms can occur at any time during that period, and a hasty retreat should be undertaken during such conditions. Because so many desire to climb the highest peak in the continental United States, and competition for permits is so fierce, many attempts occur outside of this window of usually fair and mild weather. Spring trips face the added obstacles of unstable weather and icy conditions, oftentimes requiring the use of ice axes and crampons. Autumn climbers must be fully prepared for sudden storms with the possibility of heavy snowfall and freezing temperatures.

Finding the Trail

From Lone Pine, head west from US 395 on the Whitney Portal Road and drive 13 miles to Whitney Portal, parking your vehicle either in the day-use or overnight parking lots. Whitney Portal Campground (fee, flush toilets, running water, bear boxes, and phone) and Whitney Trailhead Campground (walk-in, one-night limit, fee, flush toilets, running water, bear boxes, and phone) are close by. Whitney Portal also has a picnic area, restrooms, store, and café.

Logistics

All hikers in the Mount Whitney Zone must obtain a wilderness day-hiking permit, and backpackers must obtain a permit for all overnight visits. Due to Mount Whitney's popularity, hikers must enter a lottery at the beginning of the year or try for a walk-in permit. See page 318 for more details.

Trail Description

▶1 Your departure from Whitney Portal onto the Mount Whitney Trail is heralded by an abundance of trailhead signs that may easily result in temporary sensory overload. Nearby is the receptacle for disposal of your waste pack-out kit upon the conclusion of your journey into the Whitney Zone. Away from this trailhead hoopla, the well-beaten path winds up the hillside through a mixed forest of red firs, Jeffrey pines, and mountain mahogany to the first switchback. Heading roughly east, cross chaparral-covered slopes with a fine view up the canyon of a falls on Lone Pine Creek. Cross an unnamed stream lined with lush vegetation and then follow a quarter-mile, ascending traverse to a boulder-hop of North Fork Lone Pine Creek. A steep mountaineer's route ascends this drainage to Iceberg Lake and technical routes on Whitney's east face. Farther up the trail, you cross the signed John Muir Wilderness boundary.

A mostly shadeless and steady climb ensues, incorporating numerous switchbacks on the climb up the canyon. If hot temperatures are forecast,

Lone Pine Lake

OPTIONS

Late-starting backpackers or day hikers not up to the full-scale assault on Mount Whitney can find a haven at lovely Lone Pine Lake. Turn left from the junction and head northeast about 200 yards to the east shore of the lake. Perched at the very edge of steep Lone Pine Creek canyon, the roughly oval lake is blessed with fine views down-canyon across the open, boulder-strewn shore. With no permanent inlet, the lake level is dependent on snowmelt from the previous winter's snowpack. Anglers can test their skill on a resident population of rainbow and brook trout, while campers can find spots to pitch their tents beneath foxtail pines above the southwest shore.

try to avoid this 1.5-mile section of trail during the afternoon. Welcome relief comes in the form of a lodgepole-pine forest on the approach to a ford of Lone Pine Creek. Shortly beyond the ford is a junction ▶2 with the short spur trail to Lone Pine Lake.

Remaining on the Mount Whitney Trail, you veer right at the Lone Pine Lake junction and gently stroll through a rocky wash beneath a light covering of pine into the Whitney Zone. Soon the stiff climb resumes on a series of switchbacks leading up and over a rocky slope to Bighorn Park, a large, willow-lined meadow sprinkled with colorful wildflowers. A gently graded path skirts the meadow to the south side and then turns north to a crossing of Lone Pine Creek. Just beyond the crossing, near a waterfall, is **Outpost Camp**, ▶3 with a number of slightly sloping, pine-shaded campsites.

Away from Outpost Camp, the trail immediately crosses Mirror Creek and ascends steep switchbacks alongside a wildflower-lined, tumbling stream. At the top of the climb, you boulder-hop back over the creek and pass through head-high willows to the southeast shore of Mirror Lake. ▶4

 Camping

 Wildflowers

 Lake

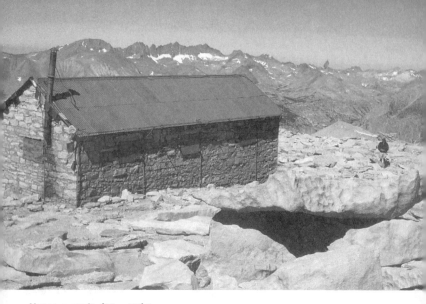

Hut at summit *of Mount Whitney*

The lake is quite attractive, set in a deep cirque below the steep cliffs of Thor Peak. Anglers can test their skill on the brook trout rumored to live here, but campers will have to continue to Trail Camp because camping has been banned here since 1972 due to severe overuse. Although camping is not allowed, the lovely surroundings of Mirror Lake make a fine rest or lunch stop.

More switchbacks lead out of Mirror Lake's basin on a stiff climb to the top of a ridge near timberline. Soon the rugged east wall of the Whitney massif appears over the top of Pinnacle Ridge. A more moderate climb leads across boulders and rocks, the rugged landscape broken intermittently by small pockets of soil with widely scattered wildflowers and tiny shrubs. A series of rock steps leads closer to Lone Pine Creek, as the trail eventually leads to a crossing of the creek on a rock bridge. Beyond the bridge, you continue to beautiful Trailside Meadows, where a colorful profusion of shooting stars, paintbrush, and columbine accents the deep-green meadow grass lining the stream. Beyond this small

Wildflowers ❀

oasis, you climb a nearly endless sea of rock, cross back over the creek, and continue to the vicinity of Consultation Lake, backdropped dramatically by Mount Irvine and Mount McAdie. Continue climbing steadily upward, weaving around boulders and over rock steps, before a stretch of gently graded trail heralds your approach to Trail Camp. ►5 A short climb leads into the well-used camp.

 Camping

Although the vast number and variety of campers may lend a circuslike atmosphere to Trail Camp, the setting, below the rugged east face of the High Sierra, is spectacular. To the north lies Wotans Throne, with Pinnacle Ridge behind, while to the south, 13,680-foot Mount McAdie and 13,770-foot Mount Irvine form an amphitheater for the icy waters of Consultation Lake. Directly above the camp, 100 switchbacks lead to the low gap in the crest known as Trail Crest. This ever-present obstacle looms over prospective climbers hunkered down at Trail Camp, resulting in a restless night's sleep for many of them.

Leaving Trail Camp behind, increasingly steep trail leads to the bottom of the 100 switchbacks. Zigzag up the slope with ever-expanding views to the east (Mount Whitney becomes hidden behind the Needles). About halfway up the slope, you climb across a shaded rock wall, where a seep may help create icy conditions; old iron railings add a wary sense of safety. The interminable switchbacks continue, as lingering snowfields may impede

Outpost Camp

In olden days, Outpost Camp bustled with a slightly different sort of activity—a packer's wife rented tents and sold meals to travelers bound for Mount Whitney and the backcountry beyond, and stock grazed in the nearby meadows of Bighorn Park, named for the previous, native inhabitants.

Trail Camp

On just about any summer day, Trail Camp assumes the atmosphere of an expedition base camp. While multicolored tents flap in the breeze, expectant mountaineers sort their gear and check equipment, while others gaze at the route above, or check the skies for any hints at the weather. Still others wait trailside, querying returning summiteers about their experience higher up on the mountain. Not surprisingly, Trail Camp is not the place for isolationists in search of a solitary wilderness experience. Plenty of level campsites have been groomed by repeated use on the nearly barren soil surrounding the camp, but campers should not expect anything close to privacy.

With a maximum of 100 day hikers and 60 backpackers departing from Whitney Portal each day, combined with an additional number of returnees and a handful of people finishing up their John Muir Trail thru-hikes, the potential exists for hundreds of people to pass through the camp on any given day. Some backpackers seek campsites in slightly less crowded areas away from the trail around Consultation Lake, but usually without much relief from the crush of visitors.

Great Views 🔭

straightforward travel below the crest. Eventually, Trail Crest ►6 is reached, where staggering views of the Great Western Divide appear to the west, encompassing a broad section of Sequoia National Park. Directly below, in a barren basin, lie the shimmering waters of Hitchcock Lakes. A short descent from Trail Crest leads to a junction with the John Muir Trail (JMT). ►7

Turn right and head north toward the summit of Mount Whitney on a steady climb that follows the JMT along an airy ridge. The trail periodically dips into notches in the ridge that provide acrophobic vistas straight down the east face. Proceeding up the trail, you may notice the sunlight glinting off the metal roof of the research hut near the summit, built by the Smithsonian Institution in 1909. Approaching the final slope below the top, the grade increases and a variety of paths head toward the summit. Despite the number of routes, the way is obvious—head for the highest spot. Soon the roof of the hut appears over the horizon, and you stand atop the highest summit in the Lower 48. ▶8 The top of the peak is a broad, sloping plateau composed of jumbled slabs and boulders. Any adjective that attempts to capture the magnificence of the summit view seems inadequate. Suffice to say, it's a complete, 360-degree panorama, with each bearing of the compass offering something extraordinary to discover—a more than just reward for the toil necessary to reach this spectacular point. After fully enjoying the summit experience, retrace your steps back to Whitney Portal.

🚶	**MILESTONES**	
▶1	0.0	Start at Whitney Portal
▶2	2.75	Right at Lone Pine Lake junction
▶3	3.8	Outpost Camp
▶4	4.5	Mirror Lake
▶5	6.0	Trail Camp
▶6	8.2	Trail Crest
▶7	8.3	Right at John Muir Trail junction
▶8	11.0	Mount Whitney

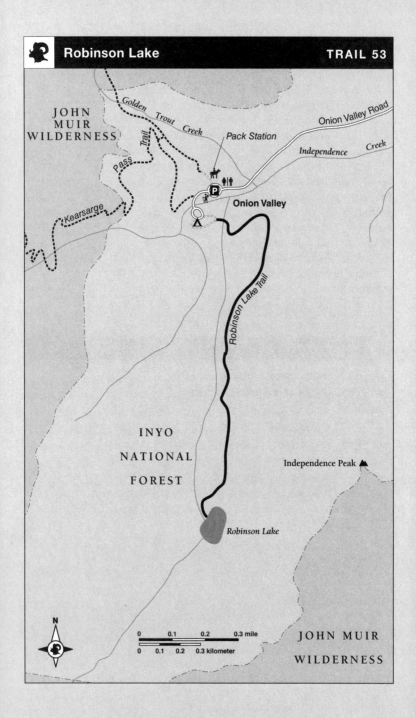

JOHN
MUIR
WILDERNESS

Golden Trout Creek

Pass Trail

Kearsarge

Pack Station

Onion Valley Road

Independence Creek

P

Onion Valley

Robinson Lake Trail

INYO

NATIONAL

FOREST

Independence Peak ▲

Robinson Lake

N

| 0 | 0.1 | 0.2 | 0.3 mile |
| 0 | 0.1 | 0.2 | 0.3 kilometer |

JOHN MUIR

WILDERNESS

Robinson Lake

A short but sometimes steep hike leads to alpine splendor at Robinson Lake in the shadow of University and Independence Peaks. Backpackers planning to overnight in the area, which is just outside the John Muir Wilderness, need not obtain a wilderness permit—a definite bonus for anyone who has been denied a permit for trails into the popular areas nearby.

Best Time

Snow blankets the area until mid-July following winters of average snowfall. The snow usually returns sometime in late October.

Finding the Trail

From the town of Independence, turn west from US 395 onto Market Street and head west following signs to Onion Valley. Drive 12.5 miles on Onion Valley Road to the end and leave your vehicle in the expansive parking lot. Restrooms, running water, and a campground (fee, vault toilets, running water, and bear boxes) are available near the trailhead. Do not leave food or scented items in your car; bears are active in Onion Valley.

Trail Description

▶1 Follow directions, given on a small sign near the parking area, into the adjacent campground and continue along the access road to the start of the trail near Campsite 8. ▶2 From there, walk up

TRAIL USE
Day Hike, Backpack, Run, Dogs Allowed
LENGTH
3.0 miles, 2 hours
VERTICAL FEET
+1325/±2650
DIFFICULTY
– 1 2 **3** 4 5 +
TRAIL TYPE
Out-and-back

FEATURES
Mountain
Lake
Stream
Camping
Swimming
Fishing
Steep

FACILITIES
Campground
Restrooms
Water
Stables

Additional Challenges

OPTIONS

From Robinson Lake, off-trail enthusiasts can follow a difficult, Class 2 cross-country route over University Pass into Center Basin, while mountaineers can follow a similarly rated route up 13,632-foot University Peak.

Nestled in a steep, horseshoe-shaped, glacier-scoured basin, sapphire-blue Robinson Lake emanates a bold, alpine presence.

Lake ≋

a stone path, which doubles as a seasonal stream in early season, to sandy tread above, and then switchback through aspens, whitebark pines, and foxtail pines on a moderately steep climb to a small, sloping basin sprinkled with scattered timber, site of some previous avalanches. Beyond the sloping basin, the grade eases to a more moderate ascent that leads near the west bank of Robinson Creek. Proceeding up the drainage, the grade increases again near a large patch of willows. Above the willows, you climb beside and then across a small stream, wind through a field of large boulders, and then crest the lip of the lake's basin. From there, a short stroll through an open area of rock, sand, and dwarf pines leads to the north shore of 10,535-foot Robinson Lake. ▶3

Nestled in a steep, horseshoe-shaped, glacier-scoured basin, sapphire-blue Robinson Lake emanates a bold, alpine presence, with steep granite walls and talus slopes rising up from the lakeshore

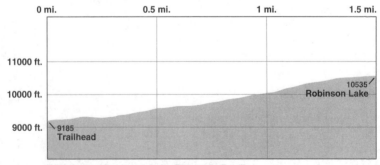

TRAIL 53 Robinson Lake Elevation Profile

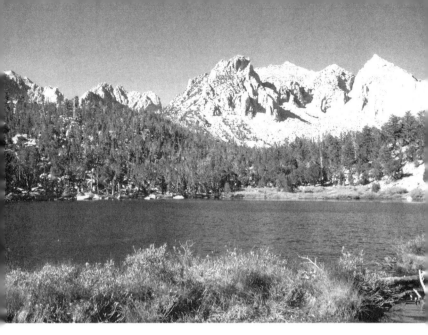

Robinson Lake

toward the summits of University and Independence Peaks. Foxtail pines along the west shore
shade a number of pleasant campsites. Rainbow and
brook trout will tempt the angler.

Camping

Fishing

🚶	**MILESTONES**	
▶1	0.0	Start at parking area
▶2	0.1	Start of trail
▶3	1.5	Robinson Lake

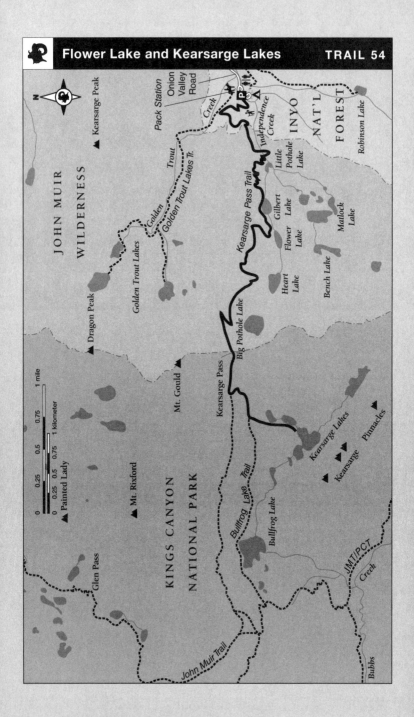

Flower Lake and Kearsarge Lakes

TRAIL 54

Kearsarge Peak

Pack Station

Onion Valley Road

Independence Creek

Creek

INYO

NAT'L

FOREST

Robinson Lake

Little Pothole Lake

Golden Trout Lakes Tr.

Gilbert Lake

Flower Lake

Matlock Lake

JOHN MUIR

WILDERNESS

Golden Trout Lakes

Bench Lake

Heart Lake

Dragon Peak

Big Pothole Lake

Mt. Gould

Kearsarge Pass

Kearsarge Lakes

Kearsarge Pinnacles

1 mile

0.75

1 kilometer

0.5

0.75

0.25

0.5

Painted Lady

0.25

Mt. Rixford

KINGS CANYON

NATIONAL PARK

Bullfrog Lake Trail

Bullfrog Lake

JMT/PCT

Creek

Glen Pass

John Muir Trail

Bubbs

Flower Lake and Kearsarge Lakes

Kearsarge Pass provides one of the least difficult eastern gateways into the High Sierra, as the climb is fairly short and rarely at more than a moderate grade. That ease is relative, though, because the trail still gains more than 2,500 feet in 5 miles at high altitude. The trail is heavily used and wilderness permits are at a premium, not only because of the relative ease but also due to the absolutely stunning terrain. Serrated peaks, subalpine lakes, flower-filled meadows, rushing streams, and incredible views are the real attractions of this part of the High Sierra. A string of five pretty lakes in the upper reaches of Independence Creek canyon offers scenic destinations for both day hikers and overnighters. Those willing to go farther afield will find sweeping vistas from Kearsarge Pass and beautiful settings around Kearsarge Lakes below.

Best Time

Snow generally leaves the trail to Flower Lake by early July. Kearsarge Pass is usually free of snow by mid-July following winters of average snowfall. Wildflowers reach their peak from mid-July to early August.

Finding the Trail

From the town of Independence, turn west from US 395 onto Market Street and head west following signs to Onion Valley. Drive 12.5 miles on Onion Valley Road to the end and leave your vehicle in the expansive parking lot. A campground (fee, vault

TRAIL USE
Day Hike, Backpack,
Run, Horse, Dogs
Allowed in Wilderness
LENGTH
5.0 miles, 2 hours to
Flower Lake
12.2 miles, 6–7 hours to
Kearsarge Lakes
VERTICAL FEET
+1325/-1325/±2650
+2675/-1425/±8200
DIFFICULTY
– 1 2 **3-4** 5 +
TRAIL TYPE
Out-and-back

FEATURES
Mountain
Lakes
Wildflowers
Great Views
Camping
Swimming
Fishing

FACILITIES
Campground
Restrooms
Water
Stables

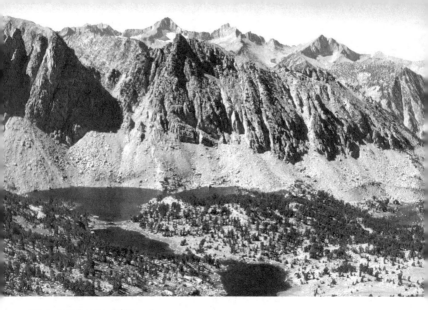

Kearsarge Lakes *and Pinnacles*

toilets, running water, and bear boxes), restrooms, and running water are available near the trailhead. Do not leave food or scented items in your car; bears are active in Onion Valley.

Logistics

Backpackers must obtain a wilderness permit for all overnight visits. See page 318 for more details on how to obtain one. Due to previous overuse, a

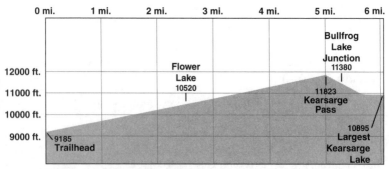

TRAIL 54 Flower Lake and Kearsarge Lakes Elevation Profile

one-night camping limit at Kearsarge Lakes and an outright ban around Bullfrog Lake are in effect. Bear canisters are required in the John Muir Wilderness east of Kearsarge Pass.

Trail Description

▶1 The trail begins near the restrooms, climbing a sagebrush-covered hillside above to the first of many switchbacks to come. Nearing the drainage of Golden Trout Creek, you reach a junction with a short connector to the Golden Trout Lakes Trail. ▶2 Remaining on the Kearsarge Pass Trail, proceed upslope through manzanita, mountain mahogany, and widely scattered red firs and limber pines toward the canyon of Independence Creek. Cross over the John Muir Wilderness boundary and continue to zigzag up the canyon, playing a game of hide and seek with the creek along the way. At one point during the climb, the stream is close enough for a thirst-slaking break. Continuing up the hillside, you have fine views down the canyon and across Owens Valley of the Inyo Mountains and south to the looming hulk of University Peak. A gently graded set of switchbacks leads to the first of the five lakes below Kearsarge Pass, Little Pothole Lake. ▶3 The willow-lined lake is attractively set in a diminutive, half moon–shaped basin, with waterfalls pouring down cliffs and flowing briefly through a patch of willows before entering the lake. A few overused campsites can be found around the shoreline beneath foxtail pines.

 Great Views

 Lake

Additional switchbacks lead away from Little Pothole Lake and farther up the canyon. After crossing a long talus slope, you draw near to willow-lined Independence Creek again and soon reach Gilbert Lake. ▶4 Gilbert is an oval-shaped lake with a pleasant-looking backdrop of craggy peaks. Grassy meadows dotted with clumps of willow provide

 Lake

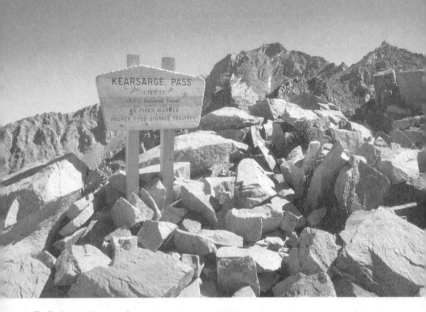

Trail sign *at Kearsarge Pass*

Fishing

Swimming

Lake

Camping

straightforward access for anglers seeking to catch the resident brook and brown trout. However, the easy access and short distance from the trailhead mean that the lake may be fished out by midseason. Hot and dusty hikers will find the water well suited for an afternoon swim. As with Little Pothole Lake, a number of overused campsites ring the shoreline.

Kearsarge Pass Trail follows a gently graded course along the north side of Gilbert Lake before resuming the climb alongside the creek through light pine forest. Soon you reach the vicinity of Flower Lake, ►5 where a very short path heads down to the shoreline and a number of pleasant, pine-sheltered campsites. The lake hosts a population of brook trout, but, similar to Gilbert Lake, the easy access may limit the catch by midseason. If you wish to visit Heart Lake, head upstream cross-country from the west end of Flower Lake, as the Kearsarge Pass Trail climbs well away from this lake. After fully enjoying the surroundings of Flower Lake, day hikers and backpackers not bound for the pass and points beyond should retrace their steps to the trailhead.

From Flower Lake, the Kearsarge Pass Trail ascends stark, shalelike terrain via some long-legged switchbacks on the way toward the broad notch of Kearsarge Pass. Gnarled, dwarf whitebark pines defy the elements, appearing to cling desperately to small pockets of soil, and look more like wind-blasted shrubs than trees. The moderate, upward traverse culminates in a sweeping vista from 11,823-foot Kearsarge Pass, ►6 with Kearsarge and Bullfrog Lakes shimmering in the customary Sierra sunshine below. Above the lakes lie the rugged Kearsarge Pinnacles and the serrated crest of the Kings-Kern Divide farther west. The high peak dominating the westward view is 11,868-foot Mount Bago. A number of signs at the pass welcome travelers to Kings Canyon National Park.

 Great Views

A moderately steep descent from the pass leads you high above the basin and down toward more-hospitable-looking terrain below. Near timberline is a junction ►7 between the Bullfrog Lake and Kearsarge Pass Trails.

Turn left and follow the Bullfrog Lake Trail on a switchbacking descent toward Kearsarge Lakes. After 0.25 mile, reach an unmarked junction ►8 with a use trail to the lakes. The U.S. Forest Service chose long ago to abandon maintenance of this path to the overused lakes, but frequent use has kept it well defined. Head south across a granite basin through widely scattered clumps of whitebark pines and past some delightful tarns to the largest of the lakes (10,895'). ►9 Tucked beneath the rugged wall of Kearsarge Pinnacles, the lakes are quite picturesque. Backpackers are limited to a one-night stay at the lakes, where a couple of bear boxes are provided for storing food and scented items. Anglers may find the fishing for rainbow trout a bit challenging.

 Lake

 Camping

 Fishing

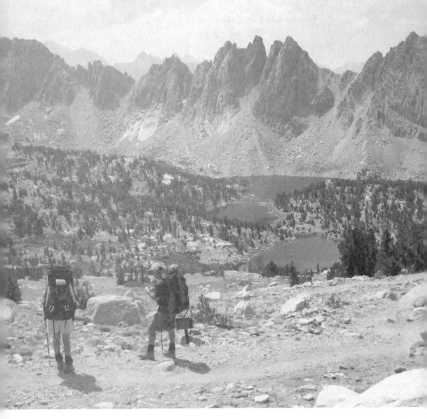

Kearsarge Lakes *backdropped by Kearsarge Pinnacles*

Bullfrog Lake

Bullfrog Lake is quite attractive, so overnighters staying at Kearsarge Lakes should avail themselves of the opportunity to take the short hike to the lake. Head back to Bullfrog Lake Trail and travel west through stunted pines and pockets of meadow on a moderate descent, hopping over numerous seasonal rivulets along the way. Soon the trail draws nearer to the main branch of the creek and proceeds through delightful open meadowlands on the way to Bullfrog Lake. Near the shore of this bluish-green lake, you quickly realize why this area was formerly such a popular camping destination—the meadow-rimmed lake rivals any in the Sierra for outstanding scenery. Across the deep trench of Bubbs Creek, the pyramidal summit of East Vidette rises sharply into the deep-blue sky, providing a dramatic counterpoint to the usually placid waters. Above the shoreline, clumps of pine shelter former campsites graced with splendid views—these days fine spots for a picnic lunch.

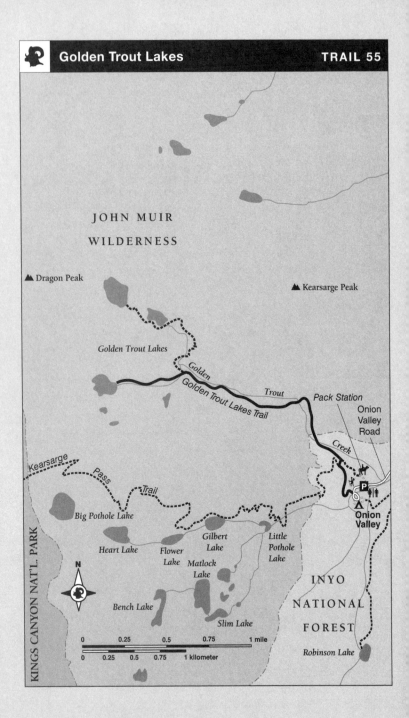

JOHN MUIR

WILDERNESS

▲ Dragon Peak

▲ Kearsarge Peak

Golden Trout Lakes

Golden

Golden Trout Lakes Trail

Trout

Pack Station

Onion
Valley
Road

Creek

Kearsarge

Pass

Trail

P

Onion
Valley

Big Pothole Lake

Gilbert
Lake

Little
Pothole
Lake

Heart Lake

Flower
Lake

Matlock
Lake

INYO

KINGS CANYON NAT'L. PARK

Bench Lake

Slim Lake

NATIONAL

FOREST

N

| 0 | 0.25 | 0.5 | 0.75 | 1 mile |
| 0 | 0.25 | 0.5 | 0.75 | 1 kilometer |

Robinson Lake

Golden Trout Lakes

The three lakes generally referred to as the Golden Trout Lakes (only the southernmost lake has the official name) provide fine destinations for either a pleasant day hike or an overnight backpack. The lakes are cradled in talus-filled cirques just below the Sierra Crest in the shadow of Mount Gould and Dragon Peak. Very few trails allow hikers into such an austere alpine environment with so little effort. Although the Kearsarge Pass Trail in the next canyon south is one of the most popular eastside trails in the High Sierra, relatively few hikers find their way up the unmaintained Golden Trout Lakes Trail. The trail is not in the best of shape, but, despite the condition, the route to the lakes is straightforward and the extraordinary scenery more than makes up for a few indistinct sections.

Best Time

Most of the trail is generally snow-free by early July, but the east-facing cirques that hold the lakes may cling to snow until mid-month. Wildflowers are best from mid-July to early August.

Finding the Trail

From the town of Independence, turn west from US 395 onto Market Street and head west following signs to Onion Valley. Drive 12.5 miles on Onion Valley Road to the end and leave your vehicle in the expansive parking lot. Restrooms, running water, and a campground (fee, vault toilets, running water,

TRAIL USE
Day Hike, Backpack, Run, Horse, Dogs Allowed

LENGTH
4.4 miles, 2–3 hours

VERTICAL FEET
+2300/-100/±4800

DIFFICULTY
– 1 2 **3** 4 5 +

TRAIL TYPE
Out-and-back

FEATURES
Mountain
Lake
Wildflowers
Camping
Swimming
Fishing

FACILITIES
Campground
Restrooms
Water
Stables

and bear boxes) are available near the trailhead. Do not leave food or scented items in your car; bears are active in Onion Valley.

Logistics

Backpackers must obtain a wilderness permit for all overnight visits. See page 318 for more details about how to obtain one.

Trail Description

▶1 The trail begins near the restrooms, climbing a sagebrush-covered hillside above to a switchback. Nearing the drainage of Golden Trout Creek, you reach a junction with a short connector to the Golden Trout Lakes Trail. ▶2

Leave the Kearsarge Pass Trail and drop shortly to a junction ▶3 with a trail from the pack station; head upstream along Golden Trout Creek through open pinyon pine and sagebrush terrain. Views up-canyon include Golden Trout Fall. Riparian vegetation appears where the trail closely follows a stretch of the creek, crosses the creek, and immediately enters the John Muir Wilderness.

Continue up the canyon on a winding climb through loose rock that leads above the waterfall.

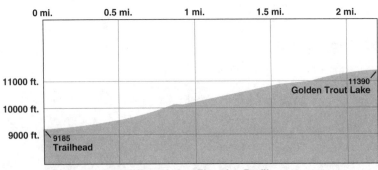

TRAIL 55 Golden Trout Lakes Elevation Profile

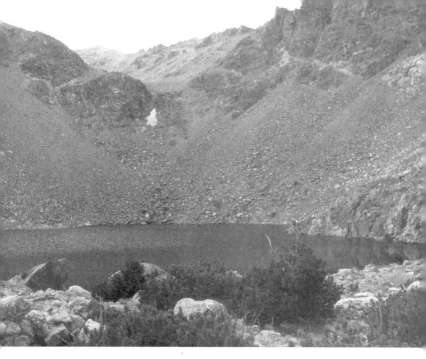

One of the *Golden Trout Lakes*

From there, pass through a flower-filled gully and cross back over Golden Trout Creek. Beyond the second creek crossing, the tread becomes faint and a little hard to follow in places, especially in areas filled with talus and boulders. However, the route is obvious—head upstream through the narrow canyon. The trail makes two close fords of the creek, but the tread is so faint here that these crossings are easily missed. Eventually, you climb less-steep terrain on the way to a lush meadow near where the creek forks into two branches. Passable campsites are nearby on a low rise. ▶4

To reach Golden Trout Lake, the southernmost lake bearing the official name, cross the left-hand branch of the creek and head west along the north bank through gnarled whitebark pines and a few foxtail pines. Once again, the tread is a bit sketchy, but the route is obvious. Continue up the creek to the east shore of Golden Trout Lake,

 Wildflowers

 Camping

 Lake

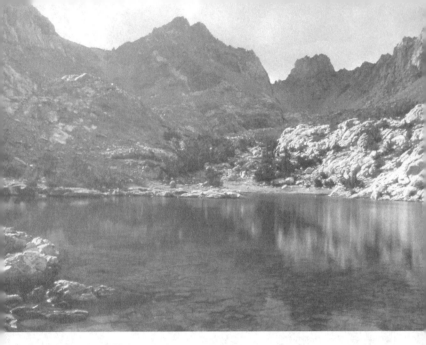

Another of the *Golden Trout Lakes*

►5 where a few matted shrubs and some widely scattered dwarf whitebark pines vainly attempt to soften the boulder- and talus-filled, glacier-carved amphitheater. The apex of this rugged amphitheater is 13,005-foot Mount Gould. A pair of fine campsites near the outlet may tempt backpackers, while anglers can test their skill on brook trout and the lake's namesake fish. Experienced off-trail enthusiasts can continue up-canyon, scrambling over boulders to Dragon Pass, a 12,800-foot notch halfway between Mount Gould and Dragon Peak.

Camping

Fishing

Unnamed Lakes

OPTIONS

The U.S. Geological Survey 7.5-minute map shows a trail that follows the right-hand branch of **Golden Trout Creek** to a pair of unnamed tarns east of **Dragon Peak**. Although this path has mostly disappeared over time, the route is an easily managed cross-country trek. From where the creek forks, follow the right-hand branch around a meadow, over the creek, and up the canyon to the lower lake. From there, the route to the upper lake is just as straightforward. Both tarns are quite scenic, picturesquely back-dropped by the multihued flanks of Dragon Peak. A few campsites can be found at both lakes.

MILESTONES

▶1   0.0   Start at Onion Valley Trailhead
▶2   0.3   Right at junction of connector
▶3   0.35 Left at junction of Golden Trout Lakes Trail
▶4   1.7   Left at fork of Golden Trout Creek
▶5   2.2   Golden Trout Lake

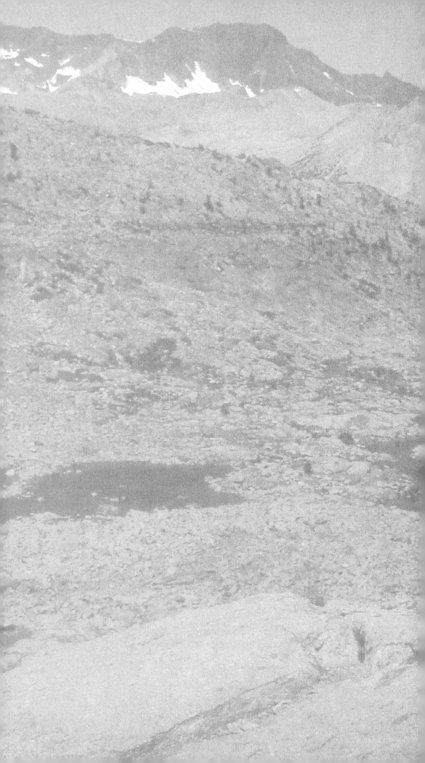

CHAPTER 7

Eastern Sierra: White Mountain Ranger District

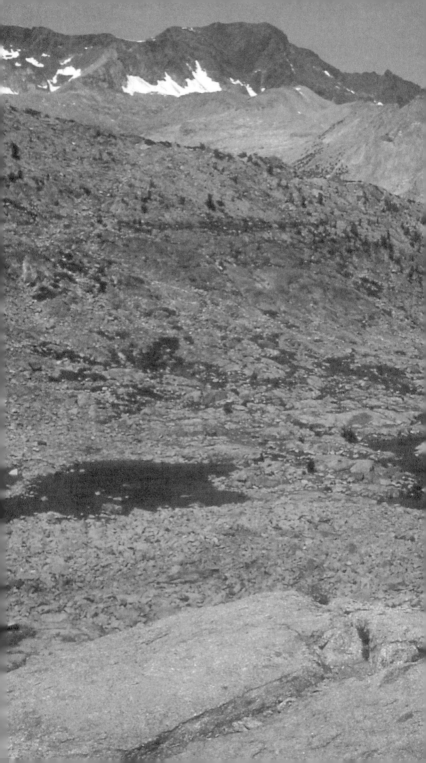

Eastern Sierra: White Mountain Ranger District

Continuing the topography found to the south, this section of the eastern Sierra within the White Mountain Ranger District rises abruptly and dramatically from the plain of Owens Valley to its high crest. Rugged mountains tower thousands of feet over the valley and the small communities dotting the plain. Trails in this area either dead-end at the base of impenetrable walls at the head of steep canyons, or they climb stiffly to high-elevation passes in the Sierra crest. The magnificent beauty found in these mountains is well known to a host of recreationists, including hikers, backpackers, climbers, equestrians, photographers, and anglers. Dramatic-looking peaks, glacier-carved cirques, flower-bedecked meadows, shimmering alpine lakes, and deeply cleft canyons are all present in abundance, just waiting to be explored.

US 395 provides the principal access to trailheads in this area. Similar to the area covered in the previous chapter, no roads or highways cross the Sierra crest through these lands. The nearest trans-Sierra road, the seasonally open Tioga Pass Road, lies well to the north in Yosemite National Park. Consequently, the combined backcountry of Sequoia and Kings Canyon National Parks and the surrounding wilderness areas creates one of the largest roadless areas in the country.

All of the trails included in this chapter involve stiff climbs at high elevations. Trail users should be in good condition and well acclimatized to the altitude to fully enjoy the experience these trails offer. Every one of the trails described here travels to at least one beautiful subalpine or alpine lake, with several trips taking in multiple lakes, and all enjoy the presence of the rugged spine of the High Sierra. Midseason visits offer the added bonus of copious wildflowers gracing the meadows and lining the stream banks.

Overleaf and opposite: *Palisade Basin*

375

Trails 56 and 57 ascend spectacular canyons of Big Pine Creek to stunning scenery in the shadow of the world-renowned Palisades, an alpine mecca of 14,000-foot peaks and icy glaciers. The remaining trips all depart from trailheads above the town of Bishop from a trio of lakes—Bishop, Sabrina, and North.

Permits

Wilderness permits are required for all overnight stays in the backcountry of John Muir Wilderness and Kings Canyon National Park. Trailhead quotas are in effect from May 1 to November 1 for eastside entry into John Muir Wilderness. Sixty percent of the daily quota is available by advance reservation with a $6 reservation fee and a $5 per-person fee. To make an advance reservation for trails described in this chapter, go to **recreation.gov** and enter "Inyo National Forest wilderness permit" in the search window. The remaining 40% of the daily quota is available as walk-in permits. These free permits can be picked up the day before the start of a trip at U.S. Forest Service offices during normal business hours. All permits can be picked up at either the Eastern Sierra Interagency Visitor Center (Lone Pine), White Mountain Ranger Station (Bishop), Mammoth Ranger Station (Mammoth Lakes), or Mono Basin Scenic Area Visitor Center (Lee Vining). For more information, call the wilderness permit information line at 760-873-2483 between 8 a.m. and 4:30 p.m.

Maps

For the White Mountain Ranger District, the U.S. Geological Survey 7.5-minute (1:24,000 scale) topographic maps are listed below, corresponding to the trails described in this section. Trail users also may want to consider using Tom Harrison's maps, *Sequoia & Kings Canyon National Parks* (1:125,000), *The Palisades* (1:31,680), or *Bishop Pass-North Lake/South Lake* (1:47,520).

> Trail 56: *Coyote Flat, Split Mountain*
>
> Trail 57: *Coyote Flat, Split Mountain, Mt. Thompson, North Palisade*
>
> Trail 58: *Mt. Thompson, North Palisade*
>
> Trails 59–61: *Mt. Thompson*
>
> Trail 62: *Mt. Thompson, Mt. Darwin*
>
> Trail 63: *Mt. Darwin*
>
> Trail 64: *Mt. Darwin, Mt. Tom*

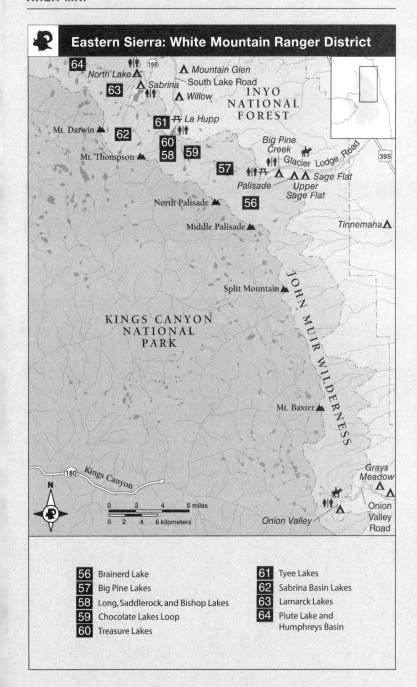

Eastern Sierra: White Mountain Ranger District

64 North Lake
63 Sabrina
168
Mountain Glen
South Lake Road
Willow

INYO NATIONAL FOREST

61 La Hupp
Mt. Darwin 62
60
58 59
Mt. Thompson

Big Pine Creek
Glacier Lodge Road
395
57 Palisade
Sage Flat
Upper Sage Flat

North Palisade 56

Middle Palisade

Tinnemaha

Split Mountain

KINGS CANYON NATIONAL PARK

JOHN MUIR WILDERNESS

Mt. Baxter

180 Kings Canyon

N

0   2   4   6 miles
0 2   4   6 kilometers

Grays Meadow

Onion Valley Road

Onion Valley

56 Brainerd Lake
57 Big Pine Lakes
58 Long, Saddlerock, and Bishop Lakes
59 Chocolate Lakes Loop
60 Treasure Lakes

61 Tyee Lakes
62 Sabrina Basin Lakes
63 Lamarck Lakes
64 Piute Lake and Humphreys Basin

Eastern Sierra: White Mountain Ranger District

TRAIL	DIFFICULTY	LENGTH	TYPE	USES & ACCESS	TERRAIN	FLORA & FAUNA	OTHER
56	4	10.0	Out-and-back	🥾🎒🏃🐕🐎	⛰️🌊	🌸	👀⛺🏊🎣
57	4	11.4	Loop	🥾🎒🏃🐕🐎	⛰️🌊	🌸	👀⛺🏊🎣🏠
58	3	8.6	Out-and-back	🥾🎒🏃🐕🐎	⛰️🌊	🌸	⛺🏊🎣
59	3	7.2	Loop	🥾🎒🏃🐕	⛰️🌊	🌸	⛺🏊🎣
60	3	7.6	Out-and-back	🥾🎒🏃🐕🐎	⛰️🌊	🌸	⛺🏊🎣
61	3	6.5	Out-and-back	🎒🏃🐕🐎	⛰️🌊	🌸	⛺🏊🎣
62	3	13.6	Out-and-back	🥾🎒🏃🐕🐎	⛰️🌊	🌸	👀⛺🏊🎣
63	4	5.4	Out-and-back	🥾🎒🏃🐕🐎	⛰️🌊	🌸	⛺🏊🎣
64	3 and 4	6.6, 14.4	Loop	🥾🎒🏃🐕🐎	⛰️🌊	🌸	👀⛺🏊🎣

USES & ACCESS	TYPE	TERRAIN	FLORA & FAUNA	OTHER
🥾 Day Hiking	🔄 Loop	🛡️ Canyon	🍁 Fall Colors	👀 Great Views
🎒 Backpacking	✏️ Out-and-back	⛰️ Mountain	🌸 Wildflowers	⛺ Camping
🏃 Running	🔻 Point-to-point	△ Summit	🌲 Giant Sequoias	🏊 Swimming
🐕 Horses	DIFFICULTY	🌊 Lake		🔒 Secluded
🐾 Dogs Allowed	- 1 2 3 4 5 +	🏞️ Stream		⬇️ Steep
👥 Child Friendly	less more	💧 Waterfall		🎣 Fishing
♿ Wheelchair-Access				🏠 Historical Interest

Eastern Sierra:
White Mountain Ranger District

Brainerd Lake 382

The Palisades are well known to alpinists around the globe, and this trip into the Middle Palisades rivals any in the Sierra for sheer alpine beauty. At times the trail is both steep and poorly maintained, but the awesome grandeur near Brainerd Lake more than compensates for these minor annoyances. Off-trail extensions to Finger Lake and Middle Palisade Glacier provide added bonuses.

TRAIL 56

Day Hike, Backpack,
Run, Horse, Dogs
Allowed
10.0 miles,
Out-and-back
Difficulty: 1 2 3 **4** 5

Big Pine Lakes 388

This semiloop through the Big Pine Lakes is a quintessential High Sierra trip, visiting a bevy of gorgeous lakes beneath the towering summits of the Palisades. Side trails to additional lakes, as well as Sam Mack Meadow and the Palisade Glacier, offer so many wonderful diversions that one could easily spend an entire week in the upper North Fork Big Pine Creek basin.

TRAIL 57

Day Hike, Backpack,
Run, Horse, Dogs
Allowed
11.4 miles, Semiloop
Difficulty: 1 2 3 **4** 5

TRAIL 58

Day Hike, Backpack,
Run, Horse, Dogs
Allowed

8.6 miles, Out-and-back

Difficulty: 1 2 **3** 4 5

Long, Saddlerock, and Bishop Lakes 400

South Lake is the jumping-off point for many fine Sierra adventures, and this trip along South Fork Bishop Creek is certainly no exception. The trail is popular for good reason—travelers are treated to rushing streams, verdant meadows, colorful wildflowers, sparkling lakes, and towering peaks. The trail's popularity can make obtaining a wilderness permit challenging, with trailhead parking at a premium as well.

TRAIL 59

Day Hike, Backpack,
Run, Horse, Dogs
Allowed

7.2 miles, Semiloop

Difficulty: 1 2 **3** 4 5

Chocolate Lakes Loop 406

This relatively short semiloop leads around aptly named Chocolate Peak from the well-traveled Bishop Pass Trail to a string of picturesque lakes surrounded by outstanding scenery.

TRAIL 60

Day Hike, Backpack,
Run, Horse, Dogs
Allowed

7.6 miles, Out-and-back

Difficulty: 1 2 **3** 4 5

Treasure Lakes 413

Excellent scenery and a variety of plant zones combine to make this trip to the Treasure Lakes quite desirable. The upper lakes should offer a reasonable expectation of solitude as well.

TRAIL 61

Day Hike, Backpack,
Run, Horse, Dogs
Allowed

6.5 miles, Out-and-back

Difficulty: 1 2 **3** 4 5

Tyee Lakes. 419

Whether you're looking to fish, camp, swim, or just hike, the lightly used path to the high granite basin holding Tyee Lakes fits the bill. The short distance makes this trail well suited for a straightforward trip for recreationists of all ages.

Sabrina Basin Lakes 425

The wonderfully picturesque Sabrina Basin near the headwaters of Middle Fork Bishop Creek holds a plethora of stunning lakes, which will leave day-trippers thirsty for more. There are numerous options for trip extensions to lakes off the beaten path via side trails and cross-country routes for those with more time. The scenery is magnificent, with towering peaks of the High Sierra trimming the basin.

TRAIL 62

Day Hike, Backpack, Run, Horse, Dogs Allowed

13.6 miles, Out-and-back

Difficulty: 1 2 **3** 4 5

Lamarck Lakes 433

Two distinctly different lakes set in the shadow of the eastern Sierra crest provide worthy destinations for a day hike or overnight backpack. Although the distance is minimal, the stiff climb may make the 2.7 miles to Upper Lamarck Lake seem a lot farther. The Wonder Lakes nearby offer a fine trip extension for cross-country enthusiasts.

TRAIL 63

Day Hike, Backpack, Run, Horse, Dogs Allowed

5.4 miles, Out-and-back

Difficulty: 1 2 3 **4** 5

Piute Lake and Humphreys Basin . . 439

Surrounded by craggy peaks and ridges, Humphreys Basin is one of the most picturesque spots in the High Sierra, especially in midseason when the floor of the basin is carpeted with a magnificent display of colorful wildflowers. The rigors of the stiff climb over Piute Pass are soon forgotten amid the beauty of the sprawling basin sprinkled with picturesque lakes and bisected by delightful brooks. Although reaching the majority of the lakes requires off-trail travel, the open topography is easily negotiated by all but beginning recreationists.

TRAIL 64

Day Hike, Backpack, Run, Horse, Dogs Allowed

6.6 miles, Out-and-back to Piute Lake

14.4 miles, Out-and-back to Humphreys Basin

Difficulty: 1 2 **3-4** 5

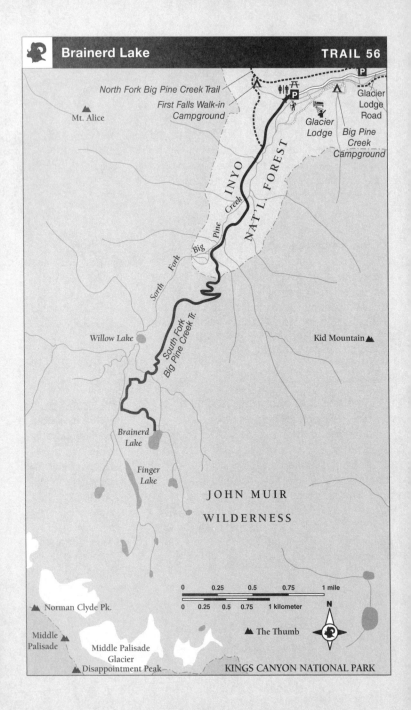

North Fork Big Pine Creek Trail

First Falls Walk-in
Campground

Mt. Alice

Glacier
Lodge

Glacier
Lodge
Road

Big Pine
Creek
Campground

INYO

NAT'L FOREST

Big

Pine

Creek

South

Fork

Willow Lake

Kid Mountain

South Fork
Big Pine Creek Tr.

Brainerd
Lake

Finger
Lake

JOHN MUIR

WILDERNESS

Norman Clyde Pk.

Middle
Palisade

Middle Palisade
Glacier

Disappointment Peak

The Thumb

| 0 | 0.25 | 0.5 | 0.75 | 1 mile |

| 0 | 0.25 | 0.5 | 0.75 | 1 kilometer |

N

KINGS CANYON NATIONAL PARK

Brainerd Lake

Alpinists from across the globe are drawn to the beauty and challenge of the bevy of 14,000-foot peaks known as the Palisades. Less-adventurous recreationists can enjoy the splendid alpine scenery found in the Middle Palisades on this journey up the canyon of South Fork Big Pine Creek to Brainerd Lake and the off-trail backcountry beyond. Although the terrain is heavenly, parts of the ascent may seem to have less divine origins. The first half of the trip climbs reasonably on well-maintained tread, but the second half climbs more steeply on rough and poorly maintained trail, which, at this altitude, may leave flatlanders perturbed and gasping for breath. Once at Brainerd Lake, the trials and tribulations are soon forgotten amid the overwhelming beauty. Those with off-trail ambitions can continue climbing to Finger Lake and an incredible view of the Middle Palisade Glacier.

Best Time

This is high-alpine country. Consequently, trails don't shed their snow in these parts until mid-summer, which is usually around mid-July following winters of average snowfall. Patches of snow may last into August in some years, especially on the north-facing slopes below the Palisades crest. Early August is generally the best time to see the wildflowers in bloom. September can be a fine time for a visit, but expect increasingly chilly nighttime temperatures as the month unfolds.

TRAIL USE
Day Hike, Backpack,
Run, Horse,
Dogs Allowed

LENGTH
10.0 miles, 5–6 hours

VERTICAL FEET
+3750/-700/±8900

DIFFICULTY
− 1 2 3 **4** 5 +

TRAIL TYPE
Out-and-back

FEATURES
Mountain
Lake
Wildflowers
Great Views
Camping
Swimming
Fishing

FACILITIES
Campground
Resort

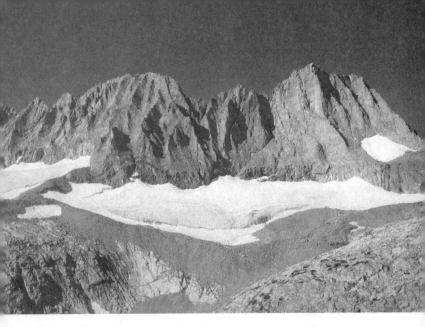

Middle Palisade *and Disappointment Peak*

Finding the Trail

From US 395 in the center of Big Pine, turn west at Crocker Street and proceed out of town, as the road becomes Glacier Lodge Road. Follow the two-lane highway past campgrounds to the overnight parking area, or continue another 0.75 mile to the day-use lot near the end of the road. Both areas are

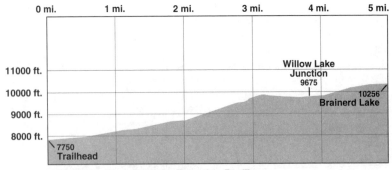

TRAIL 56 **Brainerd Lake Elevation Profile**

equipped with vault toilets. The U.S. Forest Service administers three public campgrounds (fee, vault toilets, running water, bear boxes, and phone) along Glacier Lodge Road: Upper Sage Flat, North Fork Big Pine, and Big Pine Creek. Two group campgrounds are also available by reservation. First Falls Walk-In is a no-fee campground for backpackers about a mile up the North Fork Trail, an excellent spot for those getting a late start. Although the main lodge building that housed a restaurant burned down a number of years ago, nearby Glacier Lodge continues to offer cabin rentals, guided trips, and pack trains.

> The opal-tinted, icy waters of 10,256-foot Brainerd Lake are tucked into a deep, glacier-carved bowl of granite.

Logistics

Backpackers must obtain a wilderness permit for all overnight visits. See page 376 for more details about how to obtain one.

Trail Description

▶1 From the day-use lot, stroll through shady forest next to Big Pine Creek along the continuation of the road past a few rustic cabins. Soon the road gives way to singletrack trail, as you climb a forested hillside on rock steps and then proceed across a bridge spanning North Fork Big Pine Creek. Continue past

OPTIONS

Willow Lake

At 9,565 feet, Willow Lake is just a short 0.3-mile jaunt away. Sediments are steadily transforming the lake into more of a marshy meadow, and in early summer, the standing water creates a haven for mosquitoes. However, a couple of lodgepole-shaded campsites offer overnight accommodations for backpackers who get a late start or are too pooped to carry on toward Brainerd Lake.

Finger Lake and Middle Palisade Glacier

Without question the scenery around Brainerd Lake is stunning, but to come all this way and not go beyond the lake would be missing out on some even more extraordinary scenery. With a modicum of cross-country skills, hikers can quite easily make the short journey to slender Finger Lake by following a fairly well-defined, ducked use trail that begins near the outlet of Brainerd Lake. An arcing ascent leads above the cliffs on the northwest shore and then weaves through a boulder field to Finger Lake. The 10,787-foot lake nestled into a narrow cleft of rock that arcs toward the Palisades crest evokes a miniature Norwegian fjord. Scattered pines dot the lakeshore, while tiny pockets of wildflowers soften the otherwise stark surroundings. A few campsites can be found just below the lake between the outlet and the trail. To reach the edge of the glacier, head generally south from Finger Lake on a steep cross-country route up the canyon. The ascent can by physically taxing at this altitude, but the rewards of such dramatic alpine scenery more than compensate for the effort.

the bridge to a junction with a connector to the North Fork Trail. ►2

Bear left at the junction and cross an open, sagebrush-covered slope up the canyon of the cottonwood-lined South Fork Big Pine Creek, enjoying views of Norman Clyde Peak and Middle Palisade along the way. Cross over an old road and continue up-canyon on a moderate climb, crossing a seasonal stream and a boulder-filled slope on the way to a ford of the creek. A mild ascent heads away from the ford until a steep, winding climb via rocky switchbacks leads through scattered timber to the base of some nearly vertical bluffs. Traverse the hillside and then climb steeply up a narrow cleft of rock to a crest and, after a short distance, a splendid panorama of the Palisades, stretching from Mount Sill to the Thumb, a vista rivaling any in the Sierra for stunning alpine scenery. Past this splendid vista, the trail drops into the cover of lodgepole pines, passes

Great Views

a spring-fed rivulet, and then reaches a T-junction with a short lateral to Willow Lake. ►3

 Lake

From the junction, a short descent heads down to a crossing of the lushly vegetated outlet from Brainerd Lake. From there, a winding ascent across a lodgepole-covered slope leads alongside the stream that drains Finger Lake. Turning east, the trail passes a small pond and continues uphill via switchbacks to a hump of granite that provides a fine view down-canyon of Willow Lake. Pass a second pond, make a short descent across a marshy meadow, and then swing around a granite ledge on a final climb southeast to the north shore of Brainerd Lake. ►4

The opal-tinted, icy waters of 10,256-foot Brainerd Lake are tucked into a deep, glacier-carved bowl of granite. Steep cliffs hem in the lake on virtually all sides, with snow oftentimes lingering in narrow crevices late into the summer. The craggy, glacier-clad summits of the Palisades loom over the tops of the cliffs thousands of feet above. A smattering of compact campsites near the outlet, sheltered by lodgepole and whitebark pines, offer overnighters wonderfully scenic spots to rest their heads. Anglers may wish to test their luck on the brook trout that inhabit the lake.

 Camping

 Fishing

🚶	MILESTONES	
►1	0.0	Start at day-use trailhead
►2	0.3	Left at junction with connector to North Fork Trail
►3	3.8	Ahead at Willow Lake junction
►4	5.0	Brainerd Lake

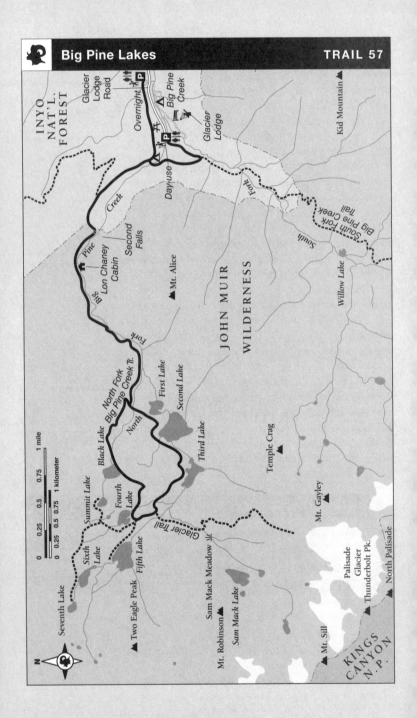

INYO
NAT'L.
FOREST

Glacier Lodge Road

Big Pine Creek

Kid Mountain ▲

Overnight

Glacier Lodge

Day-use

Creek

South Fork
Big Pine Creek Trail

Pine

Second Falls

Fork

South

Lon Chaney Cabin

Big

▲ Mt. Alice

Willow Lake

JOHN MUIR

WILDERNESS

North Fork
Big Pine Creek Tl.

First Lake

Second Lake

North

Fork

Black Lake

Third Lake

Temple Crag ▲

Summit Lake

Fourth Lake

Fifth Lake

Glacier Trail

Sam Mack Meadow ⊻

Mt. Gayley ▲

Sixth Lake

Two Eagle Peak ▲

Sam Mack Lake

Palisade Glacier

North Palisade ▲

Seventh Lake

Mt. Robinson ▲

Sam Mack Lake

Mt. Sill ▲

Thunderbolt Pk. ▲

KINGS
CANYON
N.P.

0   0.25   0.5   0.75   1 mile

0   0.25 0.5 0.75 1 kilometer

N

Big Pine Lakes

Some of the best high-alpine scenery in the Sierra can be found on this circuit through Big Pine Lakes basin in the North Fork Big Pine Creek drainage. Piercing the rarefied air near the upper height of the range, the group of peaks known as the Palisades composes a craggy spine of summits robed in scenic splendor as picturesque and dramatic as any in California, if not the entire western United States. Clinging beneath the north face of these rugged peaks, a handful of glaciers, including the Palisade Glacier (the Sierra's largest), add a definite alpine ambience to the area. Even the lower peaks, such as Temple Crag, cast a bold and rugged presence offering climbers a technical challenge and hikers a spectacular profile when viewed from a variety of vantage points along the trail. Nestled beneath the shadow of these towering peaks are the glacier-scoured basins holding the scenic Big Pine Lakes, the milky-turquoise color revealing the glacial origin of their waters. The shorelines of these lakes offer exceptional views of the surrounding wonders, as well as fine campsites.

Such spectacular scenery is bound to attract a large number of visitors, placing a high demand on the limited number of wilderness permits for those who desire to spend at least one night in the backcountry. Because the trail climbs stiffly from the trailhead to the lake's basin, most overnighters seek campsites near the first lakes along the trail, allowing a higher possibility for solitude at the more-far-flung lakes. Most day hikers should find the 11.4-mile semiloop to be plenty challenging, but extremely strong hikers, as well as backpackers,

TRAIL USE
Day Hike, Backpack,
Run, Horse,
Dogs Allowed
LENGTH
11.4 miles, 6–7 hours
VERTICAL FEET
+3175/-3175/±6350
DIFFICULTY
– 1 2 3 **4 5** +
TRAIL TYPE
Semiloop

FEATURES
Mountain
Lake
Wildflowers
Great Views
Camping
Swimming
Fishing
Historical Interest

FACILITIES
Campground
Resort

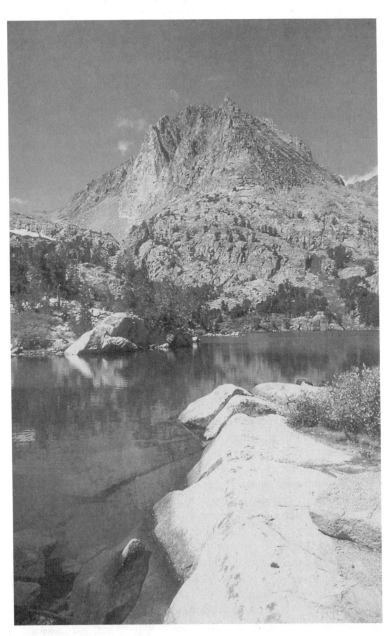

Fifth Lake *and Two Eagle Peak*

will find trip extensions to lakes beyond the loop and to the Palisade Glacier well worth the extra time and energy.

Best Time

This is high-alpine country. Consequently, trails don't shed their snow in these parts until mid-summer, which is usually around mid-July following winters of average snowfall. Patches of snow may last into August in some years, especially on the north-facing slopes below the Palisades crest. Early August is generally the best time to see the wildflowers in bloom. September can be a fine time for a visit, but nighttime temperatures become increasingly chilly as the month unfolds.

Finding the Trail

From US 395 in the center of Big Pine, turn west at Crocker Street and proceed out of town, as the road becomes Glacier Lodge Road. Follow the two-lane highway past campgrounds to the overnight parking area, or continue another 0.75 mile to the day-use lot near the end of the road. Both areas are equipped with vault toilets. The U.S. Forest Service administers

The shorelines of these lakes offer exceptional views of the surrounding wonders, as well as fine campsites.

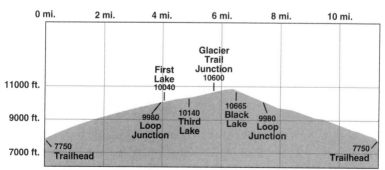

TRAIL 57 Big Pine Lakes Elevation Profile

three public campgrounds (fee, vault toilets, running water, bear boxes, and phone) along the Glacier Lodge Road: Upper Sage Flat, North Fork Big Pine, and Big Pine Creek. Two group campgrounds are also available by reservation. First Falls Walk-In is a no-fee campground for backpackers about a mile up the North Fork Trail, an excellent spot for those getting a late start. Although the main lodge building that housed a restaurant burned down a number of years ago, nearby Glacier Lodge continues to offer cabin rentals, guided trips, and pack trains.

Logistics

Backpackers must obtain a wilderness permit for all overnight visits. See page 376 for more details about how to obtain one.

Trail Description

►1 From the day-use lot, stroll through shady forest next to Big Pine Creek along the continuation of the road past a few rustic cabins. Soon the road gives way to singletrack trail, as you climb a forested hillside on rock steps and then proceed across a bridge spanning North Fork Big Pine Creek. Continue past the bridge to a junction with your connector to the North Fork Trail. ►2

Bear right at the junction and follow short switchbacks up an open slope with good views up the South Fork canyon. Back under shady forest, the grade eases on the way to a T-junction with an old road. ►3 Turn right and proceed a short distance on the roadbed to a bridge over the creek and shortly to another junction. ►4 Following a sign marked UPPER TRAIL, veer right away from the road and head east-southeast, climbing steeply, then more gradually to a junction ►5 with the trail from the overnight parking lot. Along the way, fine views of the long cascade of Second Falls should cheer you onward.

Turn left and ascend open slopes toward Second Falls. After some switchbacks, you cross into John Muir Wilderness and head up a chasm. Above the falls, the trail climbs moderately alongside the shady creek for a spell, wanders back out into the open, and then follows gently graded tread across an aspen- and lodgepole-shaded flat known as Cienega Mirth (a combination of a misspelled Spanish word and a Scottish word, both meaning "swampy place"). A number of pleasant campsites are spread about this flat.

 Camping

Beyond Lon Chaney's cabin, the trail passes through an open area with a glimpse of some of the ragged peaks at the head of the canyon. The moderate ascent resumes as the trail wanders back and forth to the creek several times through lush vegetation and light forest. Where the trail bends west, the dramatic northeast face of Temple Crag makes brief appearances. Cross willow-lined North Fork Big Pine Creek, climb more steeply via switchbacks, and then cross back over the creek, beyond which more climbing leads to a junction with the beginning of the loop section. ▶6

Lon Chaney Cabin

HISTORY

In what appears to be the middle of nowhere sits a distinguished granite fieldstone cabin with a gable roof and overhanging eaves. Used today by rangers as a wilderness cabin, the structure was originally built at the behest of silent film star Lon Chaney in the 1920s. Chaney used the cabin as a summer retreat, where he relaxed, fished, and hunted. Listed on the National Register of Historic Places, the cabin was designed by Paul Revere Williams, who holds the distinction of being the first African American granted a fellowship by the American Institute of Architects.

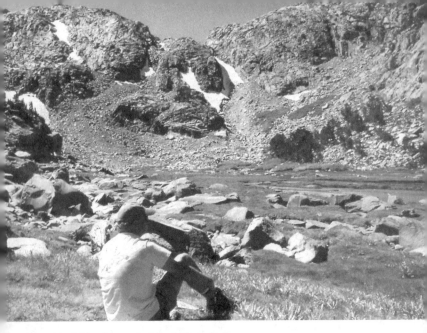

Sam Mack Meadow *on the Palisade Glacier Trail*

Camping

Lake

Camping

Fishing

Follow the left-hand trail, signed LAKES 1–7, immediately cross the creek, pass a couple of campsites, and keep climbing through scattered forest and granite slabs and around large boulders. The sound of running water from a cascade heralds the presence of nearby First Lake, ▶7 its milky-turquoise, glacier-fed waters visible through gaps in the forest. Farther on, a zigzagging descent leads to a spectacular overlook of Second Lake, with an impressive backdrop from the towering ramparts of 12,999-foot Temple Crag. Second Lake is the largest in the chain of Big Pine Lakes, but much of the shoreline is too steep to allow decent camping. Although a few isolated campsites can be found spread around the shoreline, most backpackers are more content with sites above the west shore of First Lake. Anglers can practice their craft on brook, brown, and rainbow trout in both lakes. Mildly graded trail leads well above the surface of Second Lake, where sparse forest permits stunning views of the surrounding terrain.

Beyond Second Lake, the trail follows the inlet on a climb through rocky terrain beneath a cover of lodgepole pines, before veering away from the stream on the way to the north shore of Third Lake. ▶8 Here's an even more impressive view of Temple Crag, perhaps the main reason backpackers prefer the numerous campsites sprinkled around the lightly forested shoreline. Anglers may be tempted by the brook and rainbow trout seen gliding through the chilly waters.

 Camping

Switchbacks lead away from Third Lake on a climb out of the lake's basin. Take the time to look behind you, as the view of Third Lake reposing in a rocky bowl at the base of Temple Crag and the craggy summits of the Palisades is quite impressive, along with the massive face of Mount Robinson and Aperture Peak just behind. The grade eases a bit near a small meadow, where you hop across a tiny rivulet that drains Fourth Lake. Just beyond this rivulet is a junction near a grove of pines with the Glacier Trail. ▶9

From the Glacier Trail junction, head northwest on a moderate climb through scattered pines

NOTE

Grand Views

The stunning views from the trail above Second Lake include the dramatic and precipitous flying buttresses of Temple Crag, rising high above the crystalline water. Challenging Class 5 routes on Temple Crag lure climbers from around the world. In stark contrast, the massive rock pile to the east, Mount Alice, has been dubbed "one of the ugliest peaks in the Sierra—a veritable pile of rubble" by author Steve Roper, who expressed his disdain for the peak in *Climbers Guide to the High Sierra*. Separating these two peaks is Contact Pass, where the line between the darker and lighter shades of granite is quite evident. The pass provides a cross-country route between the two canyons of Big Pine Creek.

and past rocks and boulders, with pleasant views of the Palisades to a four-way junction. ►10 The left-hand trail leads a quarter mile to Fifth Lake, while the trail straight ahead provides access to Sixth and Seventh Lakes.

BEGIN SIDE TRIP: To continue to Fifth Lake, turn left from the junction and proceed through light forest to the lake's outlet. Continue alongside the willow-lined creek on gently graded tread to the east shore of the picturesque lake, where rugged mountains, including Mount Robinson, Two Eagle Peak, and Aperture Peak, form a scenic arc around the sapphire waters. The more distant summits of Temple Crag, Mount Gayley, Mount Sill, and the Inconsolable Range provide additional visual delight. A smattering of pines dots the shoreline and the lower slopes of the basin, while grasses, sedges, and shrubs carpet the small pockets of soil between the rocky cliffs and talus slopes. Pleasant campsites near the inlet and farther around the shoreline will tempt overnighters.

Great Views 🔭

Camping ⛺

Back at the four-way junction with the trail to Sixth and Seventh Lakes, head northwest above the west shore of Fourth Lake to continue to the other lakes, and then ascend a low hill past some campsites. The grade increases where you cross a willow-lined stream flowing into Fourth Lake. Near the stream, an old and obscure path heads northwest to Sixth Lake, but the path soon deteriorates to more of a cross-country route. Traveling in the opposite direction leads very shortly to a level spot on a ridge with some campsites and an incredible view of the Palisades, spanning from Temple Crag to Mount Winchell. This excellent view was the reason the Fourth Lake Lodge was built here in the 1920s. The U.S. Forest Service removed the lodge and eight cabins after passage of the original Wilderness Act of 1964. Continue ahead from the stream to a junction, where the left-hand branch continues to Sixth and Seventh Lakes, and the right-hand trail provides access to Summit Lake.

Camping ⛺

Great Views 🔭

OPTIONS

Palisade Glacier Trail

The steep 2-mile, 1,600-foot climb to the Palisade Glacier may be well beyond the reach of most day-trippers, but those with extra time and energy will be well rewarded for the effort with absolutely outstanding scenery. From the junction, turn left and head southwest through a willow-covered meadow and across a stream draining Fifth Lake, before a zigzagging climb leads up a rocky slope through widely scattered whitebark pines. Midway up the slope is a luxuriant, spring-fed grotto carpeted with abundant wildflowers. Farther up the hillside, the path ascends alongside the creek, which is lined with more flowers, including paintbrush, buttercup, shooting star, daisy, aster, and columbine. Where the grade eases, you crest the lip of the basin holding beautiful Sam Mack Meadow and proceed across the long, thin meadowland bordered by steep walls of gray granite and bisected by a sinuous brook tinged with white glacial milk. Snow clings to the precipitous walls at the head of the canyon, lingering throughout the short summers common at this elevation. A few campsites perched on a sloping, sandy bench adjacent to the meadow and shaded by clumps of dwarf pines may tempt overnighters. Although a footpath extends to the far end of the meadow, Sam Mack Lake is most easily reached by heading cross-country up the west canyon wall and then southwest to the lakeshore.

To continue toward Palisade Glacier, ford the creek near the lower end of the meadow, where an old, small sign simply marked TRAIL points the way across the broad but shallow brook to a use trail on the far side that ascends the east wall of the canyon. Wind up the rocky hillside to the crest, and then turn south, continuing to wind around boulders and rocks amid widely scattered whitebark pines up the left-hand side of a ridge, with excellent views down to Big Pine Lakes. About a mile from Sam Mack Meadow, the route bends southeast and follows an ascending traverse to a moraine. The path becomes less discernible as you climb more steeply across talus, boulders, and slabs, but ducks should help to keep you on track. The tread completely disappears at an overlook of the Palisade Glacier, from where fortunate visitors enjoy a splendid view of the jagged Palisades.

Turn left (north) and continue toward Sixth Lake, climbing moderately steeply on rocky switchbacks; the climb is briefly interrupted where you stroll past a pond surrounded by a small meadow. Reach the top of a lightly forested rise, with a good view of the Palisades just off the trail, and then drop off the rise to the crossing of a stream in a meadow. From there, a short climb over a rock hump leads to a smaller meadow, followed by a short climb into Sixth Lake's basin. A brief descent brings you to the southeast shore. With meadows surrounding the lake and low rises dotted with whitebark pines edging the meadows, the ambience around Sixth Lake is much more pastoral than at the other Big Pine Lakes. The open terrain allows good views of Mount Robinson, Two Eagle Peak, and Cloudripper, as well as the more distant Temple Crag and Mount Gayley. Backpackers will find decent campsites scattered about the low rises around the lake.

Camping ⛰

Although no maintained trail exists between Sixth and Seventh Lakes, the route is straightforward across open meadowlands dotted with clumps of willow; simply head west-northwest along the course of the stream connecting the two lakes for a quarter mile to the east shore of Seventh Lake. The lake is quite pleasant, tucked into an open basin below the slopes of Cloudripper. The few campsites sprinkled above the lakeshore seem to be more than adequate for the small number of campers who visit the lake.

Camping ⛰

Summit Lake can be reached by retracing your steps to the junction between the trails to Sixth Lake and Summit Lake. Turn left and climb moderately to the crest of a ridge, where the lake suddenly appears through the trees. A short descent leads to the roughly oval, forest-lined lake, perched on a bench above a steep drop toward Black Lake below. Campsites seem plentiful, and anglers can test their skills on the resident brook trout. **END SIDE TRIP**

Camping ⛰

Fishing 🎣

From the four-way junction, ►10 the loop portion of the trip continues by turning northeast and skirting the south shore of Fourth Lake. Gently descending trail through scattered to light forest is followed by a gentle ascent over a forested rise and a moderate descent through lodgepole pines to the south shore of Black Lake. ►11 A number of fine campsites around the lake and above the trail offer potential overnight havens. Anglers can ply the waters in search of brook and rainbow trout.

Fishing

A steep descent leads away from Black Lake, as you eventually break out of the forest to views of Mount Alice and Temple Crag across the North Fork canyon, and Mount Sill and North Palisade along the crest. Farther along, several of the Big Pine Lakes spring into view. Long-legged switchbacks lead across a sagebrush-covered slope dotted with mountain mahogany, wild rose, and an occasional whitebark or lodgepole pine. Reach the close of the loop about a mile from Black Lake, ►12 and then retrace your steps to the parking lot. ►13

Great Views

🚶	MILESTONES	
►1	0.0	Start at day-use trailhead
►2	0.3	Right at connector junction
►3	0.4	Right at road
►4	0.5	Right to Upper Trail
►5	0.7	Left at Upper Trail
►6	3.9	Left at loop junction
►7	4.1	First Lake
►8	4.9	Third Lake
►9	5.7	Glacier Trail junction
►10	5.9	Right at Fifth Lake junction
►11	6.6	Black Lake
►12	7.5	Left at loop junction
►13	11.4	Return to trailhead

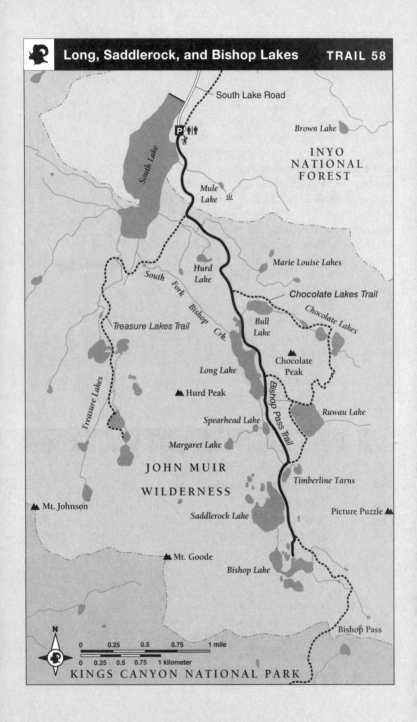

South Lake Road

Brown Lake

INYO
NATIONAL
FOREST

Mule
Lake

South Lake

Marie Louise Lakes

Hurd
Lake

Chocolate Lakes Trail

Chocolate Lakes

South Fork Bishop Crk.

Treasure Lakes Trail

Bull
Lake

Long Lake

Chocolate
Peak

Treasure Lakes

Hurd Peak

Ruwau Lake

Bishop Pass Trail

Spearhead Lake

Margaret Lake

JOHN MUIR

WILDERNESS

Timberline Tarns

Mt. Johnson

Picture Puzzle

Saddlerock Lake

Mt. Goode

Bishop Lake

N

0   0.25   0.5   0.75   1 mile
0   0.25   0.5   0.75   1 kilometer

Bishop Pass

KINGS CANYON NATIONAL PARK

Long, Saddlerock, and Bishop Lakes

The terrain in the upper reaches of South Fork Bishop Creek drainage is highly popular with a wide range of recreationists, making securing a wilderness permit or a parking place a dubious proposition on summer weekends. Unless you're willing to step off the trail, solitude is an elusive commodity. Nonetheless, a bounty of picturesque lakes, rugged peaks, rushing streams, vibrant wildflowers, verdant meadows, and groves of pines all lure you to this classic eastern Sierra journey. Adding a 2.5-mile side excursion to the Chocolate Lakes creates a fine semiloop trip (see Trail 59).

Best Time

The South Fork Bishop Creek drainage tends to shed most of its snow by early July, and wildflowers reach their peak from mid-July into early August. The water temperature of these high mountain lakes is always a bit chilly, but swimmers will find the conditions at their best from mid- to late August. Late summer and early autumn can be a great time for a trip, when the crowds have diminished and the weather is cooler but usually sunny. By late October or early November the area has usually seen the first significant storm of the season.

Finding the Trail

Turn west from US 395 in the center of Bishop at Line Drive and proceed out of town, as the road becomes South Lake Road (CA 168). Proceed 15 miles to a junction and turn left toward South Lake.

TRAIL USE
Day Hike, Backpack,
Run, Horse,
Dogs Allowed

LENGTH
8.6 miles, 4–5 hours

VERTICAL FEET
+1750/-250/±4000

DIFFICULTY
– 1 2 **3** 4 5 +

TRAIL TYPE
Out-and-back

FEATURES
Mountain
Lake
Wildflowers
Camping
Swimming
Fishing

FACILITIES
Campground
Resort

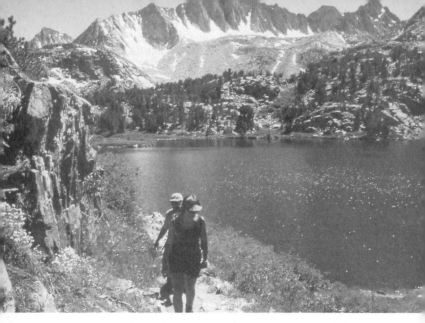

Hiking along Long Lake *with Mount Goode in the background*

Continue another 6.75 miles to the end of the road near the South Lake Dam. Backpackers must park in the overnight lot—when this lot is full, additional overnight parking is usually available 1.3 miles back down the road near Parchers Resort (a footpath connects the upper and lower lots). Day-use parking is available just below the overnight lot. Vault toilets and water are available nearby. Four U.S. Forest

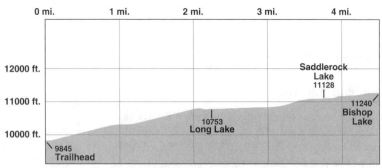

TRAIL 58 Long, Saddlerock and Bishop Lakes Elevation Profile

Service campgrounds are located along South Lake Road: Forks (fee, flush toilets, running water, and phone); Four Jeffrey (fee, flush toilets, and running water); Mountain Glen (vault toilets and fee); and Willow (vault toilets and fee). Resorts strung along South Lake Road include Bishop Creek Lodge, Cardinal Village Resort, and Parchers Resort.

> Nestled in a glacier-scoured basin at the foot of the towering northeast buttress of Mount Goode, Saddlerock Lake offers an austere haven for backpackers.

Logistics

Backpackers must obtain a wilderness permit for all overnight visits. See page 376 for more details about how to obtain one.

Trail Description

►1 The well-marked trail begins near the south end of the overnight parking lot, immediately making a very short and steep descent through lush trailside vegetation. A mild climb leads well above the east shore of South Lake through young aspens and lodgepole pines before the trail breaks out into the open to fine views up-canyon of South Fork Bishop Creek. Soon a steeper ascent heads up the hillside past the John Muir Wilderness boundary and to a Y-junction with the Treasure Lakes Trail. ►2 Veer left and head southeast through light lodgepole-pine forest to a plank bridge across a small, flower-lined stream, followed by a moderate climb to an unmarked junction with the partly cross-country route to the seldom-visited Marie Louise Lakes. Just past this faint junction, you briefly come alongside and cross another small creek before climbing over granite outcrops and around boulders via switchbacks to a Y-junction with the lower end of the Chocolate Lakes Trail. ►3

 Wildflowers

Remaining on the Bishop Pass Trail, an easy quarter-mile stroll leads over to the north shore of aptly named Long Lake. The elongated lake is

Chocolate Lakes Loop

Returning to the trailhead via the Chocolate Lakes Trail is a fairly straightforward endeavor, adding a mere 2.5 miles to the journey. Although returning to the upper loop junction near the south end of Long Lake is the most apparent way, the cross-country route from Timberline Tarns is more direct. From the easternmost tarn, ascend north over a low bench and drop down to scenic Ruwau Lake, sandwiched between Chocolate Peak and the Inconsolable Range. Pick up maintained trail on the north shore and climb deteriorating tread up and over the divide separating Ruwau Lake from the Chocolate Lakes. Drop down to the three Chocolate Lakes and then Bull Lake before descending steeply to the lower junction below the north end of Long Lake. From there, retrace your steps 1.9 miles to the trailhead.

bordered by verdant green meadows, granite boulders, and scattered conifers. Tiny islets sprinkle the crystal-blue waters, which reflect the craggy images of Mount Goode and Hurd Peak. Lovely scenery, close proximity to a trailhead, and a healthy population of rainbow, brook, and brown trout make this lake a very popular destination for hikers, backpackers, and anglers. Campsites abound around the overused shoreline, especially on a knoll near the south end of the lake. As you continue up the trail along the east shore, Long Lake seems to go on forever. Reach a T-junction ▶4 with the upper end of the Chocolate Lakes Trail near the far end of the lake.

From the junction, proceed ahead a short distance along the south end of Long Lake, cross the inlet from Ruwau Lake, and then resume the climb through a light to scattered forest of whitebark pines. Continue climbing through small meadows, fields of rock, and pockets of wildflowers to the east of picturesque Spearhead Lake, backdropped by the spine of the Inconsolable Range. Limited campsites are scattered around the shore, and fishing is reported to be fair for rainbow and brook trout. Straightforward cross-country travel leads west from the lake to lovely and isolated Margaret Lake.

Camping ◬

Lake ≋

Wildflowers ❀

Camping ◬

Lake ≋

A half-mile climb from Spearhead Lake on the Bishop Pass Trail ascends a rocky slope to the lovely Timberline Tarns, where sparkling waterfalls and tumbling cascades greet you along the way. While most backpackers bypass this area in favor of campsites at the larger lakes above, a handful of fine, out-of-the-way sites nearby are worthwhile overnight havens. An easy cross-country route from the easternmost tarn heads north over a low bench to Ruwau Lake.

 Camping

From Timberline Tarns, a short climb leads to the east shore of island-dotted Saddlerock Lake. ►5 Nestled in a glacier-scoured basin at the foot of the towering northeast buttress of Mount Goode, the lake offers an austere haven for backpackers. Anglers can ply the waters in search of elusive rainbow and brook trout.

 Fishing

Because the Bishop Pass Trail avoids Bishop Lake, an unmarked use trail from Saddlerock Lake heading south over a low rise is the preferred route to irregular-shaped Bishop Lake. ►6 Good campsites can be found on the low rise just north of the lake. Rainbow and brook trout are also present in Bishop Lake.

 Camping

大	**MILESTONES**
►1	0.0 Start at trailhead
►2	0.75 Left at Treasure Lakes junction
►3	1.9 Straight at Lower Chocolate Lakes junction
►4	2.7 Straight at Upper Chocolate Lakes junction
►5	3.75 Saddlerock Lake
►6	4.3 Bishop Lake

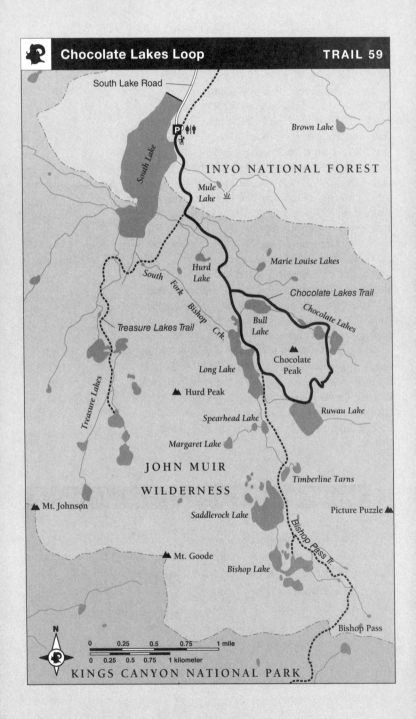

South Lake Road

Brown Lake

South Lake

INYO NATIONAL FOREST

P

Mule
Lake

Marie Louise Lakes

Hurd
Lake

Chocolate Lakes Trail

South
Fork
Bishop
Crk.

Chocolate Lakes

Treasure Lakes Trail

Bull
Lake

Chocolate
Peak

Long Lake

▲ Hurd Peak

Ruwau Lake

Treasure Lakes

Spearhead Lake

Margaret Lake

JOHN MUIR

WILDERNESS

Timberline Tarns

▲ Mt. Johnson

Saddlerock Lake

Picture Puzzle ▲

▲ Mt. Goode

Bishop Pass Tr.

Bishop Lake

N

0   0.25   0.5   0.75   1 mile

0   0.25   0.5   0.75   1 kilometer

Bishop Pass

KINGS CANYON NATIONAL PARK

Chocolate Lakes Loop

The short semiloop around aptly named Chocolate Peak branches off the well-traveled Bishop Pass Trail to a string of picturesque lakes. Additional rewards include not only some outstanding scenery but also a sense of relative seclusion away from the steady stream of hikers, backpackers, and equestrians headed up the canyon of South Fork Bishop Creek. Unfortunately, backpackers seeking to overnight at the Chocolate Lakes have to compete for the same number of permits issued for those bound for the more popular destinations along the Bishop Pass Trail. However, the 7.2-mile distance is well suited to day hiking, which doesn't require a permit. Sections of the trail between Chocolate Lakes and Ruwau Lake are rough—indistinct in parts and indiscernible in others—although route-finding is straightforward. Anglers may find the fishing to be quite good.

Best Time

Trail users can usually follow a snow-free trail around the Chocolate Lakes as early as the first part of July. Wildflowers should be at their peak from mid-July through early August.

Finding the Trail

Turn west from US 395 in the center of Bishop at Line Drive and proceed out of town, as the road becomes South Lake Road (CA 168). Proceed 15 miles to a junction and turn left toward South Lake. Continue another 6.75 miles to the end of the road near the South Lake Dam. Backpackers must park

TRAIL USE
Day Hike, Backpack,
Run, Horse,
Dogs Allowed

LENGTH
7.2 miles, 3–4 hours

VERTICAL FEET
+1690/-1690/±3380

DIFFICULTY
– 1 2 **3** 4 5 +

TRAIL TYPE
Semiloop

FEATURES
Mountain
Lake
Wildflowers
Camping
Swimming
Fishing

FACILITIES
Campground
Resort

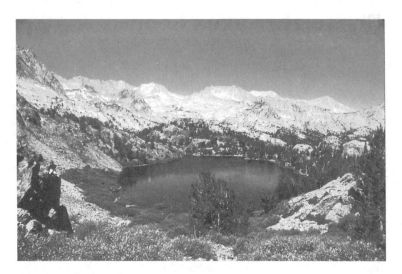

One of the *Chocolate Lakes*

in the overnight lot—when this lot is full, additional overnight parking is usually available 1.3 miles back down the road near Parchers Resort (a footpath connects the upper and lower lots). Day-use parking is available just below the overnight lot. Vault toilets and water are available nearby. Four U.S. Forest Service campgrounds are located along South Lake Road: Forks (fee, flush toilets, running water, and

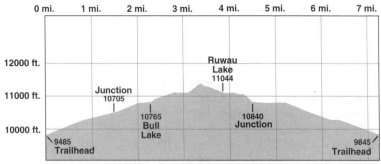

TRAIL 59   Chocolate Lakes Loop Elevation Profile

phone); Four Jeffrey (fee, flush toilets, and running water); Mountain Glen (vault toilets and fee); and Willow (vault toilets and fee). Resorts strung along South Lake Road include Bishop Creek Lodge, Cardinal Village Resort, and Parchers Resort.

Logistics

Backpackers must obtain a wilderness permit for all overnight visits. See page 376 for more details about how to obtain one.

Trail Description

►1 The well-marked trail begins near the south end of the overnight parking lot, immediately making a very short and steep descent through lush trailside vegetation. A mild climb leads well above the east shore of South Lake through young aspens and lodgepole pines before the trail breaks out into the open to fine views up the canyon of South Fork Bishop Creek. Soon a steeper ascent heads up the hillside past the John Muir Wilderness boundary and to a Y-junction with the Treasure Lakes Trail. ►2 Veer left and head southeast through light lodgepole-pine forest to a plank bridge across a small, flower-lined stream, followed by a moderate climb to an unmarked junction with the partly cross-country route to the seldom-visited Marie Louise Lakes. Just past this faint junction, you briefly come alongside and cross another small creek before climbing over granite outcrops and around boulders via switchbacks to a Y-junction with the lower end of the Chocolate Lakes Trail. ►3

Turn left at the junction, cross a talus slide, and ascend a steep draw to a meadow, soon arriving at Bull Lake. ►4 The shoreline of the picturesque lake is blanketed with a light forest of whitebark pines, wildflowers, and scattered clumps of willow. Plenty

Surrounded by grasses, shrubs, and a few pines, the largest of the three Chocolate Lakes sits at the base of a talus slope with fine views of the surrounding peaks and ridges.

 Lake

Camping

Fishing

Wildflowers

Lake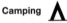

Camping

Camping

Fishing

of decent campsites are just off the trail. Anglers can test their skill on the resident brook trout.

The trail proceeds around the north shore of Bull Lake, crosses the inlet, and then climbs moderately steeply alongside the inlet through a fine display of wildflowers, including columbine, shooting star, and paintbrush. As the Inconsolable Range comes into view, ascend into a rocky basin and pass a shallow, seemingly insignificant pond, which happens to be lower Chocolate Lake. Above the lower lake, you cross the stream again and climb up to middle Chocolate Lake. ►5 Campsites spread around a hillside above the north shore will lure overnighters.

Continuing the climb, you switchback up the hillside, cross a willow-lined creek, and reach the largest of the three Chocolate Lakes. ►6 Surrounded by grasses, shrubs, and a few pines, the lake sits at the base of a talus slope with fine views of the surrounding peaks and ridges. Good campsites spread around the shoreline provide overnight havens for backpackers. All three Chocolate Lakes offer fair fishing for brook trout.

Away from the upper lake, the trail continues its circumnavigation around Chocolate Peak on a moderately steep climb across rocky terrain. The U.S. Geological Survey 7.5-minute map indicates a pair of trails leading out of the Chocolate Lakes basin and over a ridge crest to Ruwau Lake. Both trails are not maintained well and are a little rough, with sections that virtually disappear for considerable stretches. One path heads directly toward the ridge crest on a zigzagging climb up tight switchbacks, while the other path follows longer-legged switchbacks to the crest just southeast of a craggy knob. Whichever way you go, the crest offers fine views of the surrounding terrain. From the ridge crest, avoid the temptation to directly descend the talus-filled gully below. The two faint paths merge into one and then continue down a hillside above and west of this gully, becoming better defined as you descend. Eventually the north shore of Ruwau Lake is reached. ►7

Ruwau is perhaps the most scenic of the lakes along the loop, sandwiched between Chocolate Peak and the Inconsolable Range, with fine views from all angles of the neighboring craggy peaks and ridges. On warm afternoons, rock slabs on a tiny island near the north shore will entice swimmers and sunbathers willing to share the chilly, crystalline waters with the resident rainbow trout. Whitebark pines shade campsites on a low hill above the north shore not far from the outlet. Around the remainder of the shoreline, willow thickets and an assortment of wildflowers provide adornment. Although the lake is only a half mile off the well-traveled Bishop Pass Trail, the area seems just far enough off the beaten path to provide an ample helping of solitude and serenity.

 Lake

 Wildflowers

The trail heads away from lovely Ruwau Lake toward the outlet and then makes a slight descent through heather and scattered pines. Following a short ascent, the path steeply winds down toward Long Lake and meets the Bishop Pass Trail ►8 at the bottom of the descent.

Turn right and follow gently graded trail through scattered forest and wildflowers past a marshy pond. Soon aptly named Long Lake appears through the trees to the left, and Mount Goode cuts a fine profile to the southwest. Farther on, a short climb over a low hump leads directly alongside the picturesque lake. Beyond the far end of the lake, a pronounced descent through thickening forest returns you to the lower junction with the Chocolate Lakes Trail. ►9 From there, retrace your steps 1.9 miles to the trailhead. ►10

 Wildflowers

⚘ MILESTONES

▶1   0.0   Start at trailhead

▶2   0.75   Left at Treasure Lakes Trail junction

▶3   1.9   Left at lower Chocolate Lakes Trail junction

▶4   2.25   Bull Lake

▶5   2.8   Middle Chocolate Lake

▶6   3.0   Upper Chocolate Lake

▶7   3.9   Ruwau Lake

▶8   4.5   Right at Bishop Pass junction

▶9   5.3   Straight at lower Chocolate Lakes Trail junction

▶10   7.2   Return to trailhead

Treasure Lakes

While the Bishop Pass Trail may be considered by some to be something of a hikers' freeway, the trail branching away toward the Treasure Lakes sees far less traffic. The trail leads to a string of lovely lakes in a secluded granite basin directly below the Sierra Crest. The lakes are quite scenic, offering campers serene surroundings and providing anglers with excellent fishing for golden trout. Along the relatively short trail, hikers experience three distinct plant zones—montane, subalpine, and alpine. Some route-finding and a bit of boulder-hopping are necessary in order to reach the higher lakes, but travel should be straightforward for most hikers and backpackers. Although equestrians are allowed to use the trail, the absence of a distinct path over rocky terrain discourages horse use above the first two lakes.

Best Time

Snow leaves the area by mid-July, and wildflowers come into season shortly after. By September temperatures have cooled, but the weather is generally favorable until the first storm of the season, usually in late October or early November.

Finding the Trail

Turn west from US 395 in the center of Bishop at Line Drive and proceed out of town, as the road becomes South Lake Road (CA 168). Proceed 15 miles to a junction and turn left toward South Lake. Continue another 6.75 miles to the end of the road near the South Lake Dam. Backpackers must park

TRAIL USE
Day Hike, Backpack,
Run, Horse,
Dogs Allowed
LENGTH
7.6 miles, 3–4 hours
VERTICAL FEET
+1775/-450/±4450
DIFFICULTY
– 1 2 **3** 4 5 +
TRAIL TYPE
Out-and-back

FEATURES
Mountain
Lake
Wildflowers
Camping
Swimming
Fishing

FACILITIES
Campground
Resort

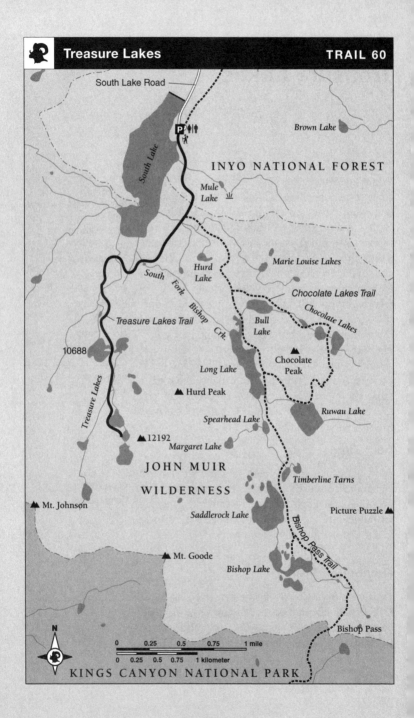

Treasure Lakes   **TRAIL 60**

South Lake Road

Brown Lake

INYO NATIONAL FOREST

Mule Lake

South Lake

Marie Louise Lakes

Hurd Lake

Chocolate Lakes Trail

Chocolate Lakes

South Fork Bishop Crk.

Treasure Lakes Trail

Bull Lake

10688

Long Lake

Chocolate Peak

▲ Hurd Peak

Treasure Lakes

Ruwau Lake

Spearhead Lake

▲12192

Margaret Lake

JOHN MUIR

Timberline Tarns

WILDERNESS

▲ Mt. Johnson

Picture Puzzle ▲

Saddlerock Lake

Bishop Pass Trail

▲ Mt. Goode

Bishop Lake

N

| 0 | 0.25 | 0.5 | 0.75 | 1 mile |

| 0 | 0.25 | 0.5 | 0.75 | 1 kilometer |

Bishop Pass

KINGS CANYON NATIONAL PARK

in the overnight lot—when this lot is full, additional overnight parking is usually available 1.3 miles back down the road near Parchers Resort (a footpath connects the upper and lower lots). Day-use parking is available just below the overnight lot. Vault toilets and water are available nearby. Four U.S. Forest Service campgrounds are located along South Lake Road: Forks (fee, flush toilets, running water, and phone); Four Jeffrey (fee, flush toilets, and running water); Mountain Glen (vault toilets and fee); and Willow (vault toilets and fee). Resorts strung along South Lake Road include Bishop Creek Lodge, Cardinal Village Resort, and Parchers Resort.

> **The trail leads to a string of lovely lakes in a secluded granite basin directly below the Sierra Crest.**

Logistics

Backpackers must obtain a wilderness permit for all overnight visits. See page 376 for more details about how to obtain one.

Trail Description

▶1 The well-marked trail begins near the south end of the overnight parking lot, immediately making a very short and steep descent through lush trailside vegetation. A mild climb leads well above the east

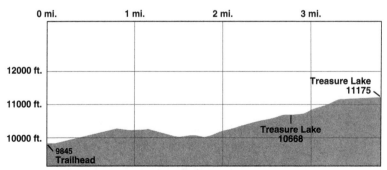

TRAIL 60 Treasure Lakes Elevation Profile

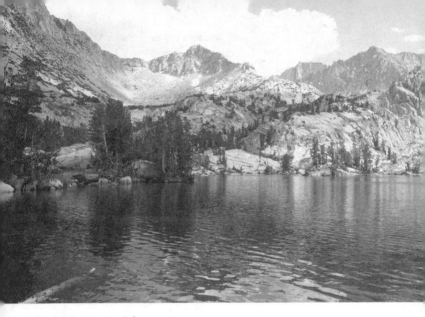

One of the *Treasure Lakes*

shore of South Lake through young aspens and lodgepole pines before the trail breaks out into the open to fine views up the canyon of South Fork Bishop Creek. Soon a steeper ascent heads up the hillside past the John Muir Wilderness boundary and to a Y-junction with the Treasure Lakes Trail. ▶2 Veer right at the junction and head through scattered to light lodgepole-pine forest to an easy crossing of a pair of small streams. A mild descent continues, as South Lake pops into view below, and Mount Johnson, Mount Gilbert, Mount Thompson, and Hurd Peak appear to the southwest. Proceed to three crossings of South Fork Bishop Creek and two tributaries, where willows, grasses, and wildflowers line the banks. Beyond the third crossing, the real climbing begins in earnest, briefly interrupted by a short descent to the crossing of Treasure Creek.

Wildflowers

Continue on a winding, moderately steep ascent beside granite boulders, over granite slabs, and through a mixed forest of lodgepole and whitebark pines. The trail winds back to another crossing of Treasure Creek and continues climbing through a diminishing cover of whitebark pines. Beyond a small pond and a switchback, you arrive at Lake 10668, ▶3 the first and largest of the Treasure Lakes. The lake is dotted with small rock islands and bordered by boggy turf along the north shore. A steep wall of rock on the far shore rises up toward Peak 12047, providing a fine backdrop to the placid waters. Gently graded tread leads around the east shore, where overnighters will find a number of exposed campsites amid clumps of pine. From the south shore, a use trail branches left to additional campsites near the lake directly east of Lake 10668.

Continuing south on the main trail, cross a stream and work your way alongside a creek coursing down a rock-filled gully, where clumps of willow and small patches of meadow sprinkled with monkeyflower soften the otherwise stark surroundings. Where the creek divides into two channels, follow the more gradual cleft on the right through large, blocky talus. Up-canyon, views of Mount Johnson and the long ridge between it and

 Lake

 Camping

 Mountain

Cross-Country Loop

Rather than retrace your steps back to the trailhead, you could vary your return by following a straightforward off-trail route over a saddle directly south of Peak 12192 and down into the canyon of South Fork Bishop Creek. From the east shore of Lake 11175, climb southeast 550 feet to the prominent saddle and then descend northeast approximately 100 yards before angling over to a tiny creek. Follow the creek briefly and then head straight toward Margaret Lake, where you can pick up a use trail near the northwest shore. Follow the use trail northeast to the south end of Long Lake, ford South Fork Bishop Creek, and shortly meet the Bishop Pass Trail. From there, head generally northwest down the Bishop Pass Trail to the Treasure Lakes Junction and then retrace your steps back to the trailhead.

OPTIONS

Lake ≋

Mount Goode add to the rugged alpine scenery. Route-finding from here is straightforward over rocky terrain, as you traverse east to a low ridge and the left-hand fork of the creek, where a trio of lakes is cradled in a deep cirque to the west of Peak 12192.

Fishing 🎣

The northwest shore of the first of the three lakes has some excellent campsites scattered among whitebark pines. All three lakes should provide anglers with good fishing for golden trout. The route ends at Lake 11175. ►4

🚶	**MILESTONES**	
►1	0.0	Start at trailhead
►2	0.75	Right at Treasure Lakes Trail junction
►3	2.8	Lake 10668
►4	3.8	Lake 11175

Tyee Lakes

The seldom-used Tyee Lakes Trail provides a steep but short route to a string of delightful lakes set in a high granite basin well east of the Sierra Crest. The 3-mile journey to Clara Lake is well suited for either a day hike, enhanced by a refreshing swim and a picnic lunch, or an overnight backpack. Thanks to the limited pressure, anglers should find plenty of trout in the Tyee Lakes to keep themselves occupied. A 0.75-mile, 600-foot climb to a view from the plateau of Table Mountain is a worthy trip extension.

Best Time

The area is snow-free by mid-July, and wildflowers come into season shortly after. By September temperatures have cooled, but the weather is generally favorable until the first storm of the season, usually in late October or early November.

Finding the Trail

Turn west from US 395 in the center of Bishop at Line Drive and proceed out of town, as the road becomes South Lake Road (CA 168). Proceed 15 miles to a junction and turn left toward South Lake. Continue another 5 miles to the trailhead on the right-hand side of the road and park your vehicle along the gravel shoulder nearby. Four U.S. Forest Service campgrounds are located along South Lake Road: Forks (fee, flush toilets, running water, and phone); Four Jeffrey (fee, flush toilets, and running water); Mountain Glen (vault toilets and fee); and

TRAIL USE
Day Hike, Backpack,
Run, Horse,
Dogs Allowed

LENGTH
6.5 miles, 3–4 hours

VERTICAL FEET
+2520/±5040

DIFFICULTY
– 1 2 **3** 4 5 +

TRAIL TYPE
Out-and-back

FEATURES
Mountain
Lake
Wildflowers
Camping
Swimming
Fishing

FACILITIES
Campground
Resort

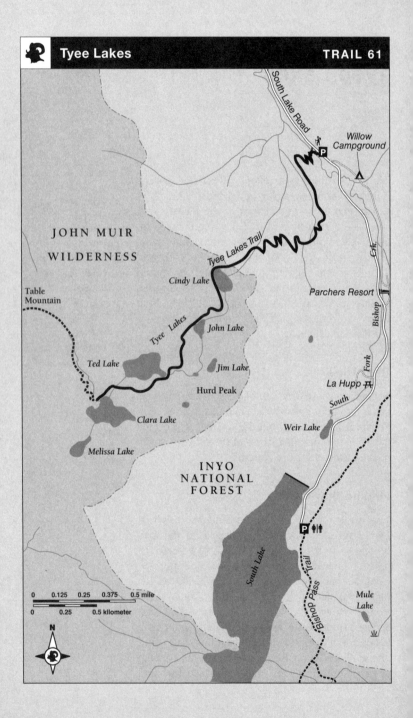

JOHN MUIR

WILDERNESS

South Lake Road

Willow
Campground

Tyee Lakes Trail

Cindy Lake

Parchers Resort

Table
Mountain

Bishop

John Lake

Tyee Lakes

Ted Lake

Jim Lake

Fork

Hurd Peak

La Hupp

South

Clara Lake

Weir Lake

Melissa Lake

INYO
NATIONAL
FOREST

South Lake

| 0 | 0.125 | 0.25 | 0.375 | 0.5 mile |

| 0 | 0.25 | 0.5 kilometer |

Bishop Pass Trail

Mule
Lake

N

Naming the Tyee Lakes

NOTE

Inexplicably, the Tyee Lakes were named for a famous brand of salmon eggs. The origin of the various first names applied to each lake (Cindy, John, Jim, Ted, Clara, and Melissa) is unknown.

Willow (vault toilets and fee). Resorts strung along South Lake Road include Bishop Creek Lodge, Cardinal Village Resort, and Parchers Resort.

Logistics

Backpackers must obtain a wilderness permit for all overnight visits. See page 376 for more details about how to obtain one.

Trail Description

▶1 Begin the hike by crossing an impressive, arched, wood bridge over South Fork Bishop Creek. From the far side of the bridge, a moderate, zigzagging climb leads up a sagebrush-covered hillside with pockets of young aspens and lodgepole pines. The steady climb continues, crossing the outlet from

Backdropped by rugged cliffs, Clara is also one of the larger Tyee Lakes, where a few whitebark pines eke out a tentative existence in the near-timberline environment.

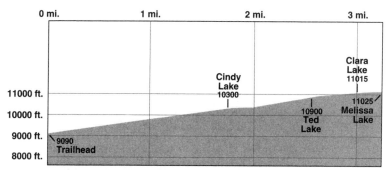

TRAIL 61 Tyee Lakes Elevation Profile

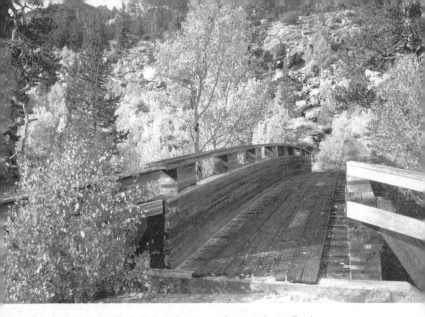

Bridge over South Fork Bishop Creek *near the Tyee Lakes Trailhead*

 Lake

Fishing

Tyee Lakes at 1.5 miles. The grade eases as you enter the John Muir Wilderness, round a hill, and approach Cindy Lake, passing a pair of fair campsites along the creek on the way to the lakeshore. ▶2 A pleasant beach on the west side invites sunbathers and swimmers, but marshy meadows, clumps of willow, and pockets of aspen border the remaining shoreline. Rising brook trout will surely tempt anglers, although much of the lakeshore is difficult to access due to the dense vegetation.

Arc around Cindy Lake, hop over the trickling inlet dribbling into the lake, and resume the climb. A number of switchbacks lead steeply uphill to grass-rimmed John Lake, the smallest and shallowest of the Tyee Lakes. Across the outlet on top of a granite hump, backpackers will find a few pine-sheltered campsites. Anglers can ply the waters for brook trout.

Leaving the west shore of John Lake, the trail makes a moderately steep climb through whitebark pines over a granite bench. Switchbacks lead to a viewpoint amid dwarf pines and scattered boulders, where you have a bird's-eye vista of John Lake below and the tiny lakes to the east of the trail (the largest is Jim Lake). From the viewpoint, a more moderate climb crosses Tyee Creek and passes by a small pond on the way to Ted Lake, ►3 one of the larger Tyee Lakes. Backpackers will find good campsites here sheltered by scattered whitebark pines. An extensive talus slope cascading down the hillside on the far side of the lake provides added scenery.

 Camping

Skirt the south side of Ted Lake and then begin a moderately steep climb up and over a talus-covered hillside to the narrow cleft holding the stream connecting Ted Lake to its upstairs neighbor. Cross this stream and climb up the cleft toward lovely Clara Lake, shown as Lake 11015 on the U.S. Geological Survey map. ►4 Backdropped by rugged cliffs, Clara is also one of the larger Tyee Lakes, where a few whitebark pines eke out a tentative existence in the near-timberline environment. Unlike at the lower lakes, rainbow trout cohabitate with the characteristic brook trout, which should provide a worthy challenge to any anglers in your group. The last lake in the chain, Melissa, ►5 is a straightforward cross-country jaunt from Clara Lake's southwest shore.

 Lake

Side Trip to Table Mountain

From Clara Lake, a 2-mile round-trip to Table Mountain will reward you with a dramatic view. Follow a winding climb up the trail through the gorge of a delightful creek that drains into Clara Lake. Near the head of the gorge, the trail becomes indistinct but the route is obvious—simply head west toward the plateau between Peaks 11684 and 11651, passing through a profusion of corn lilies on the way. With shuttle arrangements, you can continue over Table Mountain and past George Lake (good campsites) to the Lake Sabrina Trailhead.

OPTIONS

MILESTONES

►1   0.0   Start at trailhead
►2   1.75   Cindy Lake
►3   2.6   Ted Lake
►4   3.0   Clara Lake
►5   3.25   Melissa Lake

Sabrina Basin Lakes

Sabrina Basin holds so many beautiful and worthwhile lakes that deciding which ones to visit is often the most challenging part of the trip. With so many lakes to choose from, a healthy dose of solitude and serenity should be fairly easy to get. The lakes of the upper basin are particularly stunning, cradled in granite bowls and encircled by rugged cliffs, with the towering Sierra Crest providing a nearly constant backdrop. Along the way, delightful meadows, colorful wildflowers, cascading streams, and tumbling waterfalls complement the picturesque lakes, while the open nature of the basin offers striking panoramas of the surrounding terrain. Use trails and easy cross-country routes to additional lakes offer plenty of diversions away from the main trail. Whether you're out for just a day, a long weekend, or more, Sabrina Basin has much to offer.

TRAIL USE
Day Hike, Backpack,
Run, Horse,
Dogs Allowed

LENGTH
13.6 miles, 7 hours

VERTICAL FEET
+2850/-675/±7050

DIFFICULTY
– 1 2 **3** 4 5 +

TRAIL TYPE
Out-and-back

FEATURES
Mountain
Lake
Wildflowers
Great Views
Camping
Swimming
Fishing

FACILITIES
Campground
Resort

Best Time

Trails are usually snow-free by mid-July, but the lovely meadows of Sabrina Basin reach the height of wildflower season usually from late July through mid-August. Swimmers will find the chilly waters of the lakes the warmest during the month of August. September is a fine time for a visit, although nighttime temperatures may be cold. Snow generally arrives by late October or early November.

Finding the Trail

Turn west from US 395 in the center of Bishop at Line Drive and proceed out of town, as the road

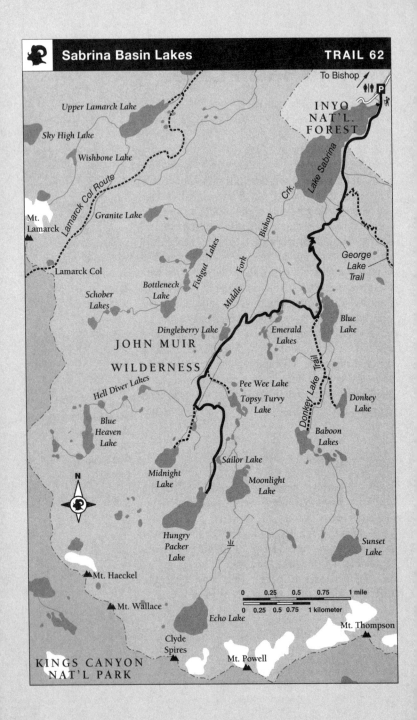

To Bishop

INYO
NAT'L.
FOREST

Upper Lamarck Lake

Sky High Lake

Wishbone Lake

Lake Sabrina

Bishop

Crk.

Mt.
Lamarck

Lamarck Col Route

Granite Lake

George
Lake
Trail

Lamarck Col

Fishgut Lakes

Middle Fork

Blue
Lake

Bottleneck
Lake

Schober
Lakes

Dingleberry Lake

Emerald
Lakes

JOHN MUIR

WILDERNESS

Hell Diver Lakes

Pee Wee Lake

Topsy Turvy
Lake

Donkey Lake Trail

Donkey
Lake

Blue
Heaven
Lake

Baboon
Lakes

Midnight
Lake

Sailor Lake

Moonlight
Lake

N

Hungry
Packer
Lake

Sunset
Lake

Mt. Haeckel

Mt. Wallace

| 0 | 0.25 | 0.5 | 0.75 | 1 mile |

| 0 | 0.25 | 0.5 | 0.75 | 1 kilometer |

Echo Lake

Mt. Thompson

Clyde
Spires

Mt. Powell

KINGS CANYON
NAT'L PARK

becomes South Lake Road (CA 168). Proceed 15 miles to a junction and continue ahead toward Lake Sabrina, passing the North Lake junction and the overnight parking area (backpackers must park here), to the day-use parking lot near the Lake Sabrina Dam, 3 miles from the South Lake junction. On the way to Lake Sabrina, you pass four U.S. Forest Service campgrounds: Big Trees (fee, flush toilets, and running water); Intake 2 (fee, flush toilets, running water, and bear boxes); Bishop Park (fee, flush toilets, running water, and bear boxes); and Sabrina (fee, flush toilets, running water, bear boxes, and phone). Nearby resorts along South Lake Road include Bishop Creek Lodge, Cardinal Village Resort, and Parchers Resort.

> Sabrina Basin holds so many beautiful and worthwhile lakes that deciding which ones to visit is often the most challenging part of the trip.

Logistics

Backpackers must obtain a wilderness permit for all overnight visits. See page 376 for more details about how to obtain one.

Trail Description

▶1 Follow the course of an old road away from the day-use parking lot through a cover of aspens

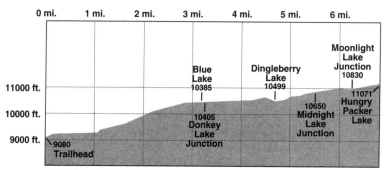

TRAIL 62 Sabrina Basin Lakes Elevation Profile

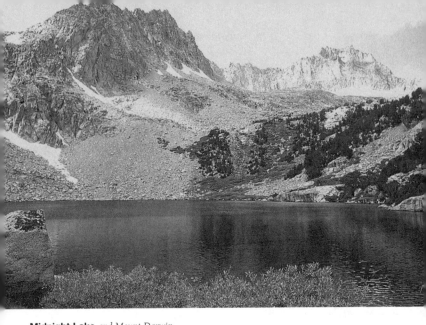

Midnight Lake *and Mount Darwin*

until singletrack trail leads to a fine vista up the canyon of Middle Fork Bishop Creek. Continue across the open slope, carpeted with sagebrush and dotted with junipers, Jeffrey pines, mountain mahogany, and a few western white pines, above the blue expanse of Lake Sabrina. Toward the far end of the lake, you have a good view of the creek cascading picturesquely into a small cove. Farther up-canyon, the rugged Sierra Crest is crowned by the 13,000-foot summits of Mount Darwin, Mount Haeckel, Mount Wallace, and Mount Powell. Cross into John Muir Wilderness near the lake's midpoint and then begin a steady climb. Reach the junction with the trail to George Lake near the far end of Lake Sabrina. ▶2

Mountain

Lake

Immediately cross George Lake's outlet and enter a light forest of lodgepole pines, switch-backing up the slope away from Lake Sabrina and crossing another stream along the way. More switchbacks interspersed with granite steps lead up a hillside, through a rocky ravine, and to a small pond, where the stiff grade abates. Near the pond, the shore of a lake appears through the trees, as you pass a couple of campsites and ford the outlet just below Blue Lake. ▶3 The lake is very photogenic, with an irregular shoreline bordered by weather-beaten lodgepole pines and granite benches, and a dramatic backdrop from the craggy, undulating crest of Thompson Ridge. Plenty of campsites are spread around the shoreline, but choose a site wisely because some are obviously too close to the water to be legal. Anglers can test their skill on brook and rainbow trout. The trail follows the west shore to a three-way junction ▶4 with the Donkey Lake Trail near the lake's midpoint.

 Lake

 Fishing

Continuing toward Sabrina Basin, turn right (northwest) from the Donkey Lake junction and follow gently graded trail over a low saddle, across a rocky slope, and then up granite ledges to a grassy vale dotted with lodgepole pines. Cross the outlet from Emerald Lakes and curve around the sometimes-marshy meadow near the lower lakes to a faint use trail on the left, which provides access to the

OPTIONS

Baboon and Donkey Lakes

A trip to these less-visited lakes is a fine way to extend your stay in the area. Head south from the junction near Blue Lake through lodgepole pines and around slabs of granite to the crossing of a seasonal stream. From there, a moderate climb leads to an unmarked junction with a faint path heading south-southwest to Baboon Lakes. The path disappears before reaching Baboon Lakes, but the route-finding is straightforward alongside the lake's outlet stream to the largest lake. To reach Donkey Lake, continue south from the unmarked junction shortly to the crossing of the creek draining Baboon Lakes, and proceed on faint tread around rock outcrops, past a small pool, and through a notch to the lake. Donkey Lake is tucked into a narrow cleft near the base of Thompson Ridge.

Side Trip to Midnight Lake

Scenic Midnight Lake offers an excellent diversion for those with extra time and energy. To reach the lake, veer right at the junction and cross the stream draining Hell Diver Lake. From there, mildly graded trail leads past a fair-sized tarn and across the creek draining Midnight Lake to steeper climbing over granite slabs. The grade eases as you crest the lip of a basin and soon stroll over to the north shore of Midnight Lake, a teardrop-shaped body of water reposing in a granite bowl surrounded by talus slopes and steep, rugged cliffs. Patches of snow cling to the shady crevices of the cliffs, and a waterfall cascades 300 feet into the lake, as 13,831-foot Mount Darwin looms in the background. Near timberline, widely scattered lodgepole pines cling tenuously to cracks in the granite hummocks lining the outlet. While the steep lakeshore inhibits camping, campsites can be found scattered along the creek between the lake and the tarn below.

Camping

Fishing

Lake

Camping

Wildflowers

larger Emerald Lakes. Fine campsites will lure overnighters at the westernmost lake, and anglers should enjoy fishing for brook and rainbow trout. Climb away from Emerald Lakes up granite steps and over granite slabs on the west side of a low ridge and then wind down the far side of the ridge to the southeast shore of Dingleberry Lake. ▶5 The lake is squeezed between the cliffs and slabs of a low ridge on one side and the steep wall of Peak 13253's east ridge on the other. Campsites can be found along the creek near both ends of the lake, but the wet meadows on the south end are a haven for mosquitoes in early season.

Beyond the south end of Dingleberry Lake, the foot and stock trails diverge for separate fords of Middle Fork Bishop Creek. The two paths reconnect beyond the ford and then climb along a tributary to a picturesque meadow, where the serpentine stream flows lazily through grasses, willows, and wildflowers. Across the valley, a dazzling waterfall plunges from Topsy Turvy Lake. In the middle of the meadow, a faint use trail heads left toward campsites near Pee Wee and Topsy Turvy Lakes. Past the upper end of the meadow, the climb resumes over numerous low granite benches to the Midnight Lake junction. ►6

From the Midnight Lake junction, head southeast across a pair of willow- and flower-lined creeks, make a mild to moderate climb around a spur ridge, and then head south through scattered whitebark pines to a sloping meadow, filled with willow, heather, and wildflowers sprinkled between glistening granite slabs. A short climb leads to a stunningly picturesque basin brimming with crystalline streams and tumbling cascades, with aptly named Picture Peak in the background. Approximately 0.75 mile from the Midnight Lake junction, you reach a junction with a use trail to Moonlight Lake. ►7

From the Moonlight Lake junction, continue south past Sailor Lake, a scenic lake nestled in an open, nearly treeless basin bordered by sloping granite shelves and slabs and pockets of verdant meadow. A number of fine, although exposed, campsites are scattered about the basin, and anglers will find brook and rainbow trout in both the lake and creek. Proceed up the main trail, with the scenic north face of Picture Peak drawing hikers like a beacon. Reach the north shore of Hungry Packer Lake, ►8 a narrow finger of water lined by steep cliffs and the towering presence of lovely Picture Peak. During snowmelt, thin ribbons of water cascade majestically down the steep face of the cliffs. A granite peninsula on the northwest shore is too close to the water for legal camping, but the slightly sloping slabs are well suited for afternoon sunbathing. Campsites are limited to a few spots around the outlet. Anglers should find fishing for rainbow trout to be challenging.

 Wildflowers

 Great Views

 Lake

 Camping

 Fishing

 Lake

OPTIONS

Moonlight Lake

Austere Moonlight Lake is best reached via a use trail below (north of) Sailor Lake, as a vast talus field inhibits access from the main trail to Hungry Packer Lake above. Following the use trail, you ford Sailor Lake's outlet, cross a meadow, and then ascend along the outlet from Moonlight Lake to the northwest shore of the rock-bound lake. Backpackers will find campsites limited to exposed patches along the outlet and the south end of a low rise above the west shore. In spite of the seemingly lifeless surroundings, the lake hosts a healthy population of brook trout.

🚶 MILESTONES

▶1   0.0   Start at trailhead
▶2   1.25 Straight at George Lake junction
▶3   3.2   Blue Lake
▶4   3.25 Right at Donkey Lake junction
▶5   4.7   Dingleberry Lake
▶6   5.5   Straight at Midnight Lake junction
▶7   6.25 Straight at Moonlight Lake junction
▶8   6.8   Hungry Packer Lake

Lamarck Lakes

Beautiful lakes and rugged mountain scenery lure hikers and backpackers up the Lamarck Lakes Trail. Although the distance is short, the elevation gain is fairly significant, requiring that visitors be in reasonable condition. Maintained trail dead-ends at Upper Lamarck Lake, which may help to explain the relatively light use the trail receives, but off-trail options to the delightful Wonder Lakes and view-packed Lamarck Col offer fine diversions for those with extra time and energy.

Best Time

Situated in the rain shadow east of the Sierra Crest, the Lamarck Lakes can be visited as early as the first part of July in years following an average snowfall. Experienced off-trail hikers planning to continue toward Lamarck Col should wait until late July for a mostly snow-free journey. Pleasant weather usually persists in this area through September, with the first snowfall occurring by late October or early November.

Finding the Trail

Turn west from US 395 in the center of Bishop at Line Drive and proceed out of town, as the road becomes South Lake Road (CA 168). Proceed 15 miles to the South Lake junction and continue ahead toward Lake Sabrina 3 miles to the North Lake junction. Turn right and follow the single-lane gravel road 1 mile to the day-use parking area, or 1.6 miles to the right-hand turn into the overnight

TRAIL USE
Day Hike, Backpack,
Run, Horse,
Dogs Allowed
LENGTH
5.4 miles, 3 hours
VERTICAL FEET
+1700/-50/±3500
DIFFICULTY
– 1 2 3 **4 5** +
TRAIL TYPE
Out-and-back

FEATURES
Mountain
Lake
Wildflowers
Camping
Swimming
Fishing

FACILITIES
Campground
Pack Station

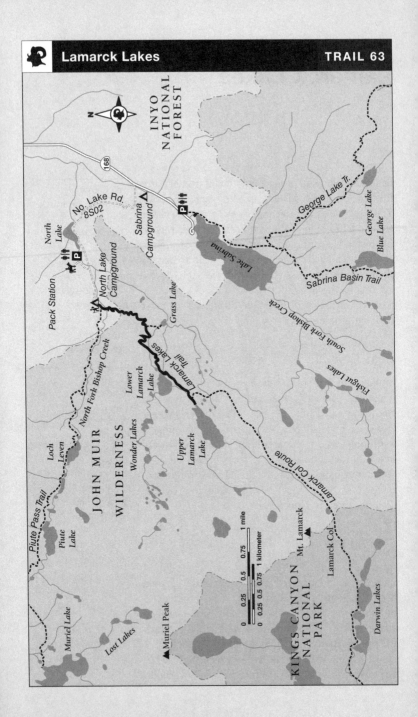

INYO NATIONAL FOREST

N

168

No. Lake Rd. 8S02

North Lake

Pack Station

North Lake Campground

Sabrina Campground

P

Lake Sabrina

George Lake Tr.

George Lake

Blue Lake

Sabrina Basin Trail

Grass Lake

South Fork Bishop Creek

North Fork Bishop Creek

Lamarck Lakes Trail

Lower Lamarck Lake

Fishgut Lakes

JOHN MUIR WILDERNESS

Loch Leven

Wonder Lakes

Upper Lamarck Lake

Lamarck Col Route

Piute Pass Trail

Piute Lake

1 mile

0.75

0.5

0.25

0

1 kilometer

0.75

0.5

0.25

0

Mt. Lamarck

Lamarck Col

Muriel Lake

Lost Lakes

Muriel Peak

KINGS CANYON NATIONAL PARK

Darwin Lakes

parking lot directly west of North Lake. Both day hikers and backpackers can be dropped at the trailhead inside North Lake Campground (fee, vault toilets, running water, and bear boxes), but drivers will have to walk the continuation of the North Lake Road from either the day-use or overnight lots to the trailhead. Nearby resorts along South Lake Road include Bishop Creek Lodge, Cardinal Village Resort, and Parchers Resort.

Lower Lamarck Lake is quite scenic, cradled beneath steep granite cliffs and backdropped by the triangular summit of Peak 12153.

Logistics

Backpackers must obtain a wilderness permit for all overnight visits. See page 376 for more details about how to obtain one.

Trail Description

▶1 From the trailhead inside North Lake Campground (1 mile from the day-use parking lot and 0.7 mile from the overnight lot), follow singletrack trail through aspens and pines a short distance to a junction ▶2 near the edge of the campground.

Veer left at the junction and cross a trio of willow-lined branches of North Fork Bishop Creek on wood-plank bridges. Past the last bridge, the

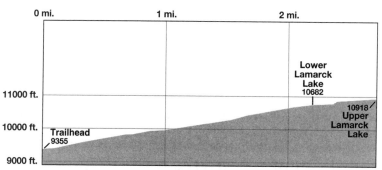

TRAIL 63 Lamarck Lakes Elevation Profile

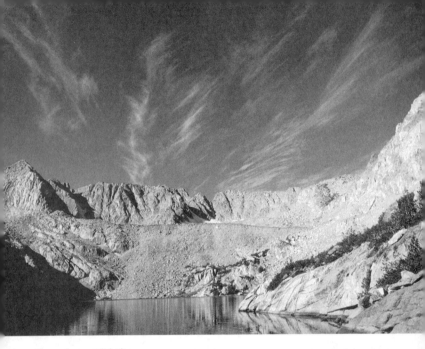

Upper Lamarck Lake

grade increases to a moderately steep, switchbacking climb through aspens and lodgepole pines. Limber pines join the forest on the way to a junction ▶3 with a short path on the left to Grass Lake, which becomes more meadow than lake as the season progresses.

Veer right at the junction and continue climbing toward Lamarck Lakes through pine forest. Switchbacks resume where the trail becomes steep, rocky, and exposed near some cliffs, from where you have down-canyon views of Grass and North Lakes. Leaving the views behind, the trail heads back into light forest and continues climbing via another set of switchbacks. Pass above a small pond on the right and soon spy the waters of the lower lake through the trees ahead. A short drop leads to a crossing of the outlet just below picturesque Lower Lamarck Lake. ▶4

Lake

Mountain

Lower Lamarck Lake is quite scenic, cradled beneath steep granite cliffs and backdropped by the triangular summit of Peak 12153. Clumps of limber pine shade several overused campsites near the outlet and slightly less-used sites above the northeast shore. Fishing in the chilly waters is reported to be fair for rainbow and brook trout.

 Fishing

From Lower Lamarck Lake, the trail proceeds up the rocky wash of Lamarck Creek, switchbacking a few times before crossing to the northwest

Cross-Country Route to Lamarck Col

OPTIONS

A boot-beaten path has been created over the years almost all the way from the vicinity of Upper Lamarck Lake to 12,920-foot Lamarck Col at the Sierra Crest. The high-elevation route is physically demanding, gaining an additional 2,800 feet in 2.6 miles, but the high-alpine scenery is a just reward. Experienced backpackers use the route over the col as a shortcut to Evolution Basin. To head toward the col, backtrack from Upper Lamarck Lake several hundred yards down the trail, cross Lamarck Creek, and make a short climb southeast on a use trail. Continue past some campsites and a small pond to a sloping meadow bisected by a gurgling stream. Follow ducks on a winding climb alongside this stream to a crossing and then continue the serpentine ascent beside boulders and rocks up a steep hillside. Reach the crest of a ridge, with good views of Grass Lake, Lamarck Lakes, North Lake, Lake Sabrina, and a section of Owens Valley and the White Mountains beyond.

The grade eases for a while on the way around the left side of the ridge through widely scattered pines and spring-fed meadows. From there, the path zigzags more steeply up an arid hillside, followed by an ascending traverse to the base of a steep hill. After surmounting the hill, the route leads into a sloping valley below the Sierra Crest. Climb up this valley toward the perennial snowfield just below the col. Depending on conditions, ascending the snowfield to the col may be difficult. The lofty aerie of Lamarck Col provides a stunning view of Mount Mendel, Mount Darwin, and the Darwin Glacier, as well as Darwin Lakes, Darwin Bench, and the deep cleft of Evolution Valley below.

Wonder Lakes

From Lower Lamarck Lake, a cross-country foray along the outlet stream to the Wonder Lakes is a straightforward enterprise. The lakes were so named after a packer was sent to plant fish in the 1930s. After some difficulty getting his stock to the lakes, he marveled that he had gotten the job done.

From the northwest shore of Lower Lamarck Lake, a steep climb leads out of the basin, where a use trail can be followed on the left-hand side of the outlet over rock slabs to the first lake. Flower-filled meadows, scattered pockets of pines, and numerous granite slabs border the lakes. Steep cliffs and glacial moraines add a decidedly alpine character to the surroundings. Less-developed campsites around the lower lakes provide a more secluded alternative to the overused sites around Lower Lamarck Lake. Anglers can fish for small brook trout in the lower lakes.

Lake

Camping

bank. Continue alongside the creek past tiny meadows dotted with pines to the east shore of Upper Lamarck Lake. ▶5 The lake, faintly reminiscent of a Norwegian fjord, is tucked into a narrow, steep-walled cirque. The starkness of the environment makes the area seem less hospitable than its lower counterpart. The only break in the cliffs and talus slopes surrounding the lake is found near some stunted pines clinging desperately to a pocket of shallow soil on a rise above the southeast shore. Fine campsites are on this rise and also near some small tarns east of the lake. The upper lake harbors brook and rainbow trout.

MILESTONES

▶1	0.0	Start at trailhead
▶2	0.05	Left at junction
▶3	1.0	Right at Grass Lake junction
▶4	2.2	Lower Lamarck Lake
▶5	2.7	Upper Lamarck Lake

Piute Lake and Humphreys Basin

Just north of Glacier Divide, which forms the northern boundary of Kings Canyon National Park, resides a large lake-dotted basin that rivals any in the High Sierra for sweeping alpine beauty. Although much effort is required for the 4.6-mile climb from North Lake (9,255 feet) to Piute Pass (11,423 feet), the stupendous scenery abounding in Humphreys Basin is more than an adequate reward. Beyond the pass, gently descending tread leads into the open basin, which has so many worthwhile lakes and tarns for those with rudimentary off-trail skills to visit that deciding where to go may be the hardest part of the whole trip. The lake-dotted basin is rimmed with dramatic peaks and unparalleled alpine scenery that even the most jaded traveler will enjoy. Day hikers and overnighters not interested in the long haul over the pass can enjoy the string of lakes on the east side. Piute Lake, in particular, is a fine place to enjoy lunch or pitch a tent.

Best Time

With elevations higher than 11,000 feet, the Piute Pass Trail usually remains snowbound until the middle of July. The wildflower display in Humphreys Basin peaks from late July into early August. September can be a fine time for a hike, but be prepared for cold nighttime temperatures as the month progresses. The first significant snowfall usually arrives by late October or early November.

TRAIL USE
Day Hike, Backpack, Run, Horse, Dogs Allowed

LENGTH
6.6 miles, 3 hours to Piute Lake
14.4 miles, 8 hours to Humphreys Basin

VERTICAL FEET
+1725/-1725/±3450
+2175/-650/±5650

DIFFICULTY
– 1 2 **3-4** 5 +

TRAIL TYPE
Out-and-back

FEATURES
Mountain
Lake
Wildflowers
Great Views
Camping
Swimming
Fishing

FACILITIES
Campground
Restrooms
Stables

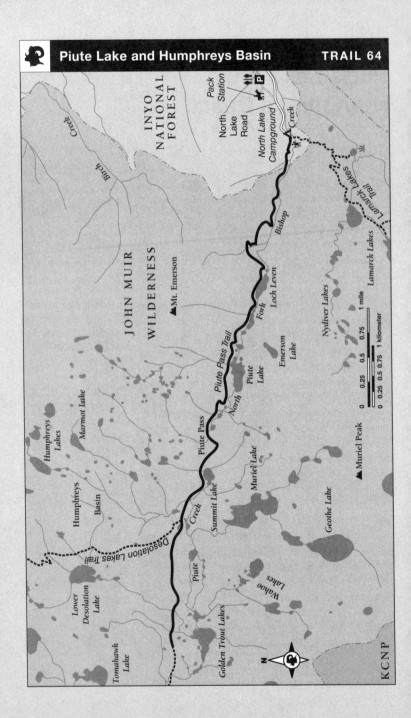

INYO NATIONAL FOREST

Pack Station

North Lake Road

North Lake Campground

Bishop Creek

Birch Creek

JOHN MUIR WILDERNESS

▲Mt. Emerson

Piute Pass Trail

Loch Leven

North Fork

Emerson Lake

Piute Lake

Lamarck Lakes

Lamarck Lakes

Nydiver Lakes

▲ Muriel Peak

Piute Pass

Marmot Lake

Humphreys Lakes

Humphreys Basin

Desolation Lakes Trail

Piute Creek

Summit Lake

Muriel Lake

Geothe Lake

Lower Desolation Lake

Piute

Wahoo Lakes

Golden Trout Lakes

Tomahawk Lake

0   0.25   0.5   0.75   1 mile
0   0.25 0.5 0.75 1 kilometer

N

KCNP

Finding the Trail

Turn west from US 395 in the center of Bishop at Line Drive and proceed out of town, as the road becomes South Lake Road (CA 168). Proceed 15 miles to the South Lake junction, and continue ahead toward Lake Sabrina 3 miles to the North Lake junction. Turn right and follow the single-lane gravel road 1 mile to the day-use parking area, or 1.6 miles to the right-hand turn into the overnight parking lot directly west of North Lake. Both day hikers and backpackers can be dropped at the trailhead inside North Lake Campground (fee, vault toilets, running water, and bear boxes), but drivers will have to walk the continuation of the North Lake Road from either the day-use or overnight lots to the trailhead. Nearby resorts along South Lake Road include Bishop Creek Lodge, Cardinal Village Resort, and Parchers Resort.

The lake-dotted basin is rimmed with dramatic peaks and unparalleled alpine scenery that even the most jaded traveler will enjoy.

Logistics

Backpackers must obtain a wilderness permit for all overnight visits. See page 376 for more details about how to obtain one.

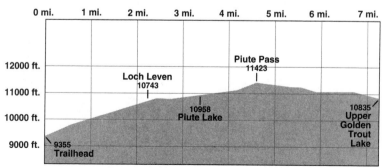

TRAIL 64 Piute Lake and Humphreys Basin Elevation Profile

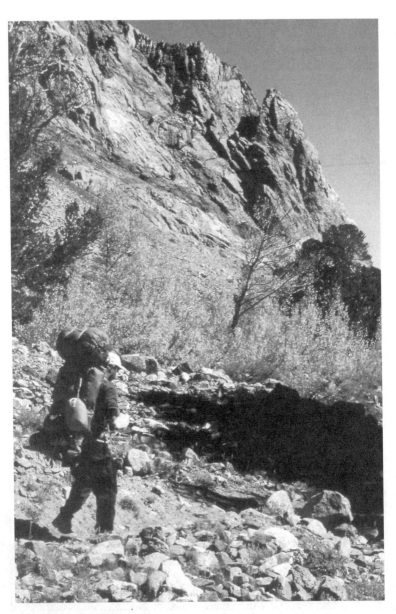

On the Piute Pass Trail

Trail Description

▶1 From the trailhead inside North Lake Campground (1 mile from the day-use parking lot and 0.7 mile from the overnight lot), follow singletrack trail through aspens and pines a short distance to a junction ▶2 near the edge of the campground.

Veer right on the Piute Pass Trail, soon entering the John Muir Wilderness, and climb gently through aspen groves, stands of lodgepole pines, and patches of flower-sprinkled meadows. Beyond a pair of log crossings of North Fork Bishop Creek, the grade increases to moderate, and the trail ascends away from the canyon floor via a series of switchbacks to a long, ascending traverse. Along the way are excellent views of a waterfall, where the waters of the North Fork plunge steeply from the basin above, as well as Peak 12961 on the left and Mount Emerson and the multihued Piute Crags on the right. Rock steps and more switchbacks lead up the canyon through diminishing amounts of lodgepole pines and then limber pines. The moderate climb eventually leads you to Loch Leven, ▶3 with delightful picnic spots and a few campsites spread around the lakeshore. Anglers should find fair fishing for brook and rainbow trout.

Leaving the lovely Loch Leven behind, the trail climbs moderately for a short time through scattered lodgepole and whitebark pines to where the grade briefly eases near some ponds. More climbing leads into the next basin and the northeast shore of Piute Lake. ▶4 Verdant meadows, patches of willow, and widely scattered stands of whitebark pine ring the lake, which is at nearly 11,000 feet, and anglers can test their skill on the resident brook and rainbow trout. Campsites near the trail at Piute Lake are badly overused; backpackers are encouraged to look for spots farther around the wind-prone lakeshore. More-remote campsites can

Wildflowers

Lake

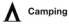
Camping

Fishing

Lake

Fishing

Camping

be found by scrambling 0.3 mile southeast up a steep slope to rockbound Emerson Lake.

From Piute Lake, follow the trail northwest toward timberline, ascending over granite slabs and passing through small meadows sliced by refreshing brooks and dotted with tiny ponds. A final ascending traverse leads to 11,423-foot Piute Pass, ►5 where a stunning view of lands both near and far is the reward for all the climbing. Immediately below and west of the pass is the broad expanse of Humphreys Basin, towered over by numerous peaks, including the rugged crest of the Glacier Divide, Muriel Peak, Mount Goethe, and the nearly 14,000-foot summit of Mount Humphreys to the north. To the west lie Pilot Peak and the deep cleft of South Fork San Joaquin River. If you're tuckered out from all the high-altitude climbing, Piute Pass makes a fine turnaround point.

 Great Views

Adventurous souls can proceed toward Humphreys Basin and a plethora of worthy destinations, where campsites are virtually unlimited, at least for those who don't mind leaving the security of a maintained trail. (Other than a ban within 500 feet of Lower Golden Trout Lake, camping is available near any of the numerous lakes and unnamed tarns.) Follow a winding descent around hummocks of granite and past tiny brooks coursing through scenic meadows on long-legged switchbacks well above Summit Lake, where interested anglers may find brook trout gliding through the pale blue waters. Continue the gently graded descent through acres and acres of wildflowers through midseason to a crossing of the outlet from Humphreys Lakes. Here, a faint use trail climbs alongside the stream toward secluded terrain around Marmot and Humphreys Lakes.

 Fishing

 Wildflowers

A short distance farther is a junction with the distinct but unmaintained trail to massive and austere Desolation Lake. Continue down the trail to a faint use trail that heads southwest a relatively short distance to Upper Golden Trout Lake, where

 Lake

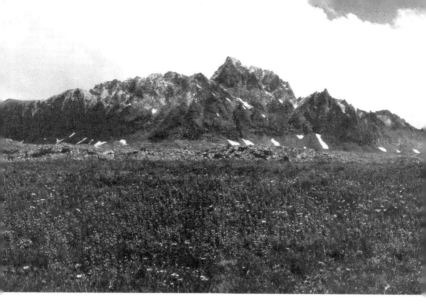

Mount Humphreys *from Humphreys Basin*

a number of scenic campsites ring the shore. ►6 The use trail may be hard to locate for first timers, but cross-country travel over open terrain to the lake is straightforward. The massive hulk of nearly 14,000-foot Mount Humphreys above the east edge of the basin dominates the landscape from just about any vantage point.

 Camping

 Mountain

🚶	**MILESTONES**	
►1	0.0	Start at trailhead
►2	0.05	Right at junction
►3	2.2	Loch Leven
►4	3.3	Piute Lake
►5	4.6	Piute Pass
►6	7.2	Upper Golden Trout Lake

Appendix 1

Top-Rated Trails

Appendix 2

Campgrounds and RV Parks

Campgrounds in the immediate vicinity of trailheads in this guide are listed below, appearing roughly in the same order as the trail descriptions (west side and then east side, south to north). Campgrounds within the national parks are mentioned first, followed by Giant Sequoia National Monument, and then a section of Inyo National Forest campgrounds, which also includes some Bureau of Land Management (BLM), county, and privately operated campgrounds. Reservations for National Park Service and U.S. Forest Service campgrounds that accept reservations can be made online at **recreation.gov**, or by calling 877-444-6777.

Sequoia and Kings Canyon National Parks

- **South Fork and Mineral King**
  South Fork
  Atwell Mill
  Cold Springs
- **Foothills**
  Potwisha
  Buckeye
- **Generals Highway**
  Lodgepole
  Dorst Creek

- **Grant Grove**
  Azalea
  Crystal Springs
  Sunset
- **Cedar Grove**
  Sentinel
  Sheep Creek
  Canyon View
  Canyon View Group
  Moraine

Giant Sequoia National Monument Campgrounds

- **Generals Highway**
  Stony Creek
  Cove Group
  Upper Stony Creek
  Fir Group
- **Big Meadows Area**
  Buck Rock
  Big Meadows

- **Hume Lake Area**
  Tenmile
  Landslide
  Logger Flat Group
  Aspen Hollow Group
  Hume Lake
  Princess

Inyo National Forest Campgrounds

- **Lone Pine Area**
  Diaz Lake (Inyo County)
  Portagee Joe (Inyo County)
  Tuttle Creek (BLM)
- **Horseshoe Meadow Road**
  Cottonwood Pass Walk-In
  Horseshoe Meadow
  Cottonwood Walk-In
- **Whitney Portal Road**
  Lone Pine
  Lone Pine Group
  Whitney Portal
  Whitney Portal Group
  Whitney Trailhead Walk-In
- **Independence**
  Independence Creek (Inyo
  County)
- **Onion Valley Road**
  Lower Grays Meadow
  Upper Grays Meadow
  Onion Valley
- **North Oak Creek Drive**
  Oak Creek
- **Independence to Big Pine**
  Goodale Creek (BLM)
  Taboose Creek (Inyo County)
  Tinemaha (Inyo County)
  Baker Creek (Inyo County)
  Glacier View (Inyo County)
- **Glacier Lodge Road**
  Sage Flat
  Upper Sage Flat
  Big Pine Creek
  Palisade Glacier and Clyde
  Glacier Group Camp

- **Baker Creek Road**
  Baker Creek
- **South Lake Road**
  Forks
  Four Jeffrey
  Creekside RV Park (privately
  operated)
  Mountain Glen
  Willow
- **CA 168**
  Big Trees
  Intake 2 Walk-In
  Intake 2 Upper
  Bishop Park Group
  Table Mountain Group
  Sabrina
- **North Lake Road**
  North Lake
- **Bishop**
  Brown's Town (privately
  operated)
  Brown's Millpond (privately
  operated)
  Horton Creek (BLM)
  Highlands RV Park (privately
  operated)
  Pleasant Valley (Inyo County)

Appendix 3

Hotels, Lodges, Motels, and Resorts

National Parks
866-875-8456, **visitsequoia.com/lodging**

Sequoia National Park
Wuksachi Lodge, 888-252-5757

Pear Lake Ski Hut, 559-565-3759
   exploresequoiakingscanyon.com/pear-lake-winter-hut

Kings Canyon National Park
John Muir Lodge, Grant Grove Cabins, Cedar Grove Lodge,
   and Bearpaw Meadow High Sierra Camp, 877-436-9615

Giant Sequoia National Monument
Hume Lake Christian Camps, 800-965-HUME, ext. 2167
   humelake.org/lodging

Kings Canyon Lodge (*damaged by 2015 Rough Fire*)

Montecito Sequoia Lodge, 800-227-9900, **mslodge.com**

Stony Creek Lodge, 877-828-1440
   sequoia-kingscanyon.com/stonycreeklodge

Private (Outside the Parks)
nps.gov/seki/planyourvisit/lodgingoutsideparks

Three Rivers
Western Holiday Lodge, 888-523-9291
   magnusonhotels.com/western-holiday-lodge-three-rivers

Buckeye Tree Lodge, 559-561-5900, **buckeyetreelodge.com**

Comfort Inn and Suites Sequoia Kings Canyon, 559-561-9010
  comfortinn.com

Cort Cottage Bed and Breakfast, 559-561-4671, **cortcottage.com**

Gateway Restaurant and Lodge, 559-561-4133, **gateway-sequoia.com**

Holiday Inn Express, 800-315-2621, **hiexpress.com**

Lake Elowin Resort, 559-561-3460, **lake-elowin.com**

Lazy J Ranch Motel, 559-561-4449, **bvilazyj.com**

The River Inn, 800-793-7309, **the-riverinn.com**

Sequoia House, 800-793-7309, **sequoiahouse.com**

Sequoia Motel, 559-561-1625, **sequoiamotel.com**

Sequoia River Dance B & B, 559-561-4411, **sequoiariverdance.com**

Sequoia Village Inn, 559-561-3652, **sequoiavillageinn.com**

Sierra Lodge, 888-575-2555, **sierra-lodge.com**

Three Rivers Motel, 559-561-4413

Mineral King Road

Silver City Resort, 559-561-3223, **silvercityresort.com**

Ranch Champagne Cabins, 559-561-3490, **ranchchampagne.com**

Appendix 4

Major Organizations

Sequoia Natural History Association

47050 Generals Highway, Unit 10
Three Rivers, CA 93271
Phone: 559-565-3759
Fax: 559-565-3728
sequoiahistory.org, snha@sequoiahistory.org

The Sequoia Fund

P.O. Box 3047
Visalia, CA 93278
Phone: 559-739-1668
Fax: 559-739-1680

National Park Foundation

1110 Vermont Ave. NW, Suite 200
Washington, D.C. 20005
Phone: 202-796-2500
Fax: 202-796-2509
nationalparks.org, ask-npf@nationalparks.org

Tehipite Chapter of the Sierra Club

P.O. Box 5396
Fresno, CA 93755-5396
559-229-4031
sierraclub.org/tehipite

Appendix 5

Useful Books

Backpacking

Beffort, Brian. *Joy of Backpacking*. Birmingham, AL: Wilderness Press, 2015.

Fletcher, Colin, and Chip Rawlins. *The Complete Walker IV*. New York, NY: Knopf, 2002.

O'Bannon, Allen, and Mike Clelland. *Allen and Mike's Really Cool Backpackin' Book: Traveling and Camping Skills for a Wilderness Environment*. Guilford, CT: Falcon Press, 2001.

Guidebooks

Arnot, Phil. *High Sierra, John Muir's Range of Light*. San Carlos, CA: Wild World Publishing/Terra, 1996.

Backpacking California: Mountain, Foothill, Coastal, and Desert Adventures in the Golden State. Berkeley, CA: Wilderness Press, 2008.

Jenkins, J. C., and Ruby Johnson Jenkins. *Exploring the Southern Sierra: East Side*. Berkeley, CA: Wilderness Press, 1992.

Morey, Kathy. *Hot Showers, Soft Beds, and Dayhikes in the Sierra: Walks and Strolls Near Lodgings*. 3rd ed. Berkeley, CA: Wilderness Press, 2008.

Morey, Kathy, Mike White, et al. *Sierra South. Backcountry Trips in California's Sierra Nevada*. 8th ed. Berkeley, CA: Wilderness Press, 2006.

———. *Sierra High Route: Traversing Timberline Country*. Seattle: The Mountaineers Books, 1997.

Schaffer, Jeffrey P., Ben Schifrin, et al. *Pacific Crest Trail: Southern California*. 6th ed. Berkeley, CA: Wilderness Press, 2003.

Secor, R. J. *The High Sierra, Peaks, Passes, and Trails.* 3rd ed. Seattle: The Mountaineers Books, 2009.

Spring, Vicky. *100 Hikes in California's Central Sierra and Coast Range.* 2nd ed. Seattle: The Mountaineers Books, 2004.

Stone, Robert. *Day Hikes in Sequoia and Kings Canyon National Parks.* 2nd ed. Red Lodge, MT: Day Hike Books, Inc., 2001.

White, Mike and Douglas Lorain. *Best Backpacking Trips in California and Nevada.* Reno, NV: University of Nevada Press, 2015.

White, Mike. *Sequoia and Kings Canyon National Parks: Your Complete Hiking Guide.* Birmingham, AL: Wilderness Press, 2012.

History and Literature

Browning, Peter. *Place Names of the Sierra Nevada.* Berkeley, CA: Wilderness Press, 1991.

Dilslayer, Larry M., and William C. Tweed. *Challenge of the Big Trees.* Three Rivers, CA: Sequoia Natural History Association, 1990.

Farquahar, Francis P. *History of the Sierra Nevada.* Berkeley, CA: University of California Press, 1965.

Jackson, Louise A. Buelah. *A Biography of the Mineral King Valley of California.* Tucson, AZ: Westernlore Press, 1988.

Strong, Douglas H. *From Pioneers to Preservationists: A Brief History of Sequoia and Kings Canyon National Parks.* Three Rivers, CA: Sequoia Natural History Association, 2000.

Tweed, William. *Beneath the Giants: A Guide to the Moro Rock-Crescent Meadow Road of Sequoia National Park.* Three Rivers, CA: Sequoia Natural History Association, 1986.

———. *Kaweah Remembered.* Three Rivers, CA: Sequoia Natural History Association, 1986.

Natural History

Johnston, Verna R. *Sierra Nevada: The Naturalist's Companion.* Revised ed. Berkeley, CA: University of California Press, 2000.

Laws, John Muir. *The Laws Field Guide to the Sierra Nevada*. Berkeley, CA: Heyday Books, 2007.

Moore, James G. *Exploring the Highest Sierra*. Stanford, CA: Stanford University Press, 2000.

Petrides, George A., and Olivia Petrides. *Western Trees*. New York: Houghton Mifflin, 1998.

Smith, Genny, ed. *Sierra East: Edge of the Great Basin*. Berkeley, CA: University of California Press, 2000.

Weeden, Norman F. *A Sierra Nevada Flora*. 4th ed. Berkeley, CA: Wilderness Press, 1996.

Index

About the Author

Mike White

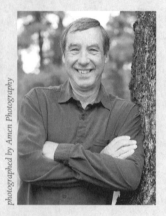

Mike White was raised in the southeast suburbs of Portland, Oregon, in the shadow of Mount Hood (whenever the Pacific Northwest skies cleared enough to allow such things as shadows). As a teenager, Mike began hiking, backpacking, and climbing in the Cascades of Oregon and Washington, and he honed his outdoor skills while attending Seattle Pacific University. After acquiring a B.A. in political science, Mike and his new wife, Robin, relocated to the high desert of Reno, Nevada, from where he discovered the joys of exploring the Sierra Nevada.

After leaving his last "real" job, Mike began a full-time writing career. He is the author or coauthor of 19 outdoor guides, including award-winning books *Top Trails Lake Tahoe* and *50 Classic Hikes in Nevada*. Mike also has contributed to *Sunset* and *Backpacker* magazines and the *Reno Gazette-Journal* newspaper. A former community college instructor, Mike is also a popular featured speaker for outdoors groups.

Series Creator

Joe Walowski

Joe Walowski conceived of the Top Trails series in 2003, and was series editor of the first three titles: *Top Trails Los Angeles*, *Top Trails San Francisco Bay Area*, and *Top Trails Lake Tahoe*. He currently lives in Seattle.